PRAISE FOR *ADVANCED PRACTICE PROVIDERS*

"This is a must-read for all healthcare organizational leaders where advanced practice registered nurses (APRNs) and physician assistants (PAs) are a part of the healthcare team. Being able to understand how to best support and utilize this workforce is crucial in the success of any healthcare delivery system. The authors of this book have brilliantly laid out a blueprint to build a strong and engaged APRN/PA staff."

–Risa Zimmerman, MBA, MPAS, PA-C, DFAAPA
Director, Office of Advanced Practice
Nebraska Medicine

"Within these pages lies a treasure trove of evidence-based tools, templates, pitfalls to avoid, and more for anyone who is interested in advanced practice in healthcare. Maria Lofgren and the Iowa team, with learnings from 15+ years creating a sustainable APP model, have given a huge gift to healthcare delivery globally. I'm especially excited about the thoughtful reflections on staying attuned to relationships between providers as well as the figures and sidebars that highlight policy implications and provide specific examples for implementation."

–Ann Williamson, PhD, RN, NEA-BC
Former Chief Nurse and Healthcare Executive

"With the rapid expansion of advanced practice providers (APPs) nationwide, new APP leaders seek guidance and insight on building a program of fully optimized providers. Lofgren et al. have accomplished this task, providing a complete and comprehensive road map for C-suites and APP leaders to follow, creating the pillars of supporting practice from student to expert for healthcare organizations."

–Bonnie Proulx, DNP, APRN, PNP-BC, FAAN
Senior Vice President Physician Enterprise
Kaufman Hall Healthcare Management and Consulting

T0293599

ADVANCED PRACTICE PROVIDERS

An Operational Guide for Workforce Integration

Maria Lofgren | Christine Gust | Douglas Van Daele

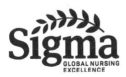

Sigma
GLOBAL NURSING
EXCELLENCE

IOWA

Sigma Theta Tau International Honor Society of Nursing (Sigma) is a nonprofit organization whose mission is developing nurse leaders anywhere to improve healthcare everywhere. Founded in 1922, Sigma has more than 135,000 active members in over 100 countries and territories. Members include practicing nurses, instructors, researchers, policymakers, entrepreneurs, and others. Sigma's more than 540 chapters are located at more than 700 institutions of higher education throughout Armenia, Australia, Botswana, Brazil, Canada, Chile, Colombia, Croatia, England, Eswatini, Finland, Ghana, Hong Kong, Ireland, Israel, Italy, Jamaica, Japan, Jordan, Kenya, Lebanon, Malawi, Mexico, the Netherlands, Nigeria, Pakistan, Philippines, Portugal, Puerto Rico, Scotland, Singapore, South Africa, South Korea, Sweden, Taiwan, Tanzania, Thailand, the United States, and Wales. Learn more at www.sigmanursing.org.

Sigma Theta Tau International
550 West North Street
Indianapolis, IN, USA 46202

To request a review copy for course adoption, order additional books, buy in bulk, or purchase for corporate use, contact Sigma Marketplace at 888.654.4968 (US/Canada toll-free), +1.317.687.2256 (International), or solutions@sigmamarketplace.org.

To request author information, or for speaker or other media requests, contact Sigma Marketing at 888.634.7575 (US/Canada toll-free) or +1.317.634.8171 (International).

ISBN: 9781646480944
EPUB ISBN: 9781646480951
PDF ISBN: 9781646480968
MOBI ISBN: 9781646481101

Library of Congress Cataloging-in-Publication Data

Names: Lofgren, Maria, author. | Gust, Christine, author. | Van Daele, Douglas, author. | Sigma Theta Tau International, publisher.

Title: Advanced practice providers : an operational guide for workforce integration / Maria Lofgren, Christine Gust, Douglas Van Daele.

Description: Indianapolis, IN : Sigma Theta Tau International, [2024] |

Includes bibliographical references and index. | Summary: "Advanced practice providers (APPs), consisting of advanced practice registered nurses (APRNs) and physician assistants (PAs), are high-demand healthcare professionals. Hospitals, clinics, and healthcare organizations are integrating these roles in their clinical operations and seek resources relating to operationalizing APPs into practice. We found a need within the profession for APP organizational practices across all disciplines, from finance to human resources to compliance, to support assimilating the uniqueness of the APP group into existing infrastructures. This book provides examples of documents and practices that can be tailored to meet an organization's specific challenges to support the efficiency, operations, and integration of the APP role.

This book adds to the literature and can guide organizations-whether academic, hospital, or clinic-based-and academic programs teaching APRNs and PAs to be leaders in healthcare where there is a need for expertise across disciplines. The book includes top-of-license practice examples that optimize APP productivity, support collaboration, focus on team-based care, and support models of independent practice. Providing APP expertise at all levels by effectively using resources within organizations will help progress healthcare toward quality patient safety goals and team care initiatives"-- Provided by publisher.

Identifiers: LCCN 2023043772 (print) | LCCN 2023043773 (ebook) | ISBN 9781646480944 (paperback) | ISBN 9781646480951 (epub) | ISBN

9781646480968 (pdf) | ISBN 9781646481101 (mobi)

Subjects: MESH: Advanced Practice Nursing--organization & administration |

Nurse Practitioners--organization & administration | Physician Assistants--organization & administration

Classification: LCC RT82.8 (print) | LCC RT82.8 (ebook) | NLM WY 128 | DDC 610.7306/92--dc23/eng/20231030

LC record available at https://lccn.loc.gov/2023043772

LC ebook record available at https://lccn.loc.gov/2023043773

Publisher: Dustin Sullivan
Acquisitions Editor: Emily Hatch
Development Editor: Jillmarie Leeper Sycamore
Cover Designer: Michael Tanamachi
Interior Design/Page Layout: Becky Batchelor
Indexer: Larry D. Sweazy

Managing Editor: Carla Hall
Publications Specialist: Todd Lothery
Project Editor: Jillmarie Leeper Sycamore
Copy Editor: Erin Geile
Proofreader: Todd Lothery

DEDICATION

This textbook is dedicated to all APRNs, PAs, and the champions that have guided the profession through their expertise, clinical knowledge, and commitment. And to our own family, friends, and mentors who offered encouragement and support throughout the writing process.

–Maria Lofgren, Christine Gust, Douglas Van Daele

ACKNOWLEDGMENTS

Thank you to the following for their valuable contributions:

Chapter 4: APRN and PA Scope of Practice

- David Asprey, PhD, PA-C, Associate Dean for Medical Education and Professional Programs, Carver College of Medicine

Chapter 9: APP Business Pro Forma

- Jason Haddy, MBA, Assistant Vice President of Finance, University of Iowa Health Care

Chapter 11: Organizational Compliance

- Randi Jelinek, CHC, CPCO, CPC, CIC, CPC-I, Compliance Associate Director, University of Iowa Health Care

Chapter 16: Patient Access Center

- Keri Semrau, MSN, BSN, RN, Director, Clinical Services, Patient Access Center, University of Iowa Health Care

Chapter 17: Organizational Initiatives

- Jason Haddy, MBA, Assistant Vice President of Finance, University of Iowa Health Care

- Rachel Kirchner, MHA, Director, UI Community Clinics & Outreach, University of Iowa Health Care, Interim CEO, UI Health Ventures

- Kate Klefstad, MHA, Associate Director of Population Health & ACO Operations, University of Iowa Health Care

- Gina Paoli, BS, CRC, Senior Project Manager, University of Iowa Health Care

The authors would like to express their gratitude for the consultative expertise to the following:

- Deanna Brennan, MBA, BSN, RN, CCDS

- Alison Bronson, MSN, RN-BC

- John Cromwell, MD, FACS, FASCRS

- Mary Greve, MPAS, PA-C, MHA
- Peggy Guither, MSN, ARNP, FNP-C, AGNP-AC
- Robert Linnell, MPAS, PA-C
- Mark Mason, MHA
- Melissa Tvedte, MSN, ARNP, FNP

We are extremely appreciative of the countless number of colleagues who have supported excelling APP practice:

- APP Lead Team
- APP Productivity Committee
- APP Steering Committee
- APP Student Placement Committee
- Clinical Staff Office
- Department of Nursing
- Finance Operations Team
- Information Systems Team
- Joint Office of Compliance
- Office of the Chief Medical Officer
- Patient Financial Services Team
- Revenue and Decision Support Team
- University of Iowa Carver College of Medicine PA Studies Program
- University of Iowa College of Nursing
- University of Iowa Hardin Library for the Health Sciences
- University of Iowa Hospital Legal Department
- University of Iowa Physicians Staff

A special thanks to Diane Crossett for her commitment to excellence, exemplary grammar, consistency, and timeliness in moving the textbook forward.

ADDITIONAL BOOK RESOURCES

For additional resources for this book, including a sample chapter, visit this book's Sigma Repository page by using the link or QR code below.

https://sigma.nursingrepository.org/handle/10755/23525

SPECIAL NOTE TO READERS

Here at Sigma, we realize that language is constantly evolving. The meaning of a word often changes over time, some words become obsolete, and some terms that were once acceptable may become controversial or even offensive, depending on the context or circumstances. We have made every effort to make language choices that are inclusive and not offensive. Should you identify words in this book that you believe negatively impact a group or groups of people, please reach out to us at Publications@SigmaNursing.org.

ABOUT THE AUTHORS

Maria Lofgren, DNP, ARNP, NNP-BC, CPNP, FAANP, is a visionary leader with over 35 years of experience spanning leadership, strategic planning, building clinical practice models, and establishing key partnerships. She is a Clinical Associate Professor and Director of Faculty Practice at the University of Iowa College of Nursing, and the Director of Advanced Practice Providers at University of Iowa Health Care. She is dually certified as a pediatric and neonatal nurse practitioner, is a Fellow of the American Association of Nurse Practitioners, and has been named one of Iowa's 100 Great Nurses. She has multiple peer-reviewed publications, book chapters, posters, and presentations and has mentored numerous APRNs and PAs. She serves on countless committees and professional organizations institutionally, statewide, and nationally. Lofgren was instrumental in leading an enterprise-wide infrastructure to maximize advanced practice providers' integration, leadership structure, and productivity. She co-leads the Certificate Program for Advanced Practice Providers and developed the course Clinical Practice Management and Leadership for Advanced Practice Providers at the University of Iowa College of Nursing.

Christine Gust, MBA, PHR, SHRM-CP, is an experienced human resources professional skilled in onboarding, training, talent acquisition, recruiting, process improvement, compliance, applicant tracking systems, leadership, interviewing, human resources information systems, and employee relations. Her work has led to aligning HR strategies to advanced practice provider organizational objectives, policies, programs, and initiatives. She is skilled at applying process improvement methodologies and is a certified Six Sigma Green Belt. She is experienced with best practices and understands the value of healthcare team optimization utilizing APPs. With over 25 years of HR experience, she serves as the human resources subject matter expert for APP-related matters within University of Iowa Health Care. Gust leads institutional metrics related to APP employment, turnover, transfers, and board specialty and has worked on special interest projects to optimize APP practice. She is well versed in APP onboarding, training, engagement, and retention. She is resource savvy and collaborates with the University of Iowa College of Nursing, Carver College of Medicine (PA Studies), and other programs for APP impact statewide.

Douglas Van Daele, MD, FACS, is a Professor in the Department of Otolaryngology, Head and Neck Surgery at the University of Iowa Roy J. and Lucille A. Carver College of Medicine and is affiliated with the Iowa City Veterans Affairs Health Care System. He is an expert in his field and is nationally and internationally known for his work.
He has multiple peer-reviewed publications, book chapters, abstracts, and presentations; has received a variety of federally funded grants; and is an acclaimed educator teaching over 100+ otolaryngology residents, fellows, and advanced practice providers.
He is a Fellow in the American Academy of Otolaryngology Head and Neck Surgery, the American College of Surgeons, the American Head and Neck Society, and the Triological Society, and he has received multiple awards for his outstanding achieve-

ments. He is the Co-chair for the Diversity, Equity, and Inclusion Task Force at UI Health Care and serves on countless committees and professional organizations institutionally, statewide, and nationally. He is a respected physician, leader, and colleague to many and has spearheaded an enterprise-wide infrastructure to maximize the integration, leadership structure, and productivity of advanced practice providers. He is an innovative leader in healthcare and has led institutional, community, and state partnerships as he has championed opportunities involving APPs in the name of patient access, quality, and collaborative teams across the healthcare continuum.

TABLE OF CONTENTS

FOREWORD

It is with great admiration and respect that we share our testament to the extraordinary journey of the visionary leaders of University of Iowa (UI) Health Care. Together, they forged a transformative path, shaping the advanced practice infrastructure within Iowa's healthcare environment. We have witnessed firsthand their dedication and unwavering commitment as leaders in the pursuit of excellence in patient care.

Advanced practice registered nurses (APRNs) and physician associates (PAs) have long collaborated to provide the very best care for their patients. Decades of outcomes have demonstrated their valuable contributions to healthcare and beyond, and the authors have captured the evidence and essence of our shared professions as we have evolved, grown, and firmly established ourselves as indispensable members of the healthcare team.

Before the advent of directors of advanced practice, and well before the idea of APRNs and PAs leading healthcare teams and occupying C-suite roles came to fruition, these professions worked together with other national leaders to create a vision for the future of advanced practice. Countless hours were spent discussing and refining best practices for PA and APRN recruitment, onboarding, orientation and training, credentialing and privileging, continuing education, professional practice evaluation, models for optimal practice and productivity, and developing centers for advanced practice.

It's amazing how far our individual professions have come and the impact they have made on patient care and the healthcare system as a whole. Equally impressive is the increasing support from the healthcare systems and policymakers that are now recognizing the importance of creating processes and systems tailored to the unique needs of advanced practice providers.

This book serves as an example to the development and implementation of a successful advanced practice program. These pages provide an excellent accounting of UI Health Care's strategic and operational endeavors over the years to strengthen relationships, organize infrastructure and supports, and optimize models of care.

As you delve into these chapters, you will gain insights into UI Health Care's journey from the collective wisdom of the authors. Together, they have articulated experiences, lessons learned, and strategies toward a successful model. We are confident you will find inspiration and practical guidance whether you are an aspiring advanced practice leader or health system executive looking to enhance your organization's infrastructure. We invite you to embark on this journey of discovery, growth, and transformation. We encourage you to embrace the wealth of knowledge they share and consider how many of these ideas might apply to your own practices and health system infrastructure.

May this book inspire and motivate all to continue the noble and wonderful mission of advancing patient care and shaping the future of healthcare.

–Jennifer M. Orozco, DMSc, PA-C, DFAA-PA
Chief Medical Officer
Senior Vice President, Clinical Affairs
American Academy of
Physician Associates
Past President, AAPA

–April N. Kapu, DNP, APRN, ACNP-BC, FAANP, FCCM, FAAN
Associate Dean, Clinical and
Community Partnerships
Professor, Vanderbilt University
School of Nursing
Past President, American Association of
Nurse Practitioners

INTRODUCTION

Welcome to *Advanced Practice Providers: An Operational Guide for Workforce Integration* from University of Iowa Health Care.

The inspiration for writing this textbook was to educate all disciplines, from finance to human resources to compliance, about the uniqueness of the APP role and the value in including their expertise at all levels across an organization. This book provides examples of documents and practices that can be tailored to any organization to support the efficiency, operations, and integration of the APP role.

For the purposes of this textbook and clarity and ease for the writing process, advanced practice provider is the term that is used to include both advanced registered nurse practitioners (ARNPs) and physician assistants (PAs). In the state of Iowa, ARNP is the licensing term that comprises certified registered nurse anesthetists (CRNAs), certified nurse midwives (CNMs), certified nurse practitioners (CNPs), and clinical nurse specialists (CNSs). PA is the licensing term for physician assistants.

The American Academy of Physician Associates adopted "physician associate" as the nationally accepted title for the profession and continues to advocate for replacing "physician assistant" in state legislation. The state of Iowa uses the term physician assistant (PA), which we use throughout this textbook. Likewise, the National Consensus Model for APRN regulation endorses the title advanced practice registered nurse (APRN). The Iowa Board of Nursing has adopted the Consensus Model except for the title change from ARNP to APRN only because of the complex reimbursement issues surrounding the titles. Third-party payer language in the state of Iowa notes that reimbursement qualifies only for licenses with the term nurse practitioner in it. Legal guidance from the ARNP professional organizations in the state of Iowa notes that changing the licensing name risks having claims denied. However, APRN is the nationally accepted term and used throughout this textbook.

This book is one example of a successful program integrating APPs into the workforce based on University of Iowa (UI) Health Care's organizational blueprint. Organizations are encouraged to use this textbook to guide their own infrastructure to optimize top-of-license practice and APP workforce integration. The nomenclature used throughout may not be in alignment with all organizations. For example, where UI Health Care uses the term "Director of APPs," other organizations may use language such as "Executive APP," "Chief APP," "VP of APPs," or nomenclature of their similar leadership structures that may be more applicable.

This book adds to the literature and can guide organizations—whether academic, hospital, or clinic-based—and academic programs teaching APRNs and PAs to be leaders in healthcare where there is a need for expertise across disciplines. The book includes top-of-license practice examples that optimize APP productivity, support collaboration, focus on team-based care, and support models of independent practice.

Chapter 1: Comparison of Medicine and Nursing Infrastructures and the Growing Advanced Practice Provider Workforce

Optimizing an APP infrastructure that can be integrated into existing leadership structures requires a concerted effort at all levels in the healthcare organization. There are multiple variables to consider while strategizing how to implement an infrastructure.

Chapter 2: Understanding the Organizational Blueprint

Leaders and providers globally, and APPs specifically, are challenged to be successful in different organizational structures. Discussing the specific enterprise blueprint helps allow for questions and concerns to be raised as well as for expectations for the working environment to be set.

Chapter 3: Establishing an Infrastructure

Having a clear appreciation and understanding of one's organizational structure has a significant impact on how to approach change. Applying an interdisciplinary steering committee or advisory board can be a positive influence in guiding projects to optimizing APP productivity in a top-of-license practice model. It is fundamental to have a solid understanding of the organization's infrastructure before making decisions that universally affect all APPs across an enterprise. Making sure decisions align with the organization's strategy and with opportunity for all interested parties to have a voice is paramount to evaluate outcomes from major decisions.

Chapter 4: APRN and PA Scope of Practice

Ensuring APPs practice to the full extent of their licensure and education has significant organizational benefits, including maximizing APP productivity and promoting a positive work environment and inclusive culture.

Chapter 5: Establishing an APP Workforce

Using a methodology for crafting an APP workforce based on many of the principles described in this chapter is fundamental to the success of integrating APPs to be part of the multidisciplinary healthcare team in a variety of clinical healthcare settings. Building APP teams from start to finish requires resource allocation and commitment like other professional hires within an organization.

Chapter 6: APP Onboarding

Organizations should plan and prepare a comprehensive onboarding program designed to incrementally bring a new APP towards full practice. Having a plan, knowing how success will be measured, and involving an interdisciplinary team in the onboarding plan will increase efficiency. This in turn sets the APP up for success and supports the APP towards full caseload, top-of-license practice, and competency.

Chapter 7: Operationalizing Telehealth

The onslaught of the COVID-19 pandemic brought rapid changes in healthcare delivery, including an unprecedented increase in telehealth, particularly in the ambulatory care setting. Organizations that successfully implemented a robust telehealth program used a number of best practices as outlined within this chapter. Telehealth has proven beneficial for patients, providers, and healthcare organizations and will continue to be an alternative method for care delivery beyond the pandemic.

Chapter 8: APRN and PA Students

Having a solid relationship between students, educational programs, and healthcare providers is essential to meet both workforce needs and the educational requirements for APRN and PA education. A well-prepared group of PAs and APRNs will be necessary to serve the healthcare needs and fill gaps in access to quality care. Organizations should commit both time and resources to educating APP students.

Chapter 9: APP Business Pro Forma

Supporting organizational infrastructures that continue to have operational growth with detailed pro formas not only aligns the organization's mission with accurately hiring the right APPs for the work effort needed but also sets the stage to support APPs entering the workforce through strategic practice questions. Pro formas specific to the APP role help organizational leadership establish relationships to align APPs with physicians, nursing staff, and other key collaborators to promote positive patient outcomes.

Chapter 10: Credentialing and Privileging

APPs entering clinical practice must undergo the credentialing and privileging process to be approved by the healthcare organization where they are employed to provide care, treat patients, and bill for the services rendered. The credentialing and privileging process ensures APPs are practicing safely and competently, protecting themselves, the organization, and most importantly the patients.

Chapter 11: Organizational Compliance

Healthcare is evolving at a rapid pace with new technology, equipment, and methods of providing services to patients. As one of the most highly regulated industries, the rules and regulations that govern it are changing at equally rapid speeds, making it difficult to stay current. An effective compliance program is vital to reduce regulatory risk, and APPs are a growing workforce and need this inclusion.

Chapter 12: Professional Development

Organizations will benefit by creating a workplace environment that supports and encourages ongoing professional development by offering a selection of professional development opportunities intended to help APPs progress through technical clinical skills, advanced knowledge, leadership opportunities, and personal growth.

Chapter 13: APP Mentoring

A formal mentoring program occurs when an organization dedicates structure, time, and resources towards pairing an APP with a colleague or peer to provide support and guidance. APPs can derive mentorship from many roles in healthcare, including peers, faculty, or other members of the collaborative healthcare team.

Chapter 14: Metrics That Matter

Organizational leaders should develop role expectations and productivity metrics to quantify the return on investment for employing APPs as part of the healthcare team. The metrics will vary based on the clinical setting, with examples provided for ambulatory, inpatient, and procedural APPs.

Chapter 15: Team-Based Care

Team-based care has become a critical approach within healthcare delivery systems, with outcomes that are beneficial across multiple dimensions. Demonstrating clear patient outcomes related to team-based care is imperative to positively influence healthcare delivery models. Through outcomes-driven research, development of new interprofessional training programs, team-based clinical practice guidelines, and health policy promoting reimbursement for team care, the overall patient experience can be transformed.

Chapter 16: Patient Access Center

A patient access center is a complex system, responsible for the first introduction to an organization's healthcare delivery system. A high-functioning access center can make a crucial difference in the healthcare delivery system and the potential for future growth of the organization.

Chapter 17: Organizational Initiatives

There are various ways that organizations address unique initiatives due to continuous changes in healthcare. Utilizing resources within a healthcare system or organization, using guiding principles to engage all team members, and promoting inclusive environments supports those unique and challenging projects where APPs are instrumental in the success.

Chapter 18: Looking to the Future

The literature continues to evolve related to not only the future of APPs but also the future of healthcare delivery systems. The more resources and knowledge that can be shared, the better we can prepare for the future from a healthcare operations perspective.

"A sign of a good leader is not how many followers you have, but how many leaders you create."
–Mahatma Gandhi

CHAPTER 1

COMPARISON OF MEDICINE AND NURSING INFRASTRUCTURES AND THE GROWING APP WORKFORCE

KEYWORDS | infrastructure, culture, interested parties, leader

Due to the variety of organizational cultures and leadership structures in healthcare organizations, a one-size-fits-all approach to advanced practice provider (APP) leadership structures is not feasible. Part of the impetus of this textbook is to share University of Iowa Health Care infrastructures to provide organizations with examples that can be adapted and changed to meet their own needs and help support APPs in their own organizations. For clarity, APP is the professional term that is used to include both advanced practice registered nurses (APRNs) and physician assistants (PAs). APRN is the licensing term that comprises certified registered nurse anesthetists (CRNAs), certified nurse midwives (CNMs), certified nurse practitioners (CNPs), and clinical nurse specialists (CNSs). PA is the licensing term for physician assistants. Together, APRN and PA are the two professional licenses that encompass the universally accepted terminology *advanced practice provider* and how these professions will be referred to throughout this textbook. This is outlined in Figure 1.1.

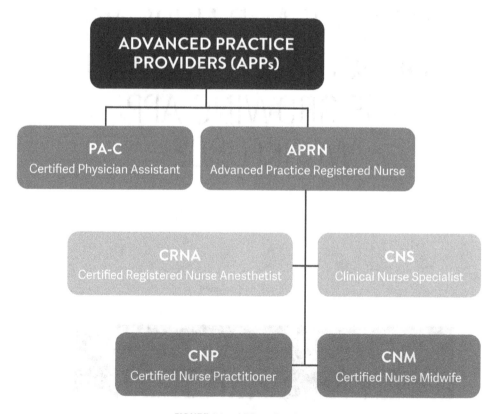

FIGURE 1.1 APP professional terms.

HEALTHCARE INFRASTRUCTURE

Medicine and nursing have historically operated within infrastructures that allow for leadership and professional resources that direct their professions. APPs are a growing workforce in the healthcare system that also require robust leadership infrastructures and need to be incorporated into the existing structures that support profession-specific issues. Understanding the traditional medicine and nursing structures will help provide perspective when designing an APP infrastructure within your organization.

Physician infrastructures often include leadership models that consist of chief medical officers, department chairs, medical directors, division directors, and, depending on the size of the organization (or in the case of an academic medical center), may include academic deans, vice presidents, and graduate medical education leaders. Nursing infrastructures consist of similar models including chief nursing executives, associate chief nursing administrators, directors of nursing, nurse managers, assistant nurse managers, and nurse educators. APPs bridge the gap between the nursing and medicine professions; thus, healthcare organizations are challenged to optimize structures and processes to best deploy and support this growing workforce. System leaders—including physicians, nursing, and other disciplines with knowledge and expertise related to APPs—are essential to operationalizing and supporting them within organizations.

APP WORKFORCE AND GROWTH

APPs can practice in nearly every clinical setting and in almost every specialty across the healthcare organization. APRN and PA academic programs have coincided in proliferation (Physician Assistant Education Association, 2020). There are more than 355,000 nurse practitioners licensed in the United States (American Association of Nurse Practitioners, 2022), with 426 DNP programs currently enrolling students at schools of nursing nationwide and an additional 70 new DNP programs in the planning stages (Rosseter, 2023). The American Academy of Physician Associates represents more than 150,000 PAs (2023), and the number of PA programs has increased substantially over the years, with the total number of accredited PA programs at 303, with estimates for potential accredited PA programs to be 322 by 2025 (Accreditation Review Commission on Education for the Physician Assistant, 2023). Many factors contribute to this increase, including the emerging demands on healthcare organizations and the anticipated shortage of physician providers in both primary and specialty care by 2033 (Association of American Medical Colleges, 2021).

Physicians, nurses, and APPs are working together to increase patient access, engage as a team for healthcare continuity, and provide value-based care that results in excellent outcomes. Patients need providers who are available and accessible for their healthcare needs. In an already taxed system, organizations should ensure that everyone on the healthcare team is equipped to practice to the full extent of their license and education. Likewise, it is imperative that all members of the healthcare team have adequate training to ensure patient safety. Academic health centers are pivotal to the research, teaching, and clinical missions sustaining healthcare systems. With changing economics, market consolidation, generational changes in the healthcare workforce, and increasing focus on chronic disease prevention and management, academic health centers need to transform their operating models and evolve into a more integrated and efficient system of care (Enders et al., 2016). One example is to define a model that will identify the types of patients who can, and should, be seen by an APP and those who should be seen by physicians to operationalize providers based on education backgrounds and knowledge.

Physicians, nurses, and APPs play a crucial role in the care of patients within multiple models of care delivery across the country. Consistent state-legislated full practice authority in all states will influence organizational practice models and encourage top-of-license practice. It is imperative to be cognizant of the issues that surround the ability to provide care to patients and become educated about the scope of practice of the APP and how these roles can add value. Today more than any other time in history, collaboration and teamwork should be at the forefront for healthcare delivery practice models. Many healthcare disciplines across the country are engaging with the Centers for Medicare & Medicaid Services (CMS) to advocate for specialty practice from an APP scope for reimbursement barriers. Currently, Medicare reimbursement rates for APPs are set at 85% of that of a physician, a practice that creates a significant institutional barrier, making it fiscally unattractive to allow APPs to practice without a physician partner underwriting documentation. Full billing authority is an essential element to actualize state-legislated full practice authority (Lofgren et al., 2017).

U.S. News and World Report has highlighted the APRN and PA professions as top-ranked positions that are gaining in popularity. In recent rankings, these healthcare occupations continue to dominate the best jobs (Ingram, 2023).

IDENTIFYING A LEADER

Over the last few years, APP infrastructures have evolved to integrate with traditional medicine and nursing leadership structures to encompass the unique needs of APPs. The success of these infrastructures and support systems for APPs are due in part to outstanding leadership in both APRN and PA professional organizations and strong support from organizational leaders as well as physician and nursing champions.

NOTE | The Triple Aim, coined in 2008 by the Institute for Healthcare Improvement, delineates policy implications for improving population health, the healthcare experience, and per capita cost (Bachynsky, 2020). The Quadruple Aim included a fourth policy implication that focuses on the care of the provider in optimizing the performance of the healthcare system. The implications of the Quadruple Aim require an exercise in balance for policymakers: how to spend resources, what coverage to provide, to whom to provide it, and how to improve the work life of the provider (Bachynsky, 2020).

As the APP workforce continues to grow, communication and accountability can be challenging. The development of lead APP roles within the department or service line has improved these challenges as well as helped connect all APPs to the organization's strategic initiatives.

A lead APP is a clinical practicing APP who takes on additional responsibility to support other APP cohorts who care for similar patient populations or service lines. They are the designated leaders responsible for daily operations which may include oversight of schedules, orientations, performance evaluations, onboarding, coordinating billing and reimbursement issues within their work group, and other matters as they arise.

Identifying leadership teams specific for APPs helps capitalize on the workforce of APRNs and PAs, optimizing infrastructures to support them as engaged and valued providers. The physician APP lead partnership emerged from the development of APP leadership infrastructures within organizations. The benefits of having a lead APP role have been discussed multiple times in the literature (Ackerman et al., 2010; Anen & McElroy, 2015, 2017). Bahouth and colleagues (2012) have described the role as one that is not intended to be hierarchical but to focus on developing strong collaborative relationships rather than authoritarian, owning, or directing. Together, the APP lead and physician colleagues can make decisions surrounding specialty patient populations based on sound clinical practice guidelines and team principles, support a strong and collaborative healthcare model, and ensure the safest and best patient outcomes by working together to lead others. Lead APPs are both practicing providers and influential leaders, and their success is due in part to the circle of support received from department, division, and unit-based colleagues.

A first step in developing an APP lead structure is defining the role and responsibilities to determine how the role will be operationalized. APP leads typically take on leadership responsibility in addition to their clinical duties. Clinical responsibilities should be offset by some level of administrative time for lead responsibilities. Each service line may determine the amount of administrative time considering some of the following criteria:

- Number of APPs in the patient cohort
- Schedule complexity, managing multiple sites/locations, 24/7 coverage, call requirements
- Projected future growth of APP cohort within work group
- Experience level of cohort, mix of experienced APPs and new graduates

The reporting structure for the lead role should be defined by the organization. The lead position may not have direct authority but rather serves as a support, mentor, lead, and communication conduit for the cohort of APPs. Some of the typical areas of responsibility are detailed in Figure 1.2.

Figure 1.3 lists examples of lead responsibilities that organizations may consider when creating the duties that may be included in the APP lead role.

UNDERSTANDING ORGANIZATIONAL CULTURE

All organizations have administrative and financial considerations that drive and form their internal workplace cultures. Understanding this cultural climate is the first step when establishing an APP leadership model. Instituting an APP director role to provide influential leadership and serve as a partner with physician, nursing, and executive leaders will support strategic initiatives across the organization. A director of APPs can help identify, mentor, grow, and develop APP leads in their role. Having an APP director at the executive level and leads surrounding patient population cohorts further facilitates communication of strategic initiatives at all levels. This ensures individual APPs have access to support and leadership even if they are the only APP within the department or division.

Executive leaders need to have a detailed understanding of where all APPs are practicing, based on patient population and location. APP leads can help develop pertinent processes, guidelines, and resources to ensure activities are aligned with the organization's overall strategic plan.

Job Title	APP Lead	
Job Title & Scope	**Reporting Structure & Authority**	**All APPs have a formal direct reporting structure to the department chair physician within their clinical department.** The APP Lead role functions under the guidance and support of the Medical Director and/or Clinical Department Administrator, which may include duties as *Administrative Supervisor*, *Functional Supervisor*, or a ***combination of both.***
		Administrative Supervisor: Has the authority and ability to exercise independent judgment regarding the supervision of employees, to include the authority to hire, evaluate, discipline and terminate, or to effectively recommend such actions.
		Functional Supervisor: Typically limited to tasks related to the assignment and distribution of work, such as training, scheduling, task assignments, and checking on work performed. While they may be asked for their input on evaluations, they may or may not be responsible for evaluating other employees.
Key Areas of Responsibility	**Provision of Care**	Supervise the care delivered by APP team and other members of the healthcare team.
	Collaboration with Care Team	Consult/collaborate with other care team members.
	Compliance/Policies Regulations Safe/Effective Care Delivery	Lead and participate in quality, safety, and process improvement initiatives. Influence others to adopt best practices. Provide leadership for and/or participate in the development of new infrastructure, program-wide quality assessments, and performance improvement initiatives.
	Education/Health/ Promotion/Research	Educate APPs and/or other members of the healthcare team. Participate in ongoing research and professional development. Serve on committees to enhance patient care and operations.
	Administration/HR Management	Lead staff performance and compliance in accordance with policies, procedures, and standards of care. Hire, develop, and manage the performance of staff. Assure team provides effective collaboration/ communications. Provide feedback and coaching to other team members to assure quality of specialized care. May have budget responsibilities.

FIGURE 1.2 APP lead roles.

APP Lead Duties May Include		
	Daily Operations	Lead resource and go-to for APPs and other assigned employees. Regularly schedule and conduct staff meetings. Troubleshoot operational issues. Assist with addressing patient concerns. Help resolve clinical issues. Communicate and resolve staffing needs in consult with medical director/CDA. Communicate provider needs. Serve as an intermediary between APPs and physicians (trainees and faculty) and other members of the care team. Ensure daily operations are in alignment with department/division initiatives including quality and safety initiatives, productivity, and growth.
	Communication	Maintain and disseminate effective communication between all members of assigned area and members of the care team (APPs, trainees, faculty, fellows, residents, nursing, ancillary, etc.).
	Productivity	Work with department leadership and individual APPs to monitor and maximize APP clinical contribution utilizing productivity metrics, ROI, top-of-license practice, and team-based care. Monitor workload and operational activity to ensure productivity expectations and top-of-license clinical practice are achieved and maintained.
	Staff Competency	Work with medical director on identifying competency requirements for specific privileges. Provide or coordinate supplemental education. Ensure staff are provided resources and training to obtain and maintain full competency and adhere to competency requirements and documentation.
	Shared Governance	Promote APP Council and ensure content is available to APPs within area of responsibility. Attend and participate in lead meetings and assist with disseminating information received from meetings as appropriate. Attend divisional or departmental meetings. Actively serve on organizational level committees as requested.
	Regulatory	Keep current on regulatory requirements at department/organizational level. Ensure work group maintains regulatory compliance. Assist with staff preparation and response during regulatory visits. Point of contact for scope of practice questions within work group in consult with CSO (Clinical Staff Office) and OAPP (Office of Advanced Practice Providers). Work with CSO and OAPP to maintain/update department list of privileges.
	Professional Growth	Work with department leadership and individual APPs to maximize APP clinical contribution utilizing productivity metrics, top-of-license practice, and team-based care. Support, facilitate, and oversight of clinical professional development and growth of APPs within clinical specialty. Ensure APPs participate in required and appropriate CME, and promote continued learning and ongoing evaluation of education gaps in APP performance.
	APP Role Development	Provide performance coaching and mentoring to assigned staff. Provide real-time feedback. Meet regularly with staff. Conduit and champion for development opportunities of staff. Recognize and reward staff performance. Actively work to promote employee engagement.
	Scheduling/Time & Attendance	Triage, schedule, and plan coverage of patient care including day-to-day work schedule and operations, cross-coverage, back-up coverage, and troubleshooting for overall consistent and appropriate care coverage. May include approval of time off requests and timecards. May have oversight of others completing these tasks.
	Hiring/Discipline/ Termination	Assist with recruiting/interviewing/selection process and provide input on hiring decisions. With department HR, provide input and attend disciplinary/termination meetings as appropriate. Monitor staffing levels and make recommendations for workforce optimization.
	Training/Education	Assess needs and provide education/training to appropriate learners. With division director determine skill needed for new hire APPs and establish and implement unit orientation, onboarding guides, and checklists. Monitor onboarding progress for new APPs.
	Performance Evaluations	Assist, provide input, or complete staff performance appraisal per organizational guidelines.
	Credentialing and Privileging	Review credentialing materials with HR and medical director to ensure APP is privileged for all appropriate procedures. With department credentialing contact, monitor progress towards privileging (i.e., know when the materials go to committees, etc.) and keep HR, preceptor, and schedulers aware of when new APP is privileged to see patients. Ensure timely completion of credentialing and privileging for new APP hires. May include coaching/instructing APP as to accurate and timely completion of all materials (credentialing form, taxonomy code, managed care billing packet, etc.).
	Orientation/Onboarding	Work with departmental leadership to determine timeline/productivity metrics for new hires. Develop detailed plan and timeline for full caseload, top-of-license practice. Communicate and implement detailed orientation schedule including calendar and IPPE competency review checklist. Identify primary preceptor and key stakeholders and make introductions. Monitor orientation/onboarding progress and make any necessary adjustments. Foster strong communication and serve as a resource/go-to for new hire.

FIGURE 1.3 APP lead duties.

APP leads work in concert with other leaders in identifying ways to ensure efficient recruitment, selection, deployment, onboarding, and retention. APP leads promote top-of-license practice, identify ways to systematically assess critical value metrics, and capture missed opportunities for revenue when APPs are involved in care. Goals include tracking APP contributions into meaningful and measurable data to gain leverage and clarity surrounding complex and multifactorial systems.

ARTICULATING EXISTING REPORTING STRUCTURES

Looking back over the centuries, physicians and other healthcare professionals had rudimentary practices, patients had modest expectations, and there were no real health systems, as clinicians were independent providers (Braithwaite et al., 2020). In 1996, the Accreditation Council for Graduate Medical Education (ACGME) limited the amount of time medical residents could spend taking care of pediatric and neonatal intensive care patients to six months of their three-year residency, including daytime rotations and night calls (Kane & Lorant, 2018). In response to this, at University of Iowa Health Care, one third of the provider workforce in the neonatal intensive care unit was ultimately replaced by neonatal and pediatric nurse practitioners. Like many organizations, this was one of the first historical changes in provider workforce when the significant need for creative infrastructures that support team-based care models was recognized. As time moved on and ongoing changes in traditional resident education by the ACGME posed restrictions, it was evident that a new model of care needed to emerge to care for patients in academic health centers that was sustainable and worked with multiple provider types, regardless of changes that occurred in medical and graduate education. Compounded by other historical issues unrelated to medical education, healthcare continued to be challenged with patient access, significant staffing shortages, high-acuity patients, and reimbursement issues.

Today, healthcare organizations are dealing with implications of the global COVID-19 pandemic, ever-changing technology, violence in the workplace, more severe staffing shortages, multiple provider types, financial challenges, and burnout, all while trying to keep providers engaged and healthy (Munn et al., 2022). Given these challenges, all organizations, regardless of size and structure, are encouraged to develop a mission statement reflective of their own desired practice expectations, organizational structures, and professional contributions. For example, University of Iowa Health Care established an infrastructure that supports APPs within the framework of a Board of Regents leadership structure and department-operated physician model based on the following mission statement:

> Provide an infrastructure for advanced practice providers that promotes
> a culture of professional practice, quality patient care, and personal

accountability that contributes to the overall success of the organization, while fostering an equitable, inclusive, and innovative environment that supports the health and well-being of patients, trainees, and ourselves. (University of Iowa Health Care, 2023, para. 3)

Providing organizational infrastructure for APPs requires leadership support to build collaborative relationships among physicians, nurses, APPs, executive leaders, and other key partners. APP leadership models involving a structure inclusive of both the APP lead and the physician division director are modeling the dyad of co-leaders at a system, hospital, or other organization and are not new models in healthcare (Hellmann, 2021). Physicians and nursing leaders are uniquely positioned to co-lead and transform healthcare delivery (Clausen et al., 2017). APP leads and physician leadership dyads function in a similar manner, working towards the safest and best patient outcomes, with decisions based on sound clinical practice guidelines and team principles and support for each other publicly to represent a strong and collaborative healthcare team. This dyad structure supports the administrative and clinical practice for seven important themes:

1. Define patient populations that should receive care from APPs as well as patient populations to receive care from physicians.

2. Structure an onboarding program for all APPs as they enter the organization, with division onboarding centered on patient-specific populations.

3. Develop clinical practice guidelines for standardization of evidence-based care practices for patient populations that are easily accessible.

4. Promote inclusivity at meetings and discussions about strategic plans and organization-wide initiatives to promote quality and safety.

5. Have well-defined caseload expectations and productivity metrics accessible through dashboards.

6. Provide professional growth opportunities to keep up to date with clinical knowledge and research.

7. Embrace opportunities to enhance visibility about the work APPs are doing.

IDENTIFYING KEY ORGANIZATIONAL LEADERS

Support from key organizational leaders that champion the work of APPs and their contribution to the mission of the organization is vital to the sustainable success of APPs. Leadership partners may include senior leaders in administration, finance, nursing, medical affairs, physician groups or faculty practice plans, and clinical operations. Leaders from support areas are equally essential to visibility and success for APPs and may include marketing, revenue cycle, human resources, compliance, legal, scheduling, credentialing and privileging, and coding and billing.

The importance in identifying all interested parties is to ensure everyone is knowledgeable about the education, certification, licensing, credentialing requirements, and scope of practice for APPs. This will alleviate any confusion and misinformation surrounding APPs and promote a common understanding to align best practices with the organization's mission. Organizations may need to develop methods and approaches for communicating ongoing and ever-changing issues specific to APPs. University of Iowa Health Care utilizes several approaches, including an APP-focused intranet site, train-the-trainer methodology using the APP leads as a communication conduit for their cohorts, and frequent communication and education through FAQs and recorded presentations that can be pushed out to large groups via targeted distribution.

As APPs are hired, it is essential they are not isolated in specialty clinical areas and are part of a clear organizational structure to ensure they are visible not only as members of the collaborative care team, within the departments and divisions, but at the highest organizational level.

Organizations should define and determine a centralized professional home, including an APP director and support staff. At University of Iowa Health Care, APPs are considered providers, and thus, the office of advanced practice providers reports to the executive director of the physician group. The APP director maintains a close relationship with the chief nursing executive for APRN matters and the College of Medicine for PA matters. Alternatively, APPs' centralized professional home may report up through the chief nursing executive and include an organizational structure with broader designated responsibilities for larger service lines such as pediatrics and adult patient populations. Regardless of the reporting structure, it is important to consider the needs, scope of practice, and support of both PAs and APRNs to be fully inclusive of both professions.

Organizations with strategic partnerships with APP educational programs (such as academic health centers) may consider an informal structure linked to leaders from the educational institutions. Figure 1.4 illustrates that the Director of Advanced Practice Providers has a dotted line to the PA Studies program and holds a dual appointment at the College of Nursing. Organizations without their own affiliated educational programs should prioritize building and sustaining positive relationships between APP leadership and appropriate educational programs.

APP structure may include dedicated support staff with subject matter expertise relating to APPs such as human resources, administrative support, data analytics, and project management. Operational oversight committees, such as the APP steering committee, should be reflected on the APP organizational chart.

From a clinical standpoint, APP oversight may be defined within the organizational bylaws and/or the Collaborative Practice Agreement or PA supervision documents (if required). This may be determined by the size and scale of the organization and the resources available, or by aligning with organizational norms for the reporting structure for other clinical leaders.

See Figure 1.4 and Figure 1.5 for organizational chart examples that reflect the structure at University of Iowa Health Care. Note that the Director of Advanced Practice Providers in this example is an influential leader in the true sense, with no direct reporting authority over APPs, but instead working as a consultative resource for all community members across the organization.

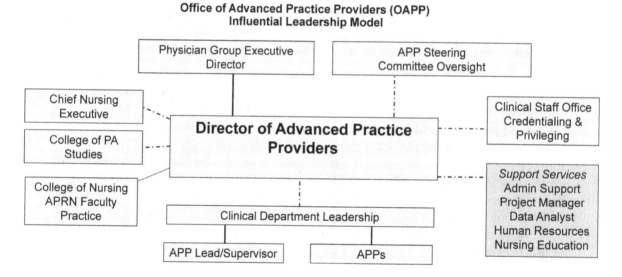

FIGURE 1.4 OAPP organizational chart.

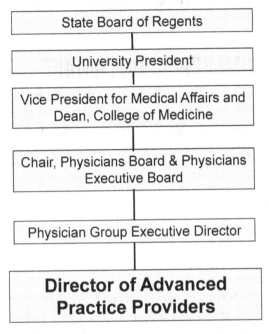

**Physician Group Organizational Chart
Including Advanced Practice Providers**

State Board of Regents

University President

Vice President for Medical Affairs and
Dean, College of Medicine

Chair, Physicians Board & Physicians
Executive Board

Physician Group Executive Director

**Director of Advanced
Practice Providers**

FIGURE 1.5   Physician group organizational chart.

IDENTIFYING ALL APPs

As APPs are employed by multiple types of organizations, including private practice, specialty departments and divisions, academic health centers, hospitals, etc., and functionally are often evaluated by physician colleagues, it is still important to provide a professional home and a sense of identity as a community with their peers. APRNs and PAs are highly educated professionals, and as graduates of their respective programs they provide quality, safe, and exceptional patient care. An article in *Forbes*, "Advanced Practice Providers Are the Key to America's Healthcare Future," states that "while these providers are distinct from each other in many ways, together they represent a healthcare workforce of certified and state-licensed medical professionals that are essential to operations in both inpatient and outpatient settings" (Corley, 2017, para. 3).

APP work effort may be difficult to identify within electronic health records (EHRs) to capture and optimize billing potential that is a direct result of APP productivity. At the very least, APP work effort needs to be able to be associated in the EHR with the patients they care for. Having a platform where all APPs are identified with accurate licensure, board certification and specialty area, as well as an accurate reporting structure, serves as a baseline tracking method for organizations as their APPs continue to grow in numbers.

ESTABLISHING A COMMUNICATION CONDUIT

Geographic and multiple practice sites, hours, and schedules make disseminating information to APPs challenging. As with any successful communication conduit, multiple pathways for distributing important information are required.

Examples of these include:

- APP council
- APP central office
- Intranet or extranet
- APP steering committee

An APP council is a platform to provide information that is pertinent to APPs (University of Iowa Health Care, 2020). Because the council includes all APPs within the organization that are credentialed and privileged, the council platform is not used for patient-population-specific education but rather all-encompassing issues affecting the greater APP disciplines including, but not limited to, changes regarding reimbursement, changes with student documentation for precepting APP students, and important quality and safety initiatives.

Organizations may have an established APP central office that represents the group of APP leaders and support staff who field, evaluate, and distribute information under the auspices of the APP council. The APP central office serves as the expert resource in the utilization of APPs across multiple environments of care and is a resource for all questions and concerns related to APPs. The central office also assists with the development of business cases for the integration of new models of care delivery using APPs. Goals include working with department leaders to establish templates and checklists to ensure documentation of orientation and identifying metrics for initial, focused, and ongoing professional performance evaluation. The APP central office establishes close relationships and collaboration with department- and division-level human resource staff, departmental clinical and administrative leadership, as well as enterprise-level departments essential to the operations of the healthcare system (i.e., information systems, clinical documentation and improvement, billing and coding). An APP central office may host an internal web-based platform, such as an intranet, used as a means to provide ongoing announcements and information pertinent for practice and host a variety of other APP resources.

An APP steering committee is one example of oversight composed of select executive-level leadership including physicians, nursing, clinical department administrators, finance, APP leads, human resources, and academic representation from the APP programs. The steering committee serves as an advisory board for all projects and initiatives that evolve from the central APP office. This is one additional avenue for communication to ensure every level of leader is engaged and aware of APP initiatives. The experience of committee members, diversity in roles, and representation from variable disciplines provide a lens towards thoughtful insight for patient satisfaction metrics, patient access and throughput, productivity and value, and provider engagement. Committee members serve as advisors to support APP productivity and top-of-license practice and vet projects and initiatives that align with the organizational strategic plan. Established as an advisory committee, the APP steering committee does not set policy or dictate how departments operationalize their APPs.

The committee serves three main purposes:

- Ensure senior leaders are aware of issues pertinent to APP practices
- Provide guidance and direction on new and existing projects
- Support the organization towards a strong APP clinical operating model

SUMMARY

Optimizing an APP infrastructure that can be integrated into existing leadership structures requires a concerted effort at all levels of the healthcare organization. There are multiple variables to consider while strategizing how to implement an infrastructure that aligns with payers and state and institutional laws and bylaws and considers how an organization's unique culture influences APP practice. Recognizing this growing group of providers as vital members of the healthcare team is first and foremost. APPs are challenged due to the variability in state practice laws, CMS and reimbursement issues, lack of CMS taxonomy codes to identify specialty practice, and poorly defined reporting structures. Today more than ever, collaboration and teamwork need to be at the forefront of healthcare delivery practice models to optimize APP practice and growth.

REFERENCES

Accreditation Review Commission on Education for the Physician Assistant. (2023). *PA programs*. http://www.arc-pa.org/accreditation/program-data/

Ackerman, M. H., Mick, D., & Witzel, P. (2010). Creating an organizational model to support advanced practice. *JONA: The Journal of Nursing Administration, 40*(2), 63–68. https://doi.org/10.1097/NNA.0b013e3181cb9f71

American Academy of Physician Associates. (2023). *About AAPA*. https://www.aapa.org/about/

American Association of Nurse Practitioners. (2022). *NP facts sheet*. https://www.aanp.org/about/all-about-NPS/np-fact-sheet

Anen, T., & McElroy, D. (2015). Infrastructure to optimize APRN practice. *Nurse Leader, 13*(2), 50–56. https://doi.org/10.1016/j.mnl.2015.01.004

Anen, T., & McElroy, D. (2017). The evolution of the new provider team: Driving cultural change through data. *Nursing Administration Quarterly, 41*(1), 4–10. https://doi.org/10.1097/naq.0000000000000202

Association of American Medical Colleges. (2021, June 11). *AAMC report reinforces mounting physician shortage*. https://www.aamc.org/news-insights/press-releases/aamc-report-reinforces-mounting-physician-shortage

Bachynsky, N. (2020). Implications for policy: The Triple Aim, Quadruple Aim, and interprofessional collaboration. *Nursing Forum, 55*(1), 54–64. https://doi.org/https://doi.org/10.1111/nuf.12382

Bahouth, M. N., Blum, K., & Simone, S. (2012). *Transitioning into hospital based practice: A guide for nurse practitioners and administrators*. Springer Publishing Company.

Braithwaite, J., Vincent, C., Garcia-Elorrio, E., Imanaka, Y., Nicklin, W., Sodzi-Tettey, S., & Bates, D. W. (2020). Transformational improvement in quality care and health systems: The next decade. *BMC Medicine, 18*(1), 340. https://doi.org/10.1186/s12916-020-01739-y

Clausen, C., Lavoie-Tremblay, M., Purden, M., Lamothe, L., Ezer, H., & McVey, L. (2017). Intentional partnering: A grounded theory study on developing effective partnerships among nurse and physician managers as they co-lead in an evolving healthcare system. *Journal of Advanced Nursing, 73*(9), 2156–2166. https://doi.org/10.1111/jan.13290

Corley, J. (2017, March 16). Advanced-practice providers are key to America's healthcare future. *Forbes*. https://www.forbes.com/sites/realspin/2017/03/16/advanced-practice-providers-are-key-to-americas-healthcare-future/?sh=491d14425998

Enders, T., Morin, A., & Pawlak, B. (2016, March 24). *Advancing healthcare transformation: A new era for academic nursing*. Manatt. https://www.manatt.com/insights/white-papers/2016/advancing-healthcare-transformation-a-new-era-for-academic-nursing.pdf

Hellmann, J. (2021, June 19). CMO-CNO partnerships can drive patient safety and quality. *Modern Healthcare*. https://www.modernhealthcare.com/providers/cmo-cno-partnerships-can-drive-patient-safety-and-quality

Ingram, J. (2023, January 10). U.S. News ranks the best jobs of 2023. *U.S. News & World Report*. https://money.usnews.com/careers/articles/u-s-news-ranks-the-best-jobs

Kane, S. K., & Lorant, D. E. (2018). The amount of supervision trainees receive during neonatal resuscitation is variable and often dependent on subjective criteria. *Journal of Perinatology, 38*(8), 1081–1086. https://doi.org/10.1038/s41372-018-0137-4

Lofgren, M. A., Berends, S. K., Reyes, J., Wycoff, C., Kinnetz, M., Frohling, A., Baker, L., Whitty, S., Dirks, M., & O'Brien, M. (2017). Scope of practice barriers for advanced practice registered nurses: A state task force to minimize barriers. *Journal of Nursing Administration, 47*(9), 465–469. https://doi.org/10.1097/NNA.0000000000000515

Munn, L. T., Huffman, C. S., Connor, C. D., Swick, M., Danhauer, S. C., & Gibbs, M. A. (2022). A qualitative exploration of the National Academy of Medicine model of well-being and resilience among healthcare workers during COVID-19. *Journal of Advanced Nursing, 78*(8), 2561–2574. https://doi.org/10.1111/jan.15215

Physician Assistant Education Association. (2020). *By the numbers: Program report 35: Data from the 2019 program survey.* https://paeaonline.org/wp-content/uploads/2020/11/program-report35-20201014.pdf

Rosseter, Robert. (2023). *Fact sheet: The Doctor of Nursing Practice (DNP).* https://www.aacnnursing.org/news-data/fact-sheets/dnp-fact-sheet

University of Iowa Health Care. (2020). *APP council.* https://uihc.org/app-council

University of Iowa Health Care. (2022, March 16). *The University of Iowa physician's guide to advanced practice providers.*

University of Iowa Health Care. (2023). *Advanced practice providers.* https://uihc.org/advanced-practice-providers

"Whatever affects one directly affects all indirectly. I can never be what I ought to be until you are what you ought to be. This is the interrelated structure of reality."

—Martin Luther King, Jr.

CHAPTER 2

UNDERSTANDING THE ORGANIZATIONAL BLUEPRINT

KEYWORDS | medical staff, private practice, health system, multi-specialty practice, academic practice

The legal, financial, and supervisory structure of the organization in which APRNs and PAs are employed significantly influences their work. While each organizational blueprint has potential benefits and pitfalls, all have the capability to provide APPs with a fulfilling practice environment. Healthcare organizational structures have evolved over time in response to changes in both the way patient care is delivered and, in many circumstances, to how revenues flow into and how expenses are assigned to groups of providers. As such, understanding the organization's structure provides insight into APP practice optimization and satisfaction and how they contribute to high-quality patient care. This chapter provides a summary of the various practice models and how the organizational blueprint can impact the way that APPs practice.

HOW PHYSICIAN GROUPS ARE ORGANIZED

A *physician group* refers to one or more physicians working together to provide patient care. These groups can be partnerships, individual or multiple associations, or corporations and tend to be organized as single or multiple subgroups based upon provider specialty training (e.g., family medicine, medical cardiology, etc.) rather than a service line model focusing on specific disease categories (e.g., primary care, cardiovascular disease, etc.). As healthcare has evolved, APPs are more frequently included in these practice groups. Practice groups contract with payers and vendors as a single entity, which can provide significant benefits because revenues minus practice expenses can be distributed directly to the providers. Group expenses and strategic investments tend to be distributed based upon consensus methodologies from all the providers or from the group leadership. The specifics of overhead allocation and its relationship to compensation can be a source of significant challenge in current fee-for-service healthcare but is even more challenging as we move into value-based or capitation contracts. Single- and multi-specialty independent groups have been common for decades; however, this is changing as practice consolidation expands due to shifts in healthcare regulation and economics.

COMPARING PRACTICE ENVIRONMENTS

There is no perfect way to organize physicians and APPs. The two major approaches are to be employed by a physician group or to be employed by a health system anchored by one or more hospitals. Each model has its own relative benefits. Physician groups tend to focus on patient access and flow and allow significant provider practice autonomy with low levels of bureaucracy. There may be significant financial investment required to buy into the practice, which translates into personal financial risk. There also tends to be less investment in shared services and continuing education. Alternatively, health systems provide little personal financial risk to the provider, but there tends to be less clinical autonomy with lower direct compensation but better employee benefits. Decision-making within larger health systems can be opaque, with onerous bureaucratic processes. A more detailed comparison between organizational structures follows.

PRIVATE PRACTICE

Private practice is one of the most straightforward structures. A specialty private practice (solo provider or provider group) tends to be a single legal corporation dedicated to providing care to a specific patient population funded by the generation of clinical revenues. An example of this would be a pediatric private practice with one or more providers. Like all corporations, private practices require a governing board with owner representation, but the makeup of that board as well as the option to buy into the practice and become an owner with corporate shares vary. Owners of a private practice may be the practicing providers or other investors. The American Medical Association (AMA) reports a steady decrease from 2012 to 2020 in the number of physicians in private practice and a corresponding decrease in the number of physicians who are practice owners (Strazewski, 2021).

One of the benefits of private practice ownership is practice profit distributions as opposed to compensation under a straightforward employment model. APP compensation may be salaried or linked to clinical productivity or quality performance. When performance-based compensation is contemplated, the metrics and expectations should be clearly outlined and transparent to the APP. Expenses such as direct patient care costs and general overhead related to patient care should be allocated among the providers in straightforward ways. In private practice, physicians and APPs tend to work closely together one-on-one with less focus on protocols for how to care for various patient populations. This means physicians and APPs focus on sharing patient panels instead of having different patient panels for each provider.

The relationship between physicians and APPs in a private practice setting should be thoughtfully evaluated to support the optimization of the practice philosophy. Examples include APPs practicing independently or a joint appointment with physician colleagues. Hospital credentialing and privileging is not required for providers practicing exclusively in ambulatory private practice. Onboarding, training opportunities, and professional advancement may be limited in private practice as they operate with fewer resources in comparison to more comprehensive health systems. The private practice structure provides the most autonomy to providers, but it comes with significant risk and responsibility for the financial performance of the company.

MULTI-SPECIALTY PRIVATE PRACTICE

Multi-specialty private practice has more complexity, especially in determining expense allocation among specialties. The practice is also most commonly a single legal corporation with the benefit of autonomy and financial risk similar to private practice. However, since revenue streams differ between specialties, with certain specialties being more lucrative than others, the distribution of clinical expense and overhead allocations can be more challenging. Malpractice premiums also may vary between specialties, requiring thoughtful approaches regarding the best way to allocate these expenses. Consideration should be given to determining whether the expense allocations are based on direct expenses, which is advantageous to higher reimbursed specialties (e.g., workers' compensation), or as a percentage of revenue, which tends to advantage lower reimbursed specialties (e.g., primary care). As primary care providers also provide referrals to specialists, a funds flow from specialists to primary care providers is commonly paid to subsidize adequate primary care compensation because the relative reimbursement is lower. APP compensation tends to be similar to single specialty practices with a strong focus on high-quality clinical care without the complexity of academic pursuits. The AMA reports the shifts toward larger practices and away from physician-owned (private) practices have accelerated. "2020 was the first year in which less than half (49.1%) of patient care physicians worked in a private practice," a drop of almost 5 percentage points from 2018. 17.2% of physicians were in practices with at least 50 physicians in 2020, up from 14.7% in 2018 (Kane, 2022, para. 3–4).

HEALTH SYSTEM MODELS

The Agency for Healthcare Research and Quality (2023, para. 6) defines a *health system* as "an organization that consists of at least one hospital and at least one group of physicians that provides comprehensive care (including primary and specialty care) who are connected with each other through common ownership."

Providers practice within a health system under either an open staff model or a closed staff model. In an *open staff model*, single and multi-specialty practices contract with hospitals or health systems to provide clinical or medical service/oversight. The hospital medical staff bylaws will define requirements for physician and APP practice within the hospital. In comparison, a *closed staff model* specifies that to obtain privileges to work within a hospital, all the providers must also be part of a specific practice group owned by or closely affiliated with the hospital.

Documentation of clinical training or certification specific to the health system is required to be part of the medical staff and is defined by the scope of practice developed by clinical service leaders or directors. There may also be specific requirements for hospital service coverage, backup, and quality oversight. Health systems may adopt state legislated practice laws or establish their own practice agreements as long they do not go beyond state legislated scope of practice. For example, in Iowa, an APRN may have a collaborative agreement with a physician or physicians if their practice so warrants, but this agreement is not a requirement of the Iowa Board of Nursing (2023). At University of Iowa Health Care, the PAs privileging document is called the PA Addendum, and APRNs are privileged under a collaborative practice agreement. It is important for there to be clear delineation of roles and responsibilities for each of the providers, and this is typically outlined in the specific service definitional privileging documents. These issues around hospital privileging, credentialing, and medical staff bylaws are explored more fully in subsequent chapters and should be part of any APP orientation to the organization. All providers should be well versed in the regulatory requirements related to their specific practice model; for example, data sharing and monetary support between private practices and hospitals is highly regulated through anti-kickback and Stark laws.

Anti-Kickback Statute [42 U.S.C. § 1320a-7b(b)] The AKS is a criminal law that prohibits the knowing and willful payment of "remuneration" to induce or reward patient referrals or the generation of business involving any item or service payable by the Federal healthcare programs (e.g., drugs, supplies, or healthcare services for Medicare or Medicaid patients). Remuneration includes anything of value and can take many forms besides cash, such as free rent, expensive hotel stays and meals, and excessive compensation for medical directorships or consultancies. In some industries, it is acceptable to reward those who refer business to you. However, in the Federal healthcare programs, paying for referrals is a crime. The statute covers the payers of kickbacks—those who offer or pay remuneration—as well as the recipients of kickbacks—those who solicit or receive remuneration. Each party's intent is a key element of their liability under the AKS.

Physician Self-Referral Law [42 U.S.C. § 1395nn] The Physician Self-Referral Law, commonly referred to as the Stark law, prohibits physicians from referring patients to receive "designated health services" payable by Medicare or Medicaid from entities with which the physician or an immediate family member has a financial relationship, unless an exception applies. Financial relationships include both ownership/investment interests and compensation arrangements. For example, if you invest in an imaging center, the Stark law requires the resulting financial relationship to fit within an exception or you may not refer patients to the facility, and the entity may not bill for the referred imaging services.

(US Department of Health & Human Services, Office of Inspector General, 2023).

The private practice of medicine is shrinking within the United States (Kane, 2019) as providers appear to prefer the employment model within a larger hospital or health system. Within this model, the provider connection to ownership of the corporation is lost, and providers are generally no longer directly at risk for the financial or regulatory performance of the practice. The main drivers of this trend are the increasingly high costs of running a practice (including technology such as EHRs), declining payer reimbursement, and the regulatory/compliance landscape. Providers employed through a health system are more insulated from business aspects of healthcare and thus less susceptible to changes required by forces outside the practice. However, less personal risk may also result in less autonomy for decision-making around practice strategy and operations and a more structured, top-down corporate model for decision-making.

A health system can exist as a series of corporations under a larger holding company or one single corporation. Having multiple professional corporations under one umbrella has implications for credentialing, payer enrollment, billing, and data sharing. In this model, each corporation must contract with all other entities within the holding corporation to seamlessly share data throughout the organization. There are circumstances when this model would be particularly beneficial for APP practice, as it would circumvent common reimbursement conflicts such as when two APPs in two separate specialties see the same patient in the same day. Compared to a single specialty practice, a multi-specialty entity model—either academic or private—does provide APPs flexibility to change their work environment between different areas or services or specialties, as long as they are practicing within the scope of their education, licensure, and board certification.

ACADEMIC PRACTICES

An academic or university-based medical center has a broader focus compared to a private practice or health system. Academic health centers' tripartite mission includes not only patient care but also education (of medical, PA, APRN, and/or other healthcare students) and research. Academic practices that are aligned with a medical school can be affiliated with, owned by, or integrated into a hospital or health system, but they rarely are stand-alone private practice corporations. Legal structures vary, but the Association of American Medical Colleges (AAMC) indicates that in 2022, 75% of medical schools in the US are either owned by the university or a separate nonprofit corporation, and a few are single or multiple separate legal corporations (AAMC, 2022a).

Working within an academic practice environment has significant implications for how APPs practice and care for patients. Each academic health system has an organized faculty practice plan that outlines the practice requirements for their medical school teaching faculty.

Academic practices must balance patient care, research, and education missions in ways purely clinical operations do not. The presence of these missions also leads to the enterprise being structured by the academic department rather than a clinical service line. For example, although the clinical service of a urology department might span from general pediatrics to adult oncology, it's the urologic faculty learner curriculum and training that drives the structure of the department. Members of the department might have alignment with their similar specialty clinical work (e.g., pediatrics vs. adults, oncology vs. urolithiasis) in their day-to-day work rather than the academic department. This may be different from other healthcare professions, which may have more focus on the clinical service rather than the academic one. Nursing in particular tends to be organized by intensity of patient care such as critical care, general inpatient, procedural, and ambulatory nursing. While these disciplines may not cross all age groups, the competencies will tend to be similar, although the patient's disease may span multiple medical or surgical specialties. The number of physician clinical track faculty involved in the clinical mission has grown over the decades, while basic science faculty have not grown to a significant degree (AAMC, 2022b; Xierali et al., 2021).

For academic practices, clinical revenues have become the major funding stream rather than tuition or research dollars. The clinical mission underwrites the other missions, as the funding streams for research and education cannot stand on their own economically (AAMC, 2014; Enders & Conroy, 2014). APPs tend to be involved primarily in the clinical mission of the organization and serve as the primary workforce to keep the clinical mission operating smoothly. However, the tripartite mission of an academic practice (patient care, education, research) invariably affects the clinical practice of the APP. All types of healthcare students, including medical students, residents, and fellows, are commonly a part of all clinical teams. APPs in an academic environment collaborate with many types of learners, alongside faculty physicians who are also involved in research and education. The expectation of all providers in an academic practice environment to keep clinical volumes high to support revenue can conflict with the departmental leadership need for faculty to write grants to fund research, write academic papers, and oversee resident and student education. An APP workforce focusing on clinical patient care supports physician faculty time and resources towards the other missions. The benefits of the academic practice model are more opportunities for continuing education, involvement in education, and higher acuity patient populations, which can be professionally fulfilling for APPs seeking this type of work environment.

MEDICAL SCHOOL AND ACADEMIC HEALTH SYSTEMS CULTURES

Freestanding academic organizations (meaning those that are not contained within a larger university) such as University of California, San Francisco; Oregon Health and Sciences University; and Medical University of South Carolina have the benefit of focusing clinical, research, and educational funds and pursuits toward healthcare activities.

Cultural issues can still exist between the school of medicine and health system in these organizations in that healthcare schools and schools of medicine tend to be federated with limited central governance with faculty seeking significant autonomy (AAMC, 2014; Enders & Conroy, 2014). Health systems tend to have significant central governance with command-and-control structures as well as extensive investments in infrastructure (AAMC, 2014; Enders & Conroy, 2014). These differences in culture can be improved by putting focus on advancing the course of the clinical mission and patient care. High-quality, safe, innovative patient care resonates with most everyone in the organization and can be a rallying cry to get beyond organizational cultural differences.

The AAMC (2022c) reports that patient care services generate the largest source of revenue for medical schools, over 40%, followed by research grants at 22%. Tuition dollars make up 3% of the revenue for medical schools.

When the healthcare system is within a larger university that includes a substantial undergraduate complement such as University of Iowa Health Care, Michigan Medicine, and Johns Hopkins Medicine, differences between the two operational initiatives must be understood by both sides so that issues resulting in competing priorities can be avoided. This is particularly true for public universities in states where legislatures have in recent years substantially reduced monetary support. The significant pressure to improve the undergraduate experience and student success is appropriate, but the cost of such improvements cannot be borne solely by tuition revenues. The larger university community then looks to the healthcare system to provide additional funds for initiatives outside patient care support, research, and education. These pressures can limit the ability of the healthcare delivery system to make the pivots and adjustments necessary to be nimble as changes occur in healthcare. These pressures outside the delivery apparatus are not present for academic health systems such as the Mayo Clinic, Cleveland Clinic, or Medical University of South Carolina, so focus can be placed squarely on healthcare workforce and investments. Healthcare delivery is a highly capital-intensive activity. Expenses such as labor and supplies continue to increase, along with capital expenditures for new technology and therapeutics coming to market, while at the same time revenue from payers is flat or declining. The cost of replacing facilities and equipment is higher than the initial outlay or depreciation. While healthcare is not a unique business in this way, being part of a larger organization such as a university is. Virtually no other ongoing business is as closely aligned with a university educational apparatus as is healthcare, specifically for these reasons. These economics can put the entire university at risk of decline should the healthcare apparatus fail and thus put at risk the entire educational mission.

There are important mutual benefits when healthcare delivery systems are contained within a larger university, such as those outlined above. The educational opportunities for students interested within healthcare majors as well as those outside healthcare are unparalleled. There is opportunity for access to shadowing, part-time jobs, practicums, and experiences for students of all types. There are also expanded opportunities for research in both the sciences and humanities compared to universities without access to healthcare delivery systems. The university community benefits of having an academic healthcare arm outweigh the risks. To be successful, however, requires clearly outlined goals, objectives, and strategic plans to advance all colleges within the university, whether directly related to healthcare or not. Trade-offs will be necessary in both long- and short-term planning, with clear and consistent communication about the reasons the trade-offs are necessary to bring leaders and frontline workers together (AAMC, 2014; Enders & Conroy, 2014).

Organizational leaders should work to address barriers to change that are unique to an academic medical center. Enders and Conroy (2014) and the AAMC (2014) describe the main challenge as alignment of all organizational cultures around the clinical mission, including the higher ed, medical center, and clinical practice cultures. Working together as a clinical system requires executive commitment to an enterprise approach, alignment around operating system finances, a shared governance approach to leadership, and awareness of the constraints of the academic medical center providing financial support to the university (AAMC, 2014; Enders & Conroy, 2014).

Academic health centers have been challenged with articulating the need for nimbleness in decision-making and with inefficient and bureaucratic structures. Much of the tension is a result of structures being put in years or decades earlier for good reason but which may be outdated. Departmental desire for autonomy can result in not only service duplication but also a real risk of activity in direct conflict with initiatives the enterprise is trying to put in place or legal/regulatory risk the enterprise is attempting to minimize. Employee and faculty satisfaction surveys commonly identify positive engagement in the local work environment but disengagement with the enterprise as a whole. This can lead to distrust between provider types, employee groups, departments, frontline workers, and administration. These cultural issues cannot be overcome in a short time period. It takes intention and a concerted effort by all teams to trust one another. Everyone within the enterprise will need to rally around the clinical mission to most efficiently and effectively care for the patients. That requires the senior leaders to provide ongoing, clear, and consistent messages to all providers and staff. The trade-off, however, is unlimited resources do not exist. The enterprise needs to be able to support the appropriate level of care for every patient, but there are limits to what is possible. Similarly, providers and staff will not be able to have unlimited assistance in providing that care. The economics of healthcare are at a tenuous balance, and institutions collectively must work across disciplines, departments, and services to provide the greatest possible care to the greatest number of patients.

UNDERSTANDING HOW PHYSICIANS MANAGE EACH OTHER

Physician groups, whether independent or within larger health systems, tend to be managed in traditional hierarchical structures. In academic organizations, the dean of the school of medicine historically represents the highest level of physician group manager, with individual physician department chairs reporting directly to the dean. Practice administrators work closely with the physician department chairs and frontline physicians to strategize and optimize the overall clinical operations of the practice. Integrating APP management into these organizations aligns with this same model, being mindful of individual state regulations that may require varying levels of supervision.

Other physician management examples include academic organizations that have aligned physician management with the associated healthcare organization. In these enterprises, it is important to develop a mechanism to coordinate and collaborate with the academic departments to ensure physician and APP practice remains synergistic. These efforts also need to be coordinated with the healthcare organizations' credentialing and privileging processes because providers need to adhere to the requirements where they will practice.

Non-academic health systems tend to have similar hierarchical structures, with a chief medical officer or chief physician executive rather than a dean who serves as the highest level of physician oversight. Department chairs in non-academic structures similarly provide leadership and oversight of all providers with privileges in the health system. In these non-academic health systems, the overall provider management structure requires credentialing and privileging with all associated hospitals.

Private practice groups also tend to have hierarchical structures with the lead physician as either the chief executive officer, chief physician executive, or the president of the governing board. This lead physician oversees department chairs as aligned by specialty. In private practice groups, there tends to be less focus on hospital credentialing and privileging and more focus on the other aspects of physician practice. APP management in these groups can be easily integrated into pre-existing management protocols.

SUMMARY

Leaders and providers globally and APPs specifically are challenged to be successful in different organizational structures. Subsequent chapters will address many of the structural ways to support APP practice. However, it is most important to determine which practice style fits the individual APP best. A complex academic enterprise with a penchant for top-down rules and regulations may not be desirable, and working directly with a hospital/health system structure or private practice physician might be a better fit. If educational opportunities and multidisciplinary team aspects of care or increased patient complexity are sources of excitement, an academic practice might be the best fit. Leaders discussing these trade-offs of their specific enterprise blueprint with the APP during recruitment and orientation helps allow for questions and concerns to be raised as well as for expectations for the working environment to be set. Once the APP has weighed their own preferences, the most important next step is to engage in a discussion with leadership about where they can be successful. This discussion provides an opportunity to explore how the organizational blueprint corresponds to the blueprints explained in this chapter.

REFERENCES

Agency for Healthcare Research and Quality. (2023). *Defining health systems.* https://www.ahrq.gov/chsp/defining-health-systems/index.html

Association of American Medical Colleges. (2014). *Advancing the academic health system for the future: A report from the AAMC advisory panel on health care.* https://www.manatt.com/uploadedFiles/Content/2_Our_People/Enders,_Thomas/AdvancingtheAcademicHealthSystemfortheFuture_AAMC_Mar2014_Paper.PDF

Association of American Medical Colleges. (2022a). *Organizational characteristics database (OCD).* https://www.aamc.org/data-reports/faculty-institutions/report/organizational-characteristics-database-ocd

Association of American Medical Colleges. (2022b). *U.S. medical school faculty trends: Counts.* https://www.aamc.org/data-reports/faculty-institutions/data/us-medical-school-faculty-trends-counts

Association of American Medical Colleges. (2022c). *U.S. medical school revenues.* https://www.aamc.org/data-reports/faculty-institutions/report/us-medical-school-revenues

Enders, T., & Conroy, J. M. (2014). *Advancing the academic health system for the future: A report from the AAMC advisory panel on health care.* https://www.aamc.org/about-us/mission-areas/health-care/advancing-future-academic-health-systems

Iowa Board of Nursing. (2023). *Advanced registered nurse practitioner – Role & scope.* https://nursing.iowa.gov/practice/advanced-registered-nurse-practitioner-role-scope

Kane, C. (2019). *Updated data on physician practice arrangements: For the first time, fewer physicians are owners than employees.* AMA 2019 Policy Research Perspectives. https://www.ama-assn.org/system/files/2019-07/prp-fewer-owners-benchmark-survey-2018.pdf

Kane, C. K. (2022). *Recent changes in physician practice arrangements: Private practice dropped to less than 50 percent of physicians in 2020.* AMA Policy Research Perspectives. https://www.ama-assn.org/system/files/2021-05/2020-prp-physician-practice-arrangements.pdf

Strazewski, L. (2021, August 9). *Practice owner or employee? Physician's specialty may tell the tale.* American Medical Association. https://www.ama-assn.org/medical-residents/transition-resident-attending/practice-owner-or-employee-physicians-specialty-may

US Department of Health and Human Services-Office of Inspector General. (2023). *Fraud & abuse laws.* https://oig.hhs.gov/compliance/physician-education/fraud-abuse-laws/

Xierali, I., Nivet, M., & Rayburn, W. (2021, April). Full-time faculty in clinical and basic science departments by sex and underrepresented in medicine status: A 40-year review. *Academic Medicine, 96*(4), 568–575. https://doi.org/10.1097/ACM.0000000000003925

CHAPTER 3

ESTABLISHING AN INFRASTRUCTURE

KEYWORDS | organizational culture, competency, leadership, support, growth, resources, APP council, taxonomy codes

Establishing an infrastructure to incorporate all healthcare team members is paramount for an engaged and productive workforce. Chapter 1 reviewed the historical healthcare infrastructures of medicine and nursing and examined the need to optimize structures and processes to best deploy the growing APP workforce. Historical barriers within an organization, such as lack of knowledge about the scope of practice of the APP role, can often interfere with initiatives towards improving infrastructures. Incorporating APPs into existing organizational infrastructures that align with strategic goals will support the overarching business operations. There are multiple resources already embedded in organizations, and integrating APPs with those resources prevents duplication. Part of that infrastructure includes effectively attributing the work effort of all providers appropriately. Aligning the work effort that APPs are performing is instrumental in supporting their professional identity and quantifying the return on investment to the organization. This chapter will detail the steps necessary for organizations to move towards a fully integrated APP infrastructure.

UNDERSTANDING ORGANIZATIONAL GEOGRAPHY

A clear appreciation and understanding of organizational structure will help define how to approach positive change. It is important to identify ways to work within the constraints of organizational structures, including labor unions, multiple healthcare-related learners, or other top-down corporate decision-making models to allow APPs to work to the top of their licenses and education. The role of the APP is rapidly expanding in healthcare, whereas the infrastructure to support it is not keeping pace (Proulx, 2021). The number of NPs required to provide patient care in an ever-growing, complex hospital environment is increasing rapidly (Bahouth et al., 2013). PAs are also expected to increase at a growth rate of approximately 35% by 2035 (Hooker et al., 2022). Ensuring that APRNs and PAs practice to the top of their licenses and education is essential to best practice and must be at the forefront of positive cultural changes to stay abreast of rapidly changing healthcare environments.

DEPARTMENTS, DIVISIONS, AND OUTREACH CLINICS

Organizational geography includes the overarching organizational structures discussed in Chapter 2 such as private practice, multi-specialty practice, health systems, and academic health systems. Substructures within an organization may also include departments, divisions, and community outreach clinics. Substructures most often are integrated into larger health and academic systems. For example, a health system that has a pediatric department may include specialty divisions such as pediatric nephrology, pediatric urology, or pediatric cardiology. This same department may include several pediatric clinics across the community or state.

Whether practicing in a department, division specialty, or outreach program, each of these substructures needs to reflect the organizational blueprint as a whole. Often there are variances in privileges for APPs from department to department or within the same department but at different locations, such as outreach clinics. Assuring APPs are competent and privileged to practice within those environments and are following the organization's delineation of privileges set forth by the clinical systems committee assures safe, quality care at every location. This is important not only for quality patient care but also for managed care billing enrollment information.

When determining competency for the same privileges in separate departments, it is important to ensure the requirements have been agreed on at the larger organizational level for consistency. Sometimes privileges for procedures vary from department to department based on clinical and diagnostic rationale for the procedure. Organizations should give thoughtful attention, focusing on safety, efficiency, and top-of-license practice when making decisions regarding variances in privileges. When making decisions regarding the same privileges for procedures that differentiate based on department or location, patient-centered practices that align with state laws and organizational bylaws should always be at the forefront. It's common to have some autonomy across divisions and departments, but having many different competency rules for the same privileges creates potentially inefficient practices and processes.

KEY LEADERSHIP SUPPORT

Healthcare has evolved into a team practice, and it is important to have key leaders surrounding and supporting APPs. Effective communication to promote a positive work culture is an important attribute for all leaders. Figure 3.1 demonstrates a circle of support for the APP regardless of how it is operationalized. Physician leadership, APP leads, the central office for APPs, and the administrative team, including human resources and clinical administrators, all play an important part in supporting the APP for success. If there is any breakdown in communication, philosophy of operation, or lack of knowledge regarding the scope of practice for the APP, it can be detrimental to the APP's successful integration into the organization.

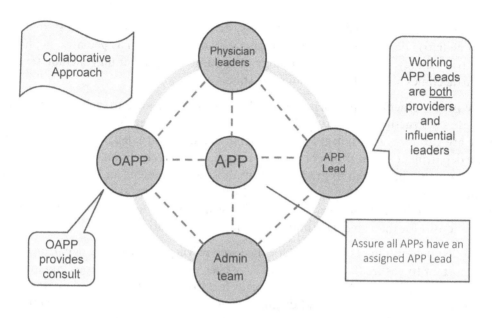

FIGURE 3.1 APP circle of support.

A thoughtful approach in building and sustaining an APP leadership infrastructure is to formulate an advisory board or enterprise steering committee to guide the organizational strategic direction for projects and initiatives associated with APPs. Interdisciplinary committees composed of key organizational leaders can support and champion a strong APP clinical operating model, leading professional practice for PAs and APRNs and capitalizing on APP productivity, retention, patient satisfaction, and safe, quality patient care. It is important to align the central APP office leadership to this committee so there is adequate resource allocation to implement and execute the initiatives that support the organization's strategic plans and to provide oversight of all projects and initiatives involving APPs. Whether an organization's structure reflects private practice, multi-specialty practice, a health system, or an academic health system, each organization operationalizes APPs in a way that fits into their own clinical practice models. An overarching enterprise committee can create recommendations for APP clinical practice models for leaders to implement where it makes sense within their organization. This is supportive of any organization where there are multiple substructures supporting APP practice to provide consistency but does not interfere with direct oversight, finances, or workflows of APPs embedded within departments or substructures.

In an academic health center model, where departments are independent in their operations, it is important to have assigned department accountability for clinical responsibilities for APPs. This includes clearly communicating information about department operations, providing overall infrastructure support, and establishing the development of clinical practice guidelines specific to patient populations. These accountable leaders can be APP leads, clinical department administrators, division directors or department chairs, or a combination of department leaders that makes sense from an organizational perspective. Utilizing an APP steering committee or advisory board to oversee APP projects and initiatives helps support and champion projects to completion and encourages the discussion and prioritization of new projects as needs develop.

Examples of project initiatives with steering committee oversight include optimizing onboarding, clarifying roles of the collaborating or supervising physician (if required), defining role expectations, providing metrics for best practices based on the clinical environment and the APP student pipeline process, and implementing a data reporting dashboard or system for ongoing productivity evaluation. Figure 3.2 lists a high-level overview of project examples that may evolve from the APP steering committee, with a solid common denominator: APP productivity and top-of-license practice. Throughout this textbook we will describe each project initiative to help others optimize the APP roles in their own organizations.

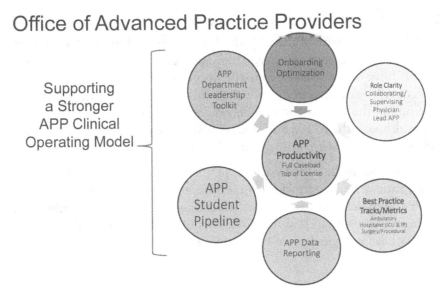

FIGURE 3.2   Supporting a stronger APP clinical operating model.

APP COUNCIL

APP councils can take on any method of governance structure that aligns with an organization's overall culture and practice philosophy. Typically, the council provides support for all APPs, regardless of license type, board certification, and specialty practice. APP councils can have formal responsibilities governed by an elected or appointed group or a more informal or general forum. At University of Iowa Health Care, the APP council is comprised of all APRNs and PAs who are credentialed and privileged. This includes nurse practitioners, clinical nurse specialists, certified registered nurse anesthetists, certified nurse midwives, and physician assistants, all from diverse clinical backgrounds including adult and pediatric ambulatory care, acute care, and critical care. The council provides a forum for discussions of relevant national, state, and organizational issues that align with the strategic plan initiatives. As the APP workforce has grown, both in numbers and geographically, a virtual, on-demand system for meetings ensures everyone can participate. Each presentation that is sent to the APP council is vetted through the APP central office for relevance to the greater APP group. As the APP workforce continues to grow exponentially, having an APP council, regardless of governance structure, serves as a collective integration of this growing workforce into the greater healthcare organization.

GROWTH OF PHYSICIANS AND APPs

In 2023, APPs at University of Iowa Health Care accounted for 30% of the entire provider workforce, including faculty, fellow, and resident physicians. The demand for the APP workforce has grown substantially over the last 10 years. Figure 3.3a shows the growth of APPs at University of Iowa Health Care. Similarly, the faculty physician workforce (minus the fellows and residents) is reflected in Figure 3.3b. It is important to note that although the APP workforce is 30% of the overall provider workforce, the faculty physician group is growing at similar rates.

When including all faculty physicians, physician fellows, and resident physicians, the provider ratio at University of Iowa Health Care is approximately 1:3 (APP to physician). APP-to-physician ratios will vary depending on the entire provider workforce, meaning those organizations that have fellows and residents included in patient care coverage may have varying degrees of provider ratio mix.

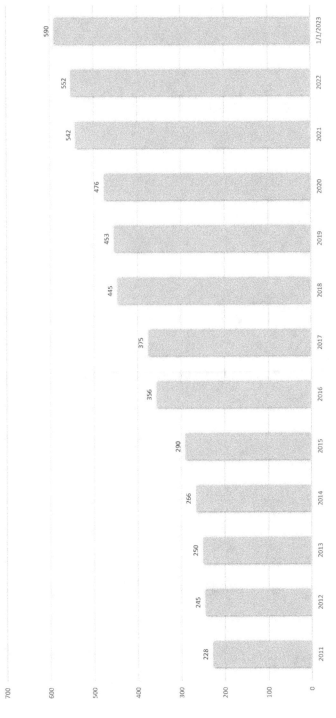

FIGURE 3.3a   Number of privileged APPs.

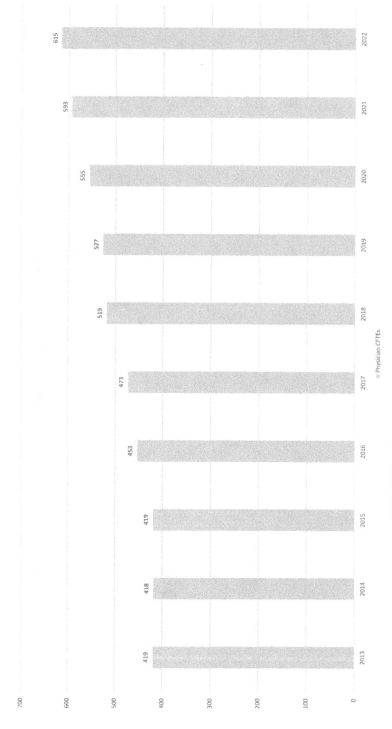

FIGURE 3.3b Number of faculty physicians (excluding residents and fellows).

HOSTING COMPREHENSIVE RESOURCES

Once an APP infrastructure is established, hosting a central platform for resources to publicize information pertinent to APPs that is valuable to multiple team members assures that everyone has the same access. Categorizing topics with specific content makes information finding user-friendly. Having multiple examples provides guidance to those team members accessing the information but does not interfere with direct oversight, finances, or workflows of APPs operationalized by their own clinical practice leaders. These resources can be distributed and implemented on any platform via an electronic toolkit to help organizations and clinical leadership operationalize and support APPs.

One example of topic content is an APP leadership toolkit that serves as a repository for a comprehensive set of resources on how to optimize and support APP leads and other organizational leaders. Topics under these categories are more directed to the leaders across the organization and may not pertain to all APPs. Organizational strategic initiatives may be another major category in the toolkit, each with relevant subject matter such as new initiatives. Additional examples include content driven from the APP steering committee to maintain transparency about projects and initiatives that pertain to all APPs and may be works in progress.

There are numerous options on how to build an intranet site for APP resources. Many of the resources developed are authored with services such as compliance, legal, and billing and coding in collaboration with the central APP office to ensure content is applicable for the entire APP workforce. Following is a list of topics and categories that University of Iowa Health Care considers valuable, and in the appendices are some of the actual documents to use as examples for development of one's own site.

Examples of toolkit categories:

- Role: Working with APPs
    - APP Recognition Best Practices
    - APP-Physician FAQ
    - Magnet® and APRN Performance Evaluation Criteria
    - PA Supervision FAQ
- APP Clinical Operating Model/Productivity
    - APP Clinical Operating Tracks
    - APP Contribution Model
    - APP Productivity Ambulatory Best Practices
    - Split/Shared Services Documentation

- Scope of Practice/Competency
  - IBON Decision-Making Algorithm
  - APRN Collaborative Practice Agreement
  - PA Addendum
- The APP Lead Role
  - APP Lead Support/Physician APP/Lead Dyad
  - APP Roles and Responsibilities
- Education and Professional Development
  - APP Expectations
  - APP Licenses and Board Certifications (Appendix A)
  - APP Professional Development Funds
  - Communication and Teamwork
  - Value-Added Professional Development
- Onboarding APPs
  - Credentialing and Privileging
  - Orientation Templates
  - APP Glossary
  - APP Job Posting Sites
  - New Hire Education and Orientation Programs
  - APP Roadmap
  - Preparing for Your New APP (Appendix B)

ELECTRONIC HEALTH RECORD

Organizations have multiple types of healthcare providers that need to be identified by name, department, provider type, specialty, or other key identifiers within the electronic health record (EHR) to effectively attribute work effort to patient care. For APPs, the baseline identifier may be isolated to their license type (PA or APRN). For a host of valid reasons—such as billing and reimbursement issues, as well as other reasons such as capturing and attributing value-based work effort—the EHR should designate the actual specialty where APPs practice. This type of data is essential as part of the overall APP infrastructure for sustainability and growth for the APP professions within an organization.

Chan et al. (2023) identified the need to be able to record and track the contributions of individual RNs to patient care and patient care outcomes. The authors further reference the National Academies report, "The Future of Nursing 2020–2030: Charting a Path to Achieve Health Equity" (2021), which underscores the need for attribution in the EHR by a unique identifier to track the collective and individual contributions to patient care outcomes. Having accurate identification in the EHR to associate the person with work effort, regardless of discipline, allows for clearer understanding of the value of all disciplines that work in various practice settings. Focusing on the accurate attribution of providers in the EHR may be considered a major strategic initiative in some organizations, as value-based programs reward organizations with incentive payments for the quality of care they give to Medicare patients (Centers for Medicare & Medicaid Services [CMS], 2022). These programs are part of University of Iowa Health Care's larger quality strategy to reform how healthcare is delivered and paid for. Therefore, the EHR serves as a significant resource for the success of the overall APP infrastructure.

TAXONOMY CODES

Taxonomy codes are CMS administrative codes set for identifying the provider type and area of specialization for healthcare providers. Each taxonomy code is a unique 10-character alphanumeric code that enables providers to identify their specialty at the claim level. To become a Medicare provider and file Medicare claims, providers must identify the taxonomy code (or codes) that reflect their classification and specialization. CMS offers a limited number of taxonomy codes for APPs, relative to the exhaustive list of taxonomy codes for physicians.

Taxonomy codes are discussed in greater detail in Chapter 10, but for the multiple benefits gained by making a reliable field for the APP's clinical specialty and board certification in the EHR and connecting the APP taxonomy code to specialty practice, it is important to discuss in this section as well. These benefits include the potential for marked improvement in revenue through accurate labeling of the APP. Documenting the APP's different clinical specialties, despite the similarity in licenses (APRN and PA), could prove fiscally beneficial when APPs care for new and established patients across an organization in different departments/specialties, as well as address the issue when more than one APP is performing services on the same day to the same patient. These types of situations in some organizations result in denied claims, but being proactive in accurate labeling of APPs in the EHR may assist with reimbursement and billing ramifications as CMS evolves and taxonomy codes are updated.

Additionally, when specifying the APP's clinical specialty and board certification in the EHR at the organizational level, there is an increased ability to evaluate efficiency within the system when comparing like providers in their clinical specialty rather than only by the APRN or PA role designation. This in turn may also provide nationally viable comparative metrics and improved internal productivity data at a specialty level. Although not a perfect fix in achieving identification at the payer level of the APP specialty and board certification, data at the organizational level potentially can influence change for optimizing reimbursement when care is rendered by the APP in those situations.

APP IDENTIFIERS IN EHR

Benefits gained by aligning APP licenses and board certifications to actual specialty practice in a reliable field in the EHR include:

- Ability to account for new and established patients across the organization as well as in specific departments/specialties when cared for by APPs. This in turn could potentially impact reimbursement in a positive way as CMS evolves and updates to align with current practice.

- Increased ability to compare efficiency within the EHR system and EHR tools when comparing to like providers in their clinical specialty rather than APRN or PA role only.

- Ability to better drill into productivity information for APPs.

Any information that can be shared and published surrounding clinical specialty definitions for APPs would be helpful as the profession continues to evolve. Supporting the movement towards clinical specialty assignment for APPs rather than just the generic taxonomy codes and/or the license designation would be very helpful for future productivity assessment. The American Association of Nurse Practitioners has advocated that CMS refine the specialty designation for APRNs and PAs because the current designation (APRN or PA) does not provide meaningful information regarding the specialty where they practice or the patient populations they serve (MedPAC, 2019).

MAJOR STRATEGIC INITIATIVES

Having a solid APP infrastructure serves as the foundation when rolling out major strategic initiatives across an organization. As discussed earlier in the chapter, part of that infrastructure is utilizing resources within an organization so as not to be duplicative. A benefit to this inclusivity is that all involved team members are invested in assuring each project or initiative will be successful.

Projects and initiatives surrounding APPs can include a multitude of topics depending on each organization's own strategic plan, professional practice model, or barriers that need to be overcome based on their own culture. One example of a major strategic initiative that requires multidimensional input is a stronger APP clinical operating model that supports top-of-license practice, resulting in improved productivity. This project example crosses over into multiple specialties, departments, and services, as well as other resource entities that may not have a direct impact but relate to the overall project success. It can be a challenge to educate department colleagues in what their role is in supporting the project. Changes in process and practice often require rigorous evidence and a thoughtful approach in identifying models that can support transformation within an organization. The *Evidence-Based Practice in Action* textbook describing comprehensive strategies, tools, and tips from the University of Iowa Hospitals and Clinics is one example that provides needed guidance about overarching steps such as identifying the problem, critiquing the evidence, selecting and implementing interventions from research and existing literature, evaluating change, and disseminating results and outcomes (Cullen et al., 2023). Because there is not a one-size-fits-all solution for optimizing project initiatives, aligning high-priority initiatives with an organization's strategic plan should be given precedence to those projects that address high-volume, high-risk, high-cost issues and improved patient outcomes (Cullen et al., 2023).

SUMMARY

It is fundamental to have a solid understanding of the organization's infrastructure before making decisions that universally affect all APPs across an enterprise. It is essential to know and appreciate the downstream effect of decisions and keep the larger view. There is a multitude of practice models utilizing APPs, and this is true not only across differing organizations but within one organizational structure. Making sure decisions align with the organization's strategy, and ensuring opportunities for all team members to have a voice, is pivotal to evaluate outcomes from major decisions. The structure of the central APP office should directly report to the key decision-makers of the organization to ensure those decisions take into consideration any unintended risk. Having a platform such as discussed in this chapter for an APP steering committee or advisory board is one of many communication channels that can provide opportunity for discussion when important and sometimes difficult decisions impact the entire enterprise.

REFERENCES

Bahouth, M. N., Ackerman, M., Ellis, E. F., Fuchs, J., McComiskey, C., Stewart, E. S., & Thomson-Smith, C. (2013). Centralized resources for nurse practitioners: Common early experiences among leaders of six large health systems. *Journal of the American Academy of Nurse Practitioners, 25*(4), 203–212. https://doi.org/10.1111/j.1745-7599.2012.00793.x

Centers for Medicare & Medicaid Services. (2022). *What are the value-based programs?* https://www.cms.gov/Medicare/Quality-Initiatives-Patient-Assessment-Instruments/Value-Based-Programs/Value-Based-Programs

Chan, G. K., Cummins, M. R., Taylor, C. S., Rambur, B., Auerbach, D. I., Meadows-Oliver, M., Cooke, C., Turek, E. A., & Pittman, P. P. (2023). An overview and policy implications of national nurse identifier systems: A call for unity and integration. *Nursing Outlook, 71*(2), 101892. https://doi.org/10.1016/j.outlook.2022.10.005

Cullen, L., Hanrahan, K., Farrington, M., Tucker, S., & Edmonds, S. (2023). *Evidence-based practice in action: Comprehensive strategies, tools, and tips from the University of Iowa Hospitals and Clinics* (2nd ed.). Sigma Theta Tau International.

Hooker, R. S., Kulo, V., Kayingo, G., Jun, H. J., & Cawley, J. F. (2022). Forecasting the physician assistant/associate workforce: 2020–2035. *Future Healthcare Journal, 9*(1), 57–63. https://doi.org/10.7861/fhj.2021-0193

MedPAC. (2019, June 14). *Report to the Congress: Medicare and the health care delivery system.* https://www.medpac.gov/document/http-www-medpac-gov-docs-default-source-reports-jun19_medpac_reporttocongress_sec-pdf/

National Academies of Sciences, Engineering, and Medicine. (2021). *The future of nursing 2020–2030: Charting a path to achieve health equity.* The National Academies Press. https://doi.org/10.17226/25982

Proulx, B. (2021). Advance practice provider transformational leadership structure: A model for change. *JONA: The Journal of Nursing Administration, 51*(6), 340–346. https://doi.org/10.1097/nna.0000000000001024

"Choose a job you love, and you will never have to work a day in your life."

—Unknown

CHAPTER 4

APRN AND PA SCOPE OF PRACTICE

KEYWORDS | APRN, PA, qualifications, practice laws, education, scope of practice

As organizations begin operationalizing APRNs and PAs within their healthcare system, consideration should be given to understanding what defines their scope of practice. *Scope of practice* describes the skills and services that APPs perform as a result of their educational preparation, state licensure, and board certification (American Medical Association [AMA], 2022). Scope of practice is determined by statutes enacted by state legislatures and by rules adopted by the appropriate state licensing entity; thus, laws, definitions, and regulations on scope of practice for APPs vary from state to state (AMA, 2022). Awareness of scope of practice is particularly important as healthcare delivery evolves in response to ever-changing patient demographics, technology, geographic provider distribution, costs, and many other environmental and societal factors (Kleinpell et al., 2012). APRNs and PAs, while licensed in adherence to their respective state-determined scopes, will often practice side by side in similar roles. In some states, APRNs and PAs serve as independent primary care providers, delivering ongoing continuous care to their own patient panels (Park et al., 2020), whereas in other states, they deliver care as part of a team. Regardless of the practice environment, the state licensing boards, professional organizations, and the organizations' clinical system committees are valuable resources surrounding APRN and PA scopes of practice for organizations.

As APRNs and PAs have become ubiquitous over the last two decades, there has been an expansion of the state-defined scope of practice afforded to the professions, with an emphasis on top-of-license (full scope) practice. Academic education programs for both APRNs and PAs have also evolved to provide their learners with the educational experiences needed, ensuring they are practice ready. Healthcare organizations can maximize APP productivity and return on investment by operationalizing top-of-license practice.

Barriers that may restrict top-of-license practice include organizational bylaws, legislative rulings, and insurance and reimbursement issues. Organizational bylaws should be reviewed and updated periodically to ensure APP practice is well aligned with state scope of practice. Including APPs in discussions and meetings at the federal, state, and organizational level when developing policies that regulate their practices can help ensure they are being appropriately utilized for optimal return on investment per their education, licensure, and certification.

REIMBURSEMENT BARRIERS

CMS reimbursement at 85% of that of a physician (Reimbursement Task Force and APRN Work Group of the WOCN Society National Public Policy Committee, 2012) creates a potential organizational barrier making it fiscally unattractive to allow APPs to practice without a physician partner underwriting documentation. Allowing for full billing authority is an essential element in actualizing state-legislated full-practice authority to capitalize on the investment of the APP workforce (Lofgren et al., 2017).

FEDERAL, STATE, AND ORGANIZATIONAL BYLAWS

Federal legislation has a direct impact on the practice of APRNs and PAs and preempts state practice laws. Professional organizations representing APRNs and PAs advocate and lobby at the federal level to ensure representation on national committees for their professional practice. The American Association of Nurse Practitioners (AANP) provides legislative leadership at the local, state, and national levels, advancing health policy; promoting excellence in practice, education, and research; and establishing standards that best serve NPs' patients and other healthcare consumers (AANP, 2022). The American Academy of Physician Associates (AAPA) advocacy engagement includes initiatives related to the federal, state, and grassroots levels (AAPA, 2021).

Healthcare organizations may also have their own staff that works closely with healthcare advocacy groups to understand legislation related to health policy that affects an organization's mission. This level of advocacy is necessary because federal statutes, regulations, and policies from the Center for Medicare & Medicaid Services (CMS) provide reimbursement for hospitals and ambulatory clinics where providers are caring for patients, and much of the language that regulates CMS was written at a time when APRNs and PAs were not recognized as providers. With the rapid growth of APPs and the expansion of scope of practice, it is important to continue to advocate for national recognition of APPs as fully reimbursable Medicare-eligible providers (CMS, 2022).

While federal and state practice laws delineate authority for practice at the state and federal level, organizational bylaws and policies define the way that APPs practice within the organization. Organizations cannot supersede state laws to expand the scope of practice, and often unintentionally limit the scope, which may interfere with their own organizational strategic plans and mission. A strong and involved APP steering committee and central APP leadership can provide the scope of practice expertise to raise awareness when bylaws are not well aligned with practice statutes. Integrating a central APP leader as part of the organization's committees and advisory boards that oversee decisions related to scope of practice can facilitate and allow for expertise at the decision-making level. Assuring APPs are familiar and have relevant access to organizational bylaws is imperative and impacts the delivery of patient care.

In addition, integrating all providers as part of the credentialing and privileging panels to balance the appropriate combination of APRNs, PAs, and physicians ensures that the process is thorough. This interprofessional panel of experts determines that the APP's training and experience are aligned with organizational requirements.

BENCHMARK SOURCES

Both the APRN and PA professions have recognized the benefit of collaboration among their respective professional organizations to establish agreed upon competencies or standards relative to education, regulation, and practice. There are four primary organizations that are associated with the physician assistant profession: PA Education Association (PAEA), the American Academy of Physician Associates (AAPA), the Accreditation Review Commission on Education for the Physician Assistant, Inc. (ARC-PA), and the National Commission on Certification of Physician Assistants (NCCPA). The four organizations worked to develop the agreed upon competencies for the PA profession in 2005, and those have since been reaffirmed and amended. The consensus competencies for the PA profession articulate the specific knowledge, skills, and aptitudes that PAs in all clinical specialties and settings should possess and be able to demonstrate throughout their careers. This set of competencies is designed to serve as a roadmap for the individual PA, for teams of providers, for healthcare systems, and for other organizations committed to promoting the development and maintenance of professional competencies among PAs. While some competencies are acquired during the PA education program, others are developed and mastered as PAs progress through their careers (AAPA, 2021).

The APRN profession established a workgroup in 2008, convened by the National Council of State Boards of Nursing and including over 40 nursing organizations representing APRNs, to develop a unified, standardized, comprehensive vision for APRN regulation (Gonzalez & Gigli, 2021). The Consensus Model for APRN Regulation, Licensure, Accreditation, Certification, and Education (LACE) was created to guide all states and jurisdictions in implementing and overseeing the uniform licensure, accreditation, certification, education, and practice of APRNs (Cahill et al., 2014). Through standardization, the consensus model aims to improve access to APRN care (Reimbursement Task Force and APRN Work Group of the WOCN Society National Public Policy Committee, 2012).

QUALIFICATIONS: EDUCATION PATHWAYS FOR APRNs AND PAs

Even though APRNs and PAs often work side by side and are categorically referenced together in many organizations, their educational pursuits are very distinct. It is important for the organizations that hire APPs to have a solid understanding of their education pathways, licensure, and board certification requirements.

PAs are educated at the master level, typically with a master's degree in physician assistant studies (MPAS). Upon completion of their degree, they are required to pass a competency and knowledge test through the national certification board to become certified, then apply for state license. State practice laws vary but may require a certain level of physician supervision. In recent years several states have enacted legislation that allows PAs to practice without direct physician supervision.

APRNs are educated with either a master of science in nursing (MSN) or doctorate in nursing practice (DNP). The educational program is specific to the patient population, and upon completion of their degree they are required to pass a competency and knowledge test through the national certification board which is specific to the patient population foci and then apply for a state license to practice. Practice laws vary for APRNs, with about half of the states and US territories adopting full practice authority (AANP, 2022).

While the educational pathways and models of education may vary significantly between APRNs and PAs, their roles and scopes of practice often have a great deal of overlap. In fact, it is common for clinical departments to have APRNs and PAs working side by side and providing care in a similar manner, with no hiring and practicing preference towards either profession. Collaboration and teamwork between these two professions has evolved, and their level of expertise in the healthcare system has been monumental in filling a gap in care.

Importantly, APRNs and PAs should understand each other's education backgrounds and preparation. APPs as shown in Table 4.1, as all members of the healthcare team, should be seen as a unified group that portrays the distinct message of mutual respect and collaboration, and that all members of the healthcare team are stronger together when bringing their individual attributes to a collective purpose to provide exceptional patient care.

TABLE 4.1 APP EDUCATION PATHWAYS

PHYSICIAN ASSISTANT	ADVANCED PRACTICE REGISTERED NURSE
Nationally certified and state licensed	Nationally certified based on patient-specific roles and state licensed
	Four roles: CNM, CRNA, CNS, CNPs with six population foci
Require bachelor's degree for acceptance	Require a bachelor's degree in nursing for acceptance
Educated at the master's degree level (27 months, three academic years)	Educated at the master's or doctoral degree level (three to four academic years)
	Two types of doctoral degrees: DNP (practice-focused) and PhD (research-focused)
State law defines scope of practice. Generally state law may require a certain level of physician supervision.	State law defines scope of practice. In most states, APRN have full practice authority and are independent providers.

In addition to understanding the education pathways and licenses, board certification programs align clinical practice specialty roles with each exam. The accredited certification programs for each specialty are listed below. APPs must keep the certification up to date by meeting the renewal requirements prior to certification expiration, as required by state regulations. The length of time a board certification is valid varies between programs; therefore, it is essential to know the certification expiration date in order to prevent any lapse.

UNIVERSITY OF IOWA HEALTH CARE APP LICENSE AND BOARD CERTIFICATIONS REQUIREMENTS

PA

1. PA License

2. PA Board Certification: National Commission on Certification of Physician Assistants (NCCPA)

APRN

1. RN License

2. APRN License

3. Board Certification (based on patient population, renewal cycles vary, certifying agencies listed below)

FNP – Family Nurse Practitioner

- American Nurses Credentialing Center (ANCC)
- American Academy of Nurse Practitioners (AANP)

PNP (acute care or primary care) – Pediatric Nurse Practitioner

- Pediatric Nursing Certification Board (PNCB), acute or primary

AGNP (acute care or primary care) – Adult/Gerontology Nurse Practitioner

- American Nurses Credentialing Center (ANCC), acute or primary
- American Association of Critical-Care Nurses (AACN), acute
- American Academy of Nurse Practitioners (AANP), primary

PMHNP – Psych Mental Health Nurse Practitioner

- American Nurses Credentialing Center (ANCC)

NNP – Neonatal Nurse Practitioner

- National Certification Corporation (NCC)

WHNP – Women's Health Nurse Practitioner

- National Certification Corporation (NCC)

CRNA – Certified Registered Nurse Anesthetist

- National Board Certification Recertification Nurse Anesthetists (CBCRNA)

CNM – Certified Nurse Midwife

- American Midwifery Certification Board (AMCB)

CNS – Clinical Nurse Specialist

- American Nurses Credentialing Center (ANCC)
- American Association of Critical-Care Nurses (AACN)

NATIONAL CONSENSUS MODEL

While PAs are broadly trained in a primary care model caring for patients across the life span, APRNs are educationally prepared to provide patient care to a specific patient population as defined by the APRN National Consensus Model (APRN Consensus Work Group & National Council of State Boards of Nursing APRN Advisory Committee, 2008). The APRN Consensus Model recognizes APRN as the state license, and further defines the four roles including the certified registered nurse anesthetists (CRNAs), certified nurse-midwives (CNMs), clinical nurse specialists (CNSs), and the certified nurse practitioners (CNPs) with their corresponding population foci (APRN Consensus Work Group, 2008; Cahill et al., 2014).

There are more than 400 academic nursing institutions in the United States that offer APRN programs, graduating more than 36,000 APRNs in 2020–2021 (American Association of Colleges of Nursing, 2020, 2021). The foundation of APRN education includes robust didactic and clinical practicums that develop and further broaden nursing expertise (AANP, 2020).

Although state practice varies, in Iowa APRNs may prescribe drugs or devices, including controlled substances, within the population foci and consistent with applicable state and federal laws, assess health status, obtain a relevant health and medical history, perform physical examinations, order preventive and diagnostic procedures, formulate a differential diagnosis, develop a treatment plan, develop a patient education plan, and promote health maintenance (Iowa Board of Nursing, 2009).

FULL PRACTICE AUTHORITY

"Full Practice Authority (FPA) is the authorization of nurse practitioners (NPs) to evaluate patients, diagnose, order and interpret diagnostic tests and initiate and manage treatments — including prescribing medications — under the exclusive licensure authority of the state board of nursing" (AANP, 2022, para. 1).

As of October 2022, the following have adopted full practice authority licensure: Alaska, Arizona, Colorado, Connecticut, Delaware, District of Columbia, Guam, Hawaii, Idaho, Iowa, Kansas, Maine, Maryland, Massachusetts, Minnesota, Montana, Nebraska, Nevada, New Hampshire, New Mexico, New York, North Dakota, Northern Mariana Islands, Oregon, Rhode Island, South Dakota, Vermont, Washington, and Wyoming.

PAs

While practicing PAs may have acquired varying degrees or certifications during their training, currently the professional standards require all PA programs to award a master's degree. PAs are broadly trained in a primary care model. Their education is traditionally fashioned in the medical model that focuses on a rigorous science background, patient interaction skills, and clinical and diagnostic reasoning. At graduation PAs are trained to take patient medical histories, perform physical examinations, order and interpret laboratory and diagnostic imaging studies, diagnose illness, provide recommendations for disease prevention, prescribe treatments including medications, and assist in surgery.

Today there are over 300 accredited PA programs nationally, and admissions to these programs is highly competitive, typically requiring a bachelor's degree and completion of prerequisite science and behavioral sciences coursework. In addition, successful applicants to PA programs generally have previous healthcare experience, averaging nearly 3,000 hours at matriculation, often having worked as EMTs, CNAs, patient care technicians, or athletic trainers. The average PA program includes didactic instruction, clinical laboratory work, simulations, procedural skills, and approximately 2,000 hours of clinical rotation in areas like pediatrics, internal medicine, family medicine, emergency medicine, women's health, surgery, and behavioral medicine. Figure 4.1 outlines licenses and certifications for both APRNs and PAs.

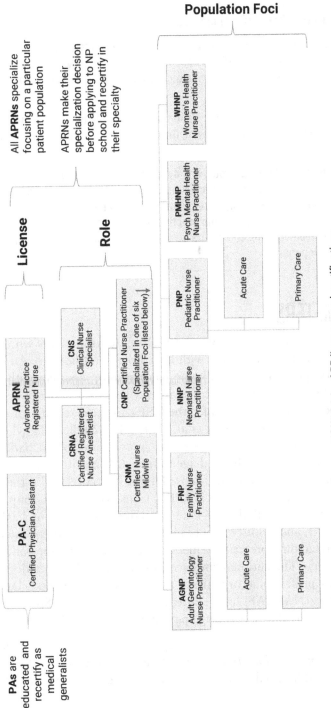

FIGURE 4.1 APP licenses and certifications.

OPTIMAL TEAM PRACTICE (OTP) LEGISLATION

In recent years, the AAPA has championed an effort to help states implement Optimal Team Practice (OTP). The AAPA defines OTP as occurring when PAs, physicians, and other healthcare professionals work together to provide quality care without administrative constraints (AAPA, 2019).

Currently, a few states have enacted legislation that eliminates the legal requirement for PAs to be directly supervised by physicians, leaving the need for a PA to have supervision to be determined at the practice level.

It will be important for healthcare systems to adopt policies, procedures and bylaws that reflect the utilization of PAs in a manner that allows them to practice at the top of their license and education. When PAs are not legally required to have formal physician supervision, PA employers (health systems, hospitals, and group practices) can be more flexible in determining the best healthcare team configurations and create new levels of efficiency in delivering the appropriate healthcare for their patients.

AGE PARAMETERS

Organizations are often challenged when APRNs care for patients who fall outside of the general age parameters that align with their board certification. An example of this is a pediatric nurse practitioner (PNP) who has cared for a patient with special healthcare needs since birth, and due to circumstances where care may not be imminently transferred to a qualified adult provider, the PNP continues to care for the patient extending into young adulthood (Heuer et al., 2019). It is challenging when APRNs have patient-specific population foci, but due to the special needs of the patients they serve, some may be outside of the traditional age ranges. APRNs often specialize in population-specific diagnoses, but are not licensed in the specialty, and rather, are licensed in one of the roles and population foci (APRN Consensus Work Group, 2008). Age parameters and patient population foci are often questioned among healthcare leaders when hiring APRNs, and priority should always be given to patient safety, including using caution surrounding prescribing medication when caring for patients outside the traditional age range. The national consensus model on APRN practice as well as position statements by professional organizations such as National Association of Pediatric Nurse Practitioners (NAPNAP) have addressed these questions. Specifically, a statement from the LACE model addresses the age parameter issue as follows:

> The *Consensus Model for APRN Regulation: Licensure, Accreditation, Certification and Education (2008)* states that APRNs be educated, certified, and licensed in one of the four roles and at least one of the six

population foci. The model also advocates for services and care to be defined by patient needs. Therefore, a rigid establishment of population age parameters is not in the best interest of patients. The definition of a population identified by specific age ranges may create barriers and limit access to care for patients with specific needs or health conditions. Circumstances exist in which a patient, by virtue of age, could fall outside the traditionally defined population focus of an APRN but, by virtue of special need, is best served by that APRN, as in the PNP example. Such patients may be identified as non-traditional patients for that APRN. In these circumstances, the APRN may manage the patient or provide expert consultation to assure the provision of evidence-based care to these patients. (LACE APRN Network, 2012, para. 2)

LIBRARY, SCHOLARSHIP, AND CLINICAL RESOURCES

Providing APPs with library resources such as scientific journals, subscriptions to current clinical information, and evidence-based data systems makes available in-depth information needed to care for patients and is important for the ongoing delivery of high-quality, evidence-based healthcare. EHR systems often have resources integrated directly into the systems. Access to resource-rich information supports learning and promotes a culture of personal accountability for ongoing knowledge.

Utilizing published resources is helpful for APPs not only as they navigate patient care questions but also as they develop new skills and experiences as their careers evolve. Having educational resources at their fingertips beyond graduation—including access to published literature that supports scope of practice, and evidence-based guidelines for specific clinical conditions to care for patients—allows APPs to advance their expertise and contribute as engaged members of the healthcare team. For example, the question regarding whether training and experience align within the scope of practice of a specific procedure or new skill is addressed in a published algorithm from the Iowa Board of Nursing illustrated in Figure 4.2. Having access to these types of resources when seeking guidance is valuable, and like other resources can guide and direct safe practices. This is an excellent resource example at the state level and duly notes that the scope of advanced practice nursing evolves and changes through experience, clinical competency, evidence-based practice and research, technology, legislation, and changes in the healthcare system (Reyes, 2017).

IOWA BOARD OF NURSING SCOPE OF PRACTICE DECISION-MAKING MODEL FOR ADVANCED REGISTERED NURSE PRACTITIONERS

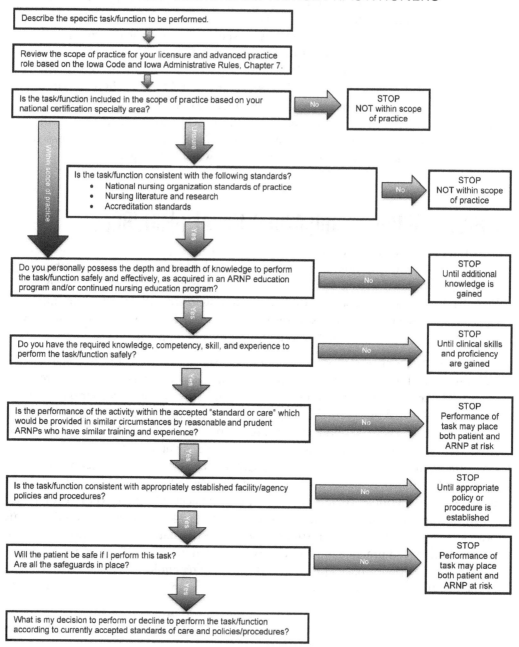

Describe the specific task/function to be performed.

Review the scope of practice for your licensure and advanced practice role based on the Iowa Code and Iowa Administrative Rules, Chapter 7.

Is the task/function included in the scope of practice based on your national certification specialty area? — **No** → STOP NOT within scope of practice

Unsure / Within scope of practice

Is the task/function consistent with the following standards?
- National nursing organization standards of practice
- Nursing literature and research
- Accreditation standards

— **No** → STOP NOT within scope of practice

Yes

Do you personally possess the depth and breadth of knowledge to perform the task/function safely and effectively, as acquired in an ARNP education program and/or continued nursing education program? — **No** → STOP Until additional knowledge is gained

Yes

Do you have the required knowledge, competency, skill, and experience to perform the task/function safely? — **No** → STOP Until clinical skills and proficiency are gained

Yes

Is the performance of the activity within the accepted "standard or care" which would be provided in similar circumstances by reasonable and prudent ARNPs who have similar training and experience? — **No** → STOP Performance of task may place both patient and ARNP at risk

Yes

Is the task/function consistent with appropriately established facility/agency policies and procedures? — **No** → STOP Until appropriate policy or procedure is established

Yes

Will the patient be safe if I perform this task? Are all the safeguards in place? — **No** → STOP Performance of task may place both patient and ARNP at risk

Yes

What is my decision to perform or decline to perform the task/function according to currently accepted standards of care and policies/procedures?

FIGURE 4.2 Iowa Scope of Practice Model. (Reyes, 2017)

SUMMARY

Understanding and assuring APPs are familiar with and have access to organizational bylaws is imperative to their ability to know the scope of practice definitions within their roles. Healthcare organizations can help to optimize appropriate scope of practice for APPs by ensuring that the committees involved in establishing their scope have sufficient representation from APP experts. Allowing APPs to practice to the full extent of their licensure and education has significant organizational benefits including maximizing APP productivity and promoting a positive work environment and inclusive culture. Iowa is one state that allows for independent practice by both APRNs and PAs. Regardless of collaborative practice agreements or other practice arrangements, APPs and physicians practicing together within the framework of their respective professional scopes of practice, whether providing independent, collaborative, or other practice requirements within their organizations, must be responsible and accountable for patients as independent members of the healthcare team in their respective specialty area and patient population.

REFERENCES

American Academy of Physician Associates. (2019, August). *Optimal team practice.* https://www.aapa.org/download/61449/

American Academy of Physician Associates. (2021). *Competencies for the PA profession.* https://www.aapa.org/download/90503/

American Association of Colleges of Nursing. (2020). *2019-2020 enrollment and graduations in baccalaureate and graduate programs in nursing.* https://www.aacnnursing.org/Portals/42/Data/Survey-Data-Highlights-2020.pdf

American Association of Colleges of Nursing. (2021). *2020-2021 enrollment and graduations in baccalaureate and graduate programs in nursing.* https://www.aacnnursing.org/Portals/42/Data/Survey-Data-Highlights-2021.pdf

American Association of Nurse Practitioners. (2020). *Position statement: Nurse practitioner education.* https://www.aanp.org/advocacy/advocacy-resource/position-statements/nurse-practitioner-education

American Association of Nurse Practitioners. (2022). *Issues at a glance: Full practice authority.* https://www.aanp.org/advocacy/advocacy-resource/policy-briefs/issues-full-practice-brief

American Medical Association. (2022). *What is scope of practice?* https://www.ama-assn.org/practice-management/scope-practice/what-scope-practice

APRN Consensus Work Group & National Council of State Boards of Nursing APRN Advisory Committee. (2008, July 7). *Consensus model for APRN regulation: Licensure, accreditation, certification, and education.* https://www.ncsbn.org/papers/consensus-model-for-aprn-regulation-licensure-accreditation-certification-and-education

Cahill, M., Alexander, M., & Gross, L. (2014). The 2014 NCSBN consensus report on APRN regulation. *Journal of Nursing Regulation, 4*(4), 5–12. https://doi.org/10.1016/S2155-8256(15)30111-3

Center for Medicare & Medicaid Services. (2022, March). *Advanced practice registered nurses, anesthesiologist assistants, & physician assistants.* https://www.cms.gov/Outreach-and-Education/Medicare-Learning-Network-MLN/MLNProducts/Downloads/Medicare-Information-for-APRNs-AAs-PAs-Booklet-ICN-901623.pdf

Gonzalez, J., & Gigli, K. (2021). Navigating population foci and implications for nurse practitioner scope of practice. *The Journal for Nurse Practitioners, 17*(7), 846–850. https://doi.org/10.1016/j.nurpra.2021.04.008

Heuer, B., Hunter, J. M., Hatton, A., Lee, A., Lofgren, M., & Reyes, I. (2019). NAPNAP position statement on age parameters for pediatric nurse practitioner practice. *Journal of Pediatric Health Care, 33*(2), A9–A11. https://doi.org/10.1016/j.pedhc.2018.10.007

Iowa Board of Nursing. (2009, July 1). *Advanced registered nurse practitioners.* https://www.legis.iowa.gov/docs/iac/chapter/03-02-2016.655.7.pdf

Kleinpell, R. M., Hudspeth, R., Scordo, K. A., & Magdic, K. (2012). Defining NP scope of practice and associated regulations: Focus on acute care. *Journal of the American Academy of Nurse Practitioners, 24*(1), 11–18. https://doi.org/10.1111/j.1745-7599.2011.00683.x

LACE APRN Network. (2012, April 24). *Clarifying statement on age parameters for APRNs.*

Lofgren, M. A., Berends, S. K., Reyes, J., Wycoff, C., Kinnetz, M., Frohling, A., Baker, L., Whitty, S., Dirks, M., & O'Brien, M. (2017). Scope of practice barriers for advanced practice registered nurses: A state task force to minimize barriers. *Journal of Nursing Administration, 47*(9), 465–469. https://doi.org/10.1097/nna.0000000000000515

Park, J., Han, X., & Pittman, P. (2020). Does expanded state scope of practice for nurse practitioners and physician assistants increase primary care utilization in community health centers? *Journal of the American Association of Nurse Practitioners, 32*(6), 447–458. https://doi.org/10.1097/jxx.0000000000000263

Reimbursement Task Force and APRN Work Group of the WOCN Society National Public Policy Committee. (2012). Reimbursement of advanced practice registered nurse services: A fact sheet. *Journal of Wound, Ostomy and Continence Nursing, 39*(2 Suppl), S7–16. https://doi.org/10.1097/WON.0b013e3182478df0

Reyes, J. A. (2017). *Scope of practice decision-making model for advanced registered nurse practitioners.* https://nursing.iowa.gov/sites/default/files/documents/2017/06/arnp_practicedecisionmakin_model_.pdf

"Be not afraid of going slowly. Be afraid of standing still."
—Chinese proverb

CHAPTER 5

ESTABLISHING AN APP WORKFORCE

KEYWORDS | APP workforce, job description, scheduling, networking, SBAR, recruitment

Creating a stable APP workforce requires methodical, strategic, and well-thought-out plans. Understanding factors such as clinical setting, patient population, the scheduling needs to serve the patient population, the type of APPs, and the productivity metrics used to evaluate return on investment all must be taken into consideration. It is important to use analogous methodology when building an APP workforce, not only within a designated unit, but across an organization for ease of replication among various organization leaders.

The healthcare provider workforce is shifting for a multitude of reasons. The Medicare policy limiting growth in physician residency positions; limitations in resident work hours by the Accreditation Council for Graduate Medical Education (ACGME); and value-based purchasing payment policies incentivizing organizations to reduce readmissions, length of stay, and improve patient experiences (Aiken et al., 2021) are all contributing factors. Likewise, the increase in patients older than 65 years of age, the acuity of critically ill patients (White et al., 2017), and the impact from the COVID-19 global pandemic further intensifies provider staffing issues. APPs are increasingly used in the management of hospitalized patients to bridge this gap in the workforce (Kleinpell et al., 2008; Pastores et al., 2011). APPs have been identified as a solution for meeting these challenges, and while the roles of APPs vary by organization and specialty within organizations (Aiken et al., 2021), implementing practice models requires thoughtful strategy.

HOW TO CREATE IT: INPATIENT

When building practice models in an academic medical center setting where there are multiple learners and provider types, it is important to build an APP practice that can function in collaboration with diverse disciplines, including residents and fellows, but at the same time be a sustainable practice model regardless of changes within the ACGME or other contributing workforce challenges. The situation, background, assessment, recommendation tool (SBAR) was originally developed by Michael Leonard, MD, a physician leader for patient safety, along with colleagues Doug Bonacum and Suzanne Graham at Kaiser Permanente of Colorado (Leonard et al., 2004). The SBAR was introduced by rapid response teams at Kaiser Permanente in Colorado in 2002 as a technique to investigate patient safety and facilitate prompt and appropriate communication (Achrekar et al., 2016). Adopting the SBAR tool provides a framework for communicating to organizational leadership and other team members the need for supplementing or adding APPs. Although the SBAR originally was used for communicating to a healthcare team about a patient condition, it is a helpful tool to concisely describe the circumstances when articulating a comprehensive plan to various leaders from different professional backgrounds, all of whom have input and authority for decisions regarding new APP hires.

Prior to building a business proposal, it is helpful to put together an SBAR describing details of what is essential to foster a successful plan. Without this thoughtful approach and comprehensive vision, organizations may hire the wrong type of APPs for the patient population, which can lead to increased turnover and poor quality. Having a thorough, visionary long-term plan helps all team members understand up front that building a sustainable APP workforce for a specified patient population requires patience and strategy.

The SBAR approach is a thoughtful process to an organized method of getting buy-in and having clear expectations when adding APPs to fill the gap in the health provider workforce.

Situation – Describe the current staffing model where there is need for additional APPs. This is important to articulate the various levels of experience of interns, residents, fellows, or their restricted and variable work hours. In addition, if there are APPs already staffing the unit, how they function in concert with each other needs to be explained. For example, APPs often pick up additional patients if residents must leave post call or for other education requirements, increasing patient caseload, which helps clarify the need for adding more APPs. Staffing a unit with providers does not always equate to standard shift work because there are multiple variables that come into play. Understanding this, especially when it comes to high-risk situations like minimizing handoffs and addressing fluctuating acuity, is important for quality patient care outcomes. Being able to describe the number of patient beds, the staffing ratios, and patient workload assignments based on benchmarking and professional organization standards—and having a detailed schedule to visually demonstrate the gaps—can enhance a clearer understanding to the decision-makers for the need to add APPs.

Background – Pertinent information that relates to the situation detailing the need for additional APPs such as growth in bed numbers, changes in acuity of the patient population, coverage challenges and descriptions of patched options when there are gaps in care, other contributory workforce challenges, as well as quality metrics impacted from staffing issues, is often not obvious. These can be used as trigger questions to look at further data that is unit specific and used as baseline metrics when additional APP FTEs (full-time equivalent) are approved.

Assessment – Highlight the analysis and consideration of options based on expert opinion that contribute to the need for additional APP FTEs. The overall occupancy rate of the unit, the average number of actual discharges and admissions, and the time of day most of the work effort takes place—all can help guide the recommendation and demonstrate a thoughtful plan based on patient care needs in the unit. Providing the general overall staff engagement of the unit is helpful as it plays an important role in patient outcomes and organizational success. Including input from professions such as nursing, pharmacy, and other frontline staff is helpful because the overall goal is to establish highly functioning teams. Explaining the board certifications and experience required, and the local market to recruit APPs, demonstrates that the plan is thoughtfully calculated. It is valuable to include graphs and charts to visually demonstrate gaps in care.

Recommendation – The recommendation (or "ask") provides details on executing the plan for the additional APPs to provide a stable workforce providing consistency and quality of care. Kapu and colleagues (2014) examined the financial impact of adding nurse practitioners to inpatient care teams and identified value by means of generating revenue, reducing length of stay, and standardizing quality care—all metrics that address the value-based payment policies incentivizing hospitals. Outcome measures to help demonstrate return on investment may include baseline data such as decreasing length of stay, timely discharges, improvement of documentation including complication or co-morbidity (CC) and major complication or comorbidity (MCC) capture, standardization of clinical practice guidelines that in turn will reduce the central-line-associated blood-stream infection (CLASBI) and catheter-associated urinary tract infection (CAUTI) rates, and optimizing appropriate utilization of labs and imaging.

Determining the number of APPs needed for a various practice model can be challenging because APPs function in unique roles. When calculating the number of APPs required for an inpatient unit, it is important to consider number of patient beds, safe caseload expectations based on patient acuity, and the number and experience of other provider types, as well as workflow in the unit at various times throughout the day. APPs may be needed for night or weekend coverage, and understanding scheduling needs is important for determining the number of FTEs needed, as well as the actual bodies of APPs needed for appropriate coverage, either part-time or full-time, for sustainability. Table 5.1 demonstrates an example for calculating the FTE needed to provide coverage for both a 12-hour, seven-day weeknight coverage and 8.5 hour weekend coverage.

TABLE 5.1 CALCULATING FTE

FTE calculation (2,080 hours per 1.0 FTE) identifying the number of APP FTE needed using a 15% benefit rate (non-work hours such as vacation time) and 85% work time (2,080 * 0.85 = 1,768 hours).

CALCULATED FTE EXAMPLE

NIGHT SHIFT; 12 HOURS; 7 DAYS WEEK	DAY SHIFT; 8.5 HOURS; SAT/SUN
12 hrs x 7 days week = 84 work hours	8.5 hrs x 2 days weekend = 17 work hours
84 x 52 weeks per year = 4,368 work hours	17 x 52 weeks per year = 884 work hours
4,368 / 1,768 (benefit time)	884 / 1,768 (benefit time)
= 2.5 FTE needed to cover	= 0.5 FTE needed to cover

Calculating FTE is helpful, but to be effective it requires understanding of the unit as a whole and the workflow of how other provider types come and go throughout the unit in any given day—for example, getting input from other disciplines for anticipated coverage issues that need to be accounted for due to gaps from other provider types. Knowing the APP workforce availability in the market is essential and impacts the overall execution of the plan. When building APP teams that address medical provider shortages, it is important to develop a practice model that is sustainable and promotes an environment where APPs can grow professionally, have longevity, and are engaged. Appendix C gives further details related to establishing APP inpatient scheduling guidelines. Inpatient APPs are often required to work shifts covering nights, weekends and holidays, and work schedules should be established based upon the needs of the clinical unit.

HOW TO CREATE IT: OUTPATIENT

Strategically utilizing APPs is important for all settings, and the SBAR can be used as a communication tool to address the need to build the APP workforce in any setting such as inpatient described above, but also in primary care and in ambulatory specialty practices. Evaluating patient scheduling backlog and methodically defining an APP's patient panel based on diagnosis and APP competency will improve patient access and ultimately get the patient seen faster. This in turn further delineates and opens availability for higher acuity patients who require a physician specialty. Although there are no regulatory guidelines surrounding this, in academic medical centers and larger organizations where there are patients frequently referred by other specialists, it is not uncommon that specialty physicians see new patients when referred by another specialty physician (e.g., an otolaryngologist to otolaryngologist). However, it is not uncommon for an APP with extensive clinical-specific education and experience in the specialty to see new patients referred to the specialty from a primary care physician or other provider to expedite care into the system. The goal, regardless of specialty, is to clearly define the patient care templates and identify patients with diagnoses where the APP can comfortably and competently get the patient the care needed in a timely manner.

Patient caseload expectations and scheduling templates are important to standardize and define as much as possible, so the APP understands the productivity expectations and goals. A consistent definition of clinical full-time equivalent (cFTE) position should be provided and allow for approximately 80% to 90% of the cFTE to be face-to-face patient care time and 10% to 20% of the time for documentation. A clinical session is traditionally defined in four-hour blocks. Appendix D outlines examples of scheduling templates for APPs that can be adopted and altered for any organization's needs.

Schedule examples can assist departments in finding a template that works best for the patient populations served. APP clinical skills and competency evolve over time; thus patient templates and scheduling guidelines should be regularly reviewed and analyzed to ensure the department is operating at optimal efficiency. Supporting the APP to allow adequate time to complete all documentation during the work hours is important and will understandably change with experience and competence. Taking time up front to standardize EHR templates for documentation is essential for efficiency. Schedules, templates, and caseload expectations will change and evolve over time and thus should be evaluated and adjusted to meet the patient population and skills level of the APP to continue to support top-of-license practice and improve patient access. Table 5.2 depicts a sample schedule for an APP in a specialty service. Additional schedule samples can be found in Appendix D.

TABLE 5.2   SAMPLE SCHEDULE (10.5 HOUR WORKDAY/4 PER WEEK; 8 CLINICAL SESSIONS)

SCHEDULE	DAY 1	DAY 2	DAY 3	DAY 4	DAY 5	WEEKLY TOTAL
0700-0800	Documentation/ Admin	Documentation/ Admin	Off	Documentation/ Admin	Documentation/ Admin	
0800-1200	Patient Care (4 hrs)	Patient Care (4 hrs)	(or rotate day off)	Patient Care (4 hrs)	Patient Care (4 hrs)	
1200-1230	Break	Break		Break	Break	
1230-1300	Documentation/ Admin	Documentation/ Admin		Documentation/ Admin	Documentation/ Admin	
1300-1700	Patient Care (4 hrs)	Patient Care (4 hrs)		Patient Care (4 hrs)	Patient Care (4 hrs)	
1700-1730	Documentation/ Admin	Documentation/ Admin		Documentation/ Admin	Documentation/ Admin	
Total Worked Hours	10	10	0	10	10	40

The goal is to improve patient access, and again, define the types of patients for which APPs have their own schedule and bill independently, as well as those patients for whom APPs have shared schedules and bill as a split/shared visit with a physician. Consistency of the cFTE allocation helps capture the work effort when the APP is practicing independently or when the APP is practicing in a team. Shared templates are an acceptable practice model, although using an APP as a physician scribe is an inefficient practice model that does not support top-of-license practice. Figure 5.1 illustrates APPs and physicians utilized effectively in two models when patient panels are clearly described.

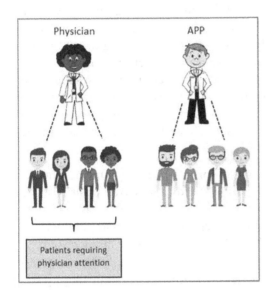
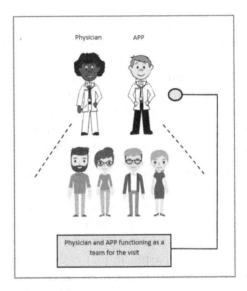

FIGURE 5.1   Practice models.

HOW TO SUSTAIN IT

Leaders should work closely with internal departments—such as finance, strategic planning, and business development—to build a long-term strategy based on hiring projections or forecasts. Knowing or anticipating future clinical needs will be helpful as hiring pipelines are established. Forecasting growth in certain clinical areas may help identify specific board certifications needed to proactively build a talent pool. For example, with known future growth in the operating room, service line efforts can be focused on future CRNA needs. Prioritization of a well-educated, competent, and diverse workforce will help meet the changing demands within the healthcare system (Snapp et al., 2021).

Hiring pipelines may include APP students who have rotated through clinical placement, attended feeder schools (i.e., an affiliated college of nursing or PA school), and current RN or other staff who are seeking to expand their career into an APP role. University of Iowa Health Care partners with their own affiliated college of nursing to provide career counseling to RNs seeking to pursue a DNP educational track so that students can make an informed decision considering post-graduation employment opportunities. Healthcare organizations without an affiliated educational program should form close partnerships with local universities to develop a hiring pipeline.

Recruitment processes include a variety of interested parties including human resources, lead APPs, department leadership, or other vested team members. The process includes understanding the APP labor market, knowing the position requirements, creating effective job postings, utilizing interviewing skills, and preparing for and welcoming the new APP. The organization's recruiter, talent acquisition specialist, or human resources department representative will likely coordinate the APP recruitment process, working closely with the department level supervisory team. A recruiter or human resources representative leading the search will ensure that internal processes and labor and employment regulations are followed. Recruiters are experienced in candidate care, have advanced knowledge of internal recruitment processes, are aware of and consider the pertinent labor and employment laws and regulations, and will oversee the process to ensure that a legal and compliant search occurs.

Each organization may have an internal approval process for recruitment, whether for a replacement position, such as after a resignation, or for a new APP position. The approval process may include those metrics identified by the organization as pertinent when hiring an APP and may require approval from department leadership, human resources, finance, and executive leadership. A workforce manager, or labor resource manager or department, may oversee this process, or it may fall to the finance, operations, or the human resources department to manage the process, but regardless, having APP expertise for input is valuable. Once the position is filled, a detailed orientation and onboarding should be prepared. Appendices B and E provide ways to prepare for the new APP and sample onboarding checklists.

Adequate expertise should be applied to the recruitment and hiring process as it impacts legal, compliance, patient safety, quality of care, and team engagement. Consider how turnover or hiring the wrong skill mix impacts the healthcare team, and how being short-staffed wears down or frustrates great employees. Some examples are listed here:

- **Apathy and resentment for staff:** This is especially important in team-based work environments, or in a work group that is based on collaboration. When a member of the team is not functioning well, it puts a larger burden on coworkers to pick up the slack, which can lead to dissatisfaction and ultimately resentment.

- **Turnover or disengagement of best staff:** Skilled and well-liked APPs will always be in high demand. It's common to lean on high performers to achieve results. Leaders should be attuned to the distribution of work so that the best staff members do not become burned out or disengaged, or even worse, leave the organization and take their talents, skills, and knowledge elsewhere.

- **Weakened employer reputation:** Being an employer of choice is a desirable goal for any organization. An organization that is well regarded can increase employee and patient satisfaction, leading to growth. Likewise, an organization with a poor reputation is not likely to attract or retain quality APPs.

- **Diminished work climate:** Many organizations contend with low morale. This can occur when the work climate is poor or dysfunctional. Bad moods and poor attitudes can be contagious within an APP team.

- **Erosion of quality patient care:** Satisfied and engaged APPs are more likely and motivated to provide good patient care and satisfaction (Greenslade & Jimmieson, 2011).

The goal in the recruitment process is to hire the APP(s) based upon their demonstrated clinical experience and sound clinical judgement, ability to adapt and learn, and fit with the organizational or department work culture (Langley et al., 2018). Interview questions should be structured, determined in advance, be related to the job duties and role, and should be consistently asked of every potential APP (Wegmeyer et al., 2022).

Table 5.3 provides examples of questions to consider and avoid.

TABLE 5.3 INTERVIEW QUESTIONS

USE SPECIFIC EXAMPLES: BEHAVIOR BASED	AVOID HYPOTHETICAL QUESTIONS
Tell me about a time when you went over and above your job responsibilities to provide exceptional care to a patient.	If you needed to, would you go over and above to provide care to a patient?
What were your specific job responsibilities? Talk me through a typical day.	Do you think you can do this job?
Describe a conflict you encountered with a coworker. How was it resolved?	Do you get along well with your coworkers?
Give me an example of a quality improvement project that you participated in. What was your specific role? What was the outcome?	Would you be willing to participate in a quality improvement project?

EFFECTIVE JOB DESCRIPTIONS

The job description should include general tasks, duties, and functions of the role, using an organization's standard template. Although the day-to-day duties for an APP position may vary by department or patient population, the general role responsibilities should be consistent. The job description will provide role clarity for the APP candidate and answer the question, "What's expected of me?" Job descriptions will also include work performance expectations, answering the question, "What does success look like?"

The APP job description should list the department, reporting structure (who supervises this position and who reports to this position), and whether classified (for pay purposes) as exempt or non-exempt under the Fair Labor Standards Act. A copy of the job description should be provided to any candidate who is interviewing for a position.

FAIR LABOR STANDARDS ACT (FLSA)

The Fair Labor Standards Act (FLSA) provides pay practice guidelines administered by the Wage and Hour Division of the US Department of Labor (2022). FLSA establishes which employees are exempt from overtime pay and those who are subject to overtime pay (non-exempt).

The APP job description will also include the required and preferred position qualifications in several core categories that should be included as part of the job posting such as education, experience, and license/certifications. It's important to note the distinction between PAs' and APRNs' licenses and board certifications as well as the varying certifying bodies for APRNs. This is further specified in Appendix A. Clearly stating the required and desired qualifications means the APP (and any incumbents) must have these items to be considered for the role. For licensing of new APP graduates, the job posting may list that active and unrestricted license is required; thus the start date for a new graduate APP may be delayed or changed to align with the issuance of their required license.

Examples of these qualification categories are listed in Table 5.4.

TABLE 5.4 QUALIFICATIONS

CATEGORY	DESCRIPTION EXAMPLES
Education	▪ Education sufficient to obtain professional license issued by the state licensing body
Experience	▪ One to three years' experience practicing as an APRN or PA in an ambulatory clinic setting, preferred ▪ Experience with adult/geriatric patient population

License/ Certification	■ Active and unrestricted APRN or PA license issued by state licensing body, required
	■ If APRN, must also maintain active and unrestricted RN license issued by the state licensing body
	■ Active and unrestricted board certification appropriate to patient population

PROFESSIONAL DEVELOPMENT AND NETWORKING

Professional networking involves shared, mutually beneficial interactions among colleagues and among an interdisciplinary network (Goolsby & Knestrick, 2017). Professional networking is career-focused within a profession or with those who have a shared expertise and clinical focus. It involves gathering and exchanging information, contacts, and experiences while developing professional resources.

Networking among APPs within the organization helps grow knowledge of other APPs' function in specialty areas and will expand their view of the profession. Growing and maintaining a strong professional network helps APPs stay informed about the latest trends and best practices, helps them grow clinically and intellectually, and promotes engagement among their peers. Networking is important to exchange information and develop professional social contacts and may initiate collaborations with experts that ultimately improve patient care (Last et al., 2021).

APPs may network within their own specialty, and among interdisciplinary colleagues, to develop meaningful professional relationships. APPs may expand their network to include local chapters and state/national organizations and groups specific to their interests and disciplines such as those focused on research, evidence-based practice, policy and advocacy, clinical practice, and education. Goolsby and Knestrick (2017) describe interdisciplinary networking as providing contacts for collaboration with the goal of improving patient care.

NETWORKING GUIDE

- Practice active listening. Reciprocate. Follow up answers with a question.
- Join APP professional groups and associations. Attend meetings and conferences.
- When meeting a new APP professional contact, get to know the person and start by asking for information about their area of expertise. Follow up after you make a new contact.
- Participate in online discussions and forums to make new APP contacts you can meet later in person at conferences or networking events.
- Stay in contact with former colleagues and employers.

SUMMARY

Using a methodology for crafting an APP workforce based on many of the principles described in this chapter is fundamental to the success of integrating APPs to be part of the multidisciplinary healthcare team in a variety of clinical healthcare settings. Building APP teams from start to finish requires resource allocation and commitment similar to other professional hires within an organization. APPs serve unique and pivotal roles within the healthcare system, and it makes sense to adopt the existing resources within organizations, apply APP expertise to those resources, and in turn meet the unique needs of how APPs function so models of care can be established and successful.

REFERENCES

Achrekar, M. S., Murthy, V., Kanan, S., Shetty, R., Nair, M., & Khattry, N. (2016). Introduction of situation, background, assessment, recommendation into nursing practice: A prospective study. *Asia-Pacific Journal of Oncology Nursing, 3*(1), 45–50. https://doi.org/10.4103/2347-5625.178171

Aiken, L. H., Sloane, D. M., Brom, H. M., Todd, B. A., Barnes, H., Cimiotti, J. P., Cunningham, R. S., & McHugh, M. D. (2021). Value of nurse practitioner inpatient hospital staffing. *Medical Care, 59*(10), 857–863. https://doi.org/10.1097/mlr.0000000000001628

Goolsby, M. J., & Knestrick, J. M. (2017). Effective professional networking. *Journal of the American Association of Nurse Practitioners, 29*(8), 441–445. https://doi.org/10.1002/2327-6924.12484

Greenslade, J. H., & Jimmieson, N. L. (2011). Organizational factors impacting on patient satisfaction: A cross sectional examination of service climate and linkages to nurses' effort and performance. *International Journal of Nursing Studies, 48*(10), 1188–1198. https://doi.org/10.1016/j.ijnurstu.2011.04.004

Kapu, A. N., Kleinpell, R., & Pilon, B. (2014). Quality and financial impact of adding nurse practitioners to inpatient care teams. *Journal of Nursing Administration, 44*(2), 87–96. https://doi.org/10.1097/nna.0000000000000031

Kleinpell, R. M., Ely, E. W., & Grabenkort, R. (2008). Nurse practitioners and physician assistants in the intensive care unit: An evidence-based review. *Critical Care Medicine, 36*(10), 2888–2897. https://doi.org/10.1097/CCM.0b013e318186ba8c

Langley, T. M., Dority, J., Fraser, J. F., & Hatton, K. W. (2018, June). A comprehensive onboarding and orientation plan for neurocritical care advanced practice providers. *Journal of Neuroscience Nursing, 50*(3), 157–169. https://doi.org/10.1097/JNN.0000000000000359. https://journals.lww.com/jnnonline/Fulltext/2018/06000/A_Comprehensive_Onboarding_and_Orientation_Plan.8.aspx

Last, K., Power, N. R., Delliere, S., Velikov, P., Sterbenc, A., Antunovic, I. A., Lopes, M. J., Schweitzer, V., & Barac, A. (2021). Future developments in training. *Clinical Microbiology & Infection, 27*(11), 1595–1600. https://doi.org/10.1016/j.cmi.2021.06.032

Leonard, M., Bonacum, D., & Graham, S. (2004). The human factor: The critical importance of effective teamwork and communication in providing safe care. *Quality & Safety in Health Care, 13*(Suppl 1), i85–i90. https://doi.org/10.1136/qshc.2004.010033

Pastores, S. M., O'Connor, M. F., Kleinpell, R. M., Napolitano, L., Ward, N., Bailey, H., Mollenkopf, F. P., Jr., & Coopersmith, C. M. (2011). The Accreditation Council for Graduate Medical Education resident duty hour new standards: History, changes, and impact on staffing of intensive care units. *Critical Care Medicine, 39*(11), 2540–2549. https://doi.org/10.1097/CCM.0b013e318225776f

Snapp, B., Moore, T. A., Wallman, C., & Staebler, S. (2021). 2020 neonatal nurse practitioner workforce survey: An executive summary. *Advances in Neonatal Care, 21*(3), 242–246. https://doi.org/10.1097/anc.0000000000000903

US Department of Labor, Wage and Hour Division. (2022). *Digital reference guide to the Fair Labor Standards Act.* https://www.dol.gov/sites/dolgov/files/WHD/legacy/files/Digital_Reference_Guide_FLSA.pdf

Wegmeyer,, L., Tenbrink, A.P., Delacruz, A., Salim, R., & Speer, A. (2022). Interviews from scratch: Individual differences in writing interview questions. *Personnel Assessment and Decisions, 8*(1), n.p. https://doi.org/10.25035/pad.2022.01.002. https://scholarworks.bgsu.edu/pad/vol8/iss1/2/

White, T., Kokiousis, J., Ensminger, S., & Shirey, M. (2017). Supplementing intensivist staffing with nurse practitioners: Literature review. *AACN Advanced Critical Care, 28*(2), 111–123. https://doi.org/10.4037/aacnacc2017949

"The beginning is the most important part of the work."
—Plato

CHAPTER 6

APP ONBOARDING

KEYWORDS | onboarding, orientation, community, role transition, resources, goals

An intentionally designed onboarding process is crucial to transitioning APPs effectively into practice. Although APPs may be well prepared from an educational standpoint, and have the necessary skills and competencies, every healthcare organization and service line requires their own onboarding program (Kapu, 2022). Expecting a new PA or APRN to jump into a busy clinical setting without a period of onboarding and acclimation can be dissatisfying to all team members (Chaney et al., 2022).

It is important to note the distinction between onboarding and orientation. *Orientation* is typically a short-term process that establishes the employment relationship. Examples include benefit enrollment, payroll direct deposit, email set up, review of employee handbook and policies, completing compliance-driven training, and gaining the appropriate computer access. *Onboarding* takes a more comprehensive view and consists of a series of educational and clinical activities planned, designed, and structured to incrementally bring a new APP towards full productivity and top-of-license practice.

Healthcare organizations may differ in their training resources, including the availability of preceptors and mentors, and are often challenged with providers simultaneously onboarding APPs while carrying their own patient load or clinical responsibilities. Having a structured, well-defined onboarding path that establishes role clarity for all colleagues will efficiently guide the new APP towards a successful experience.

BUILDING A SENSE OF COMMUNITY

Chapter 1 described the benefits of an organizational infrastructure specific to APPs, including establishing a designated leader and centralized office for APPs to provide a professional home and APP community. There are common themes or characteristics defining an employee's sense of belonging to a professional community, including caring for something larger than themselves, showing loyalty to each other and the collective work, and being part of a team atmosphere.

Proactively structuring a work setting as a professional community helps reinforce a sense of belonging and strengthens engagement and identity among group members. When planning an APP workforce, consider how APPs engage within the work environment, ensuring that the most basic needs of a professional community are met through a welcoming and supportive approach. Being intentional with activities designed to grow professional relationships among colleagues fosters a climate of open communication among team members. Plan time in the onboarding schedule for team building, introductions, and networking. Identify other APP colleagues within the work group who are willing to introduce the new APP to others in the department and set up informal meet-and-greet opportunities. Efforts to assimilate a new APP socially within the work group demonstrates a supportive work culture, which has a positive impact on engagement, retention, organizational commitment, and sense of belonging. New APPs themselves can be encouraged to strategize about building strong connections at work to be intentional about engaging with coworkers on a professional level to build camaraderie.

ENGAGING IN YOUR WORK COMMUNITY

- Think about examples of a strong work community. What did this look like? How did the leaders conduct themselves to support the community and how did colleagues behave towards each other?

- Consider prior work environments. How have you personally engaged in your work community? How did you treat others? Were you open and responsive? Did you extend yourself to new team members?

- What can you do personally to strengthen your APP work community? Consider your personal brand. How do you want to be perceived in the work environment? What can you do personally to be a positive influence in your work environment?

STRUCTURING AN ONBOARDING PROGRAM

The goal of onboarding is to guide a newly hired APP efficiently and effectively into full practice and includes incremental increases in responsibilities over time. When successful, the APP is meeting defined productivity metrics, working at top of license, and carrying a full patient case load. A structured onboarding process will ensure new APPs understand what is expected and have the support and resources necessary to succeed in their role.

Unlike physicians who undergo specialized training and residency, APPs will have varied exposure to hospital medicine, academic medicine, private practice, and specialized areas of practice (McGrath et al., 2021). PAs are board certified as medical generalists, and APRNs are board certified within a certain role and/or patient population. Clinical specialty services, beyond the designated board certifications, need to have a distinct training plan for onboarding APPs who have not previously worked or have experience in these designated specialties.

Leadership support for a structured onboarding program is considered a critical success factor (Morgan et al., 2020). Championing a methodical onboarding program will require support from organizational leaders, including assuring APPs are not being placed into independent clinical activities too early in the process. Morgan and colleagues (2020) describe the benefits and goals of onboarding as follows:

- Increase employee satisfaction
- Improve patient safety and quality of care

- Communicate organizational values and mission
- Educate on standard work process
- Verify clinical competency

WELCOMING AND PREPARING FOR YOUR NEW APP

Preparations should be taken to proactively welcome the new APP. Positive relationships with peers and leaders and demonstrating a culture of teamwork are important contributors to job satisfaction (Waltz et al., 2020). In the weeks prior to starting employment, leaders can periodically touch base with the new APP to answer any questions and provide a point of contact. A welcome email or text can be sent a few days prior to the start date, or touch base via phone to be sure the new APP knows all the first day instructions such as parking, lunch arrangements, dress code, etc. Department leaders, human resources representatives, and APP leads should develop checklists and guides to standardize pre-hire activities.

Kapu (2022) suggests that role clarity and an onboarding program designed to provide adequate time to teach, evaluate, and achieve patient-population-specific clinical competency is the single most important component of effective onboarding. Ensuring all team members have a clear understanding of the roles and responsibilities of the APP and how that position fits within the team-based care model will promote a culture of mutual respect (Chaney et al., 2022).

Onboarding should be flexible and individualized and take into consideration the APP's base knowledge coming into the role. This includes whether APPs are new or familiar with the clinical specialty. The literature supports that many APPs feel unprepared to confidently care for patients in their first year of practice, especially when caring for high-acuity patients (MacLellan et al., 2015). APPs will advance through the onboarding process at varying rates. Anglin et al. (2021) describe this as the ramp up period, which may vary depending on the new APPs previous clinical experience, previous knowledge of the EHR system, time since graduation, confidence and comfort, and achievement of certain competencies.

ROLE CLARITY

Providing role clarity during the onboarding process includes the following elements:

- Define the patient population. What types of patients and diagnosis will the APP be responsible for treating?

- What is the practice care model with other members of the healthcare team? Will the APP see patients independently or with a physician in a split/shared visit?

- How will the APP's productivity be measured and evaluated? Who will be tracking these metrics?

- Will caseload expectations change over time? If so, what is the timeline and how will progress be measured? What should be the progress at 90 days, 180 days, and one year in the role?

- What is the billing methodology?

DEVELOPING AN ONBOARDING PLAN

A well-planned onboarding roadmap like Figure 6.1 is helpful to provide to the new APP a visual of activities leading towards full caseload and top-of-license practice.

CLINICAL ONBOARDING TEMPLATE

Using a clear onboarding template ensures that all colleagues understand the priorities and activities so an APP will be practice ready when the onboarding is complete. This includes identifying the accountable leaders/mentors for the APP and setting clear, measurable onboarding goals with a specific training plan followed up with periodic check-ins. The onboarding template should be shared with the APP, department operational leaders, human resources, preceptor, mentor, lead APP, and physician mentor. Having a point person or dedicated go-to person available to answer questions, guide the APP through the process, and provide advice, feedback, and evaluation about their clinical care is one of the most important aspects of the onboarding program (Anglin et al., 2021).

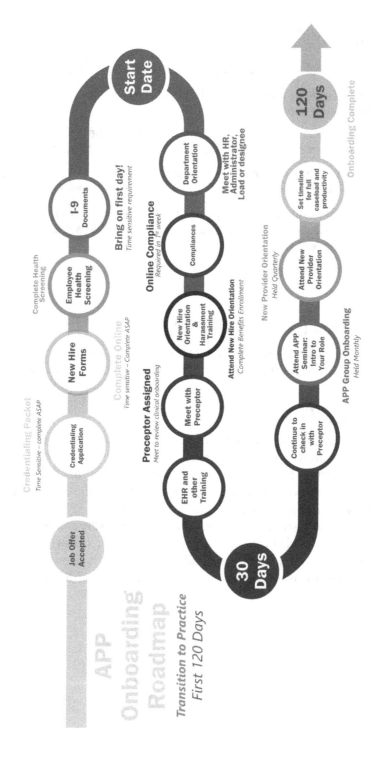

FIGURE 6.1 APP onboarding roadmap.

Figure 6.2 demonstrates an onboarding template outlining the productivity metrics with the specific training to reach those metrics. Using this example, a 30-day, 60-day, 90-day, and six-month goal is set for each metric. At each of these intervals, the APP meets with the appropriate organization leader and reviews actual versus goal metrics, and if gaps exist, the training template is revised or enhanced. Benefits to this approach include setting clear, measurable goals; having a detailed plan in place for reaching the goals; ensuring all team members are aware of the goals; and having a stake in the outcome.

APP Name: Hire Date:	Ambulatory	Training Plan	30 Days		60 Days		90 Days		6 Months, Full Productivity	
			Goal	Actual	Goal	Actual	Goal	Actual	Goal	Actual
# Clinic Sessions Per Week	8–9 (based on 1.0 FTE)									
Average Worked RVU per APP (wRVU)	At or above 65th Percentile MGMA Benchmark									
Average Patients per Session	8–10 Patients per Clinic Session									
Slot Utilization Rate	Schedule above 85% Filled									
Schedule Template Rate (unavailable/pre-allocated %)	< 10% of Template Schedule									
Facilitated Access Rate	> 90% of patients seen within 10 days from defined group									
Care Provider Mean Score	Press Ganey Patient Satisfaction at or above 96.00									
		Signatures:								
		APP:								
		Preceptor:								
		Lead APP:								
		Physician Mentor:								

FIGURE 6.2 Template for APP clinical onboarding.

ROLE TRANSITION STRATEGIES

Moving into a new APP role can bring significant and unique challenges. Providing experience, understanding, support, and resources to new APPs will allow for a smoother transition into their role (Faraz, 2019). Every APP new to their role will experience professional transition to some degree. One or more of the following types of transitions may apply:

- New department/patient population

- RN to NP

- Student to PA

- Ambulatory to inpatient/inpatient to ambulatory

- New to academic health center/hospital/clinic/private practice

- Small to large organization/large to small

- Rural to urban/urban to rural

- Private practice to healthcare system or vice versa

APP TRANSITION STRATEGIES

- Be proactive in determining your onboarding needs. Know the length of onboarding and the expectations.

- Participate in the process. Do not wait for others to create your path.

- Understand KPI (Key Performance Indicators). Know the productivity metrics for your role and take an active part in measuring success.

- Recognize and manage emotions surrounding change and ambiguity. Take care of your well-being.

- Have patience. Allow yourself transition time. Ask for appropriate timelines for being practice ready.

- Prepare. Seek journal articles, books, and other resources related to areas in which you need more knowledge.

- Network. Connect with professional colleagues to share experiences and grow professional relationships.

- Foster and strengthen your relationship with your preceptor.

- Set goals and track your progress. Check in periodically with your leaders to be sure you are on the right track.

Support during transition into clinical practice is crucial for both PAs and APRNs. PA graduates have described requiring an average of six to eight months to feel proficient in their first jobs, with one-third of PAs surveyed in primary care not feeling proficient at one year, and new APRNs report experiencing anxiety, isolation, and a lack of confidence in their new roles, despite often having experience as an RN (Morgan et al., 2020). Offering support through building a sense of community, structured onboarding, clear productivity metrics, and an open and engaged mentor or preceptor will help ease transition anxiety. Too many competing priorities and focusing efforts in too many areas may add to stress and anxiety and undermine efforts to improve efficiently. Knowing the action plan—what success looks like—is imperative with setting and ultimately achieving goals.

RESOURCES AND GETTING HELP

APPs will grow and learn at their own rate and may need to reach out to organization leaders and subject matter experts along the way for help. Providing a guide to common questions and resources will be helpful for new APPs. The onboarding plan should include resources for extra help and questions regarding the EHR, coding and billing, documentation, credentialing and privileging, and general practice information. Another helpful tool to share with your new APP is a glossary and resource list, which can be found in Appendices F and G.

APPs should be provided a department organizational chart and a list of key colleagues and resources, and introductions should be provided. Following are some common examples:

- Nurse managers
- Physician leaders
- Operational managers
- Nursing and ancillary staff
- Environmental services, facilities, food & nutrition services staff
- Administrative, support, and clerical staff
- Clinical resources: pharmacy, radiology, therapies, dietetics, chaplains, case management
- Non-clinical: finance, marketing, supply, human resources

NETWORKING AND CONNECTIONS

Networking among colleagues within the organization helps a new APP grow knowledge of other specialty areas and how their role functions and will allow for stronger collaboration in team-based care. By growing and maintaining a strong professional network APPs will develop relationships that have the potential to assist them as they integrate into the organization.

SETTING GOALS AND PRIORITIES

This chapter discussed transitioning to a new position, noting that it can be overwhelming and may lead to feeling pulled in many directions with competing priorities. APPs, having completed rigorous academic programs and established themselves as healthcare professionals tend to be very self-motivated and commonly exhibit traits as high achievers, willing and eager to put forth the time and effort to advance knowledge, skills, and abilities. APPs and leadership should partner in setting professional goals that are aligned with the expectations, metrics, and deliverables related to the role and also aligned with the organization's strategic goals. Above all, initial goals and priorities should be agreed upon by APPs and their leaders so that efforts and resources may be allocated towards the identified priorities.

SUMMARY

Organizations should plan and prepare a comprehensive onboarding program designed to incrementally bring a new APP towards full practice and competency. Having a plan, knowing how success will be measured, and involving an interdisciplinary team in the onboarding plan will increase efficiency. Refer to Appendix H for a case study developing an APP onboarding program. From a new hire perspective, a clear, structured onboarding plan helps to create a smooth transition into the role and promote a professional home. As most healthcare organizations have limited resources, and preceptors, mentors, and physician leaders carry their own patient load or clinical responsibilities, having a well-defined onboarding path with role clarity will benefit the team and ultimately allow for efficiently guiding the new APP towards full case load, top-of-license practice, and competency.

REFERENCES

Anglin, L., Sanchez, M., Butterfield, R., Rana, R., Everett, C. M., & Morgan, P. (2021). Emerging practices in onboarding programs for PAs: Strategies for onboarding. *Journal of the American Association of Nurse Practitioners, 34*(1), 32–38. https://doi.org/10.1097/01.Jaa.0000723932.21395.74

Chaney, A., Martin, A., Cardona, K., & Presutti, R. J. (2022). Nurse practitioner and physician assistant onboarding in a family medicine practice. *Journal of the American Association of Nurse Practitioners, 34*(3), 522–528. https://doi.org/10.1097/JXX.0000000000000611

Faraz, A. (2019). Facilitators and barriers to the novice nurse practitioner workforce transition in primary care. *Journal of the American Association of Nurse Practitioners, 31*(6), 364–370. https://doi.org/10.1097/jxx.0000000000000158

Kapu, A. (2022). Nurse practitioner leadership essential: Ensuring a positive onboarding experience for new nurse practitioners. *JONA: The Journal of Nursing Administration, 52*(9), 447–448. https://doi.org/10.1097/NNA.0000000000001180

MacLellan, L., Levett-Jones, T., & Higgins, I. (2015, July). Nurse practitioner role transition: A concept analysis. *Journal of the American Association of Nurse Practitioners, 27*(7), 389–397. https://doi.org/10.1002/2327-6924.12165

McGrath, B., Konold, V., Forbes, M., Murphy, E., Cerasale, M., & Schram, A. (2021). The 90-day orientation: An onboarding strategy for hospitalist PAs and NPs. *Journal of the American Academy of Physician Associates, 34*(9), 52–55. https://doi.org/10.1097/01.JAA.0000758228.45700.9c

Morgan, P., Sanchez, M., Anglin, L., Rana, R., Butterfield, R., & Everett, C. M. (2020, March). Emerging practices in onboarding programs for PAs and NPs. *Journal of the American Academy of Physician Associates, 33*(3), 40–46. https://doi.org/10.1097/01.JAA.0000654016.94204.2e

Waltz, L. A., Munoz, L., Weber Johnson, H., & Rodriguez, T. (2020). Exploring job satisfaction and workplace engagement in millennial nurses. *Journal of Nursing Management, 28*(3), 673–681. https://doi.org/10.1111/jonm.12981

"Technology gives us power, but it does not and cannot tell us how to use that power. Thanks to technology, we can instantly communicate across the world, but it still doesn't help us know what to say."

—Jonathan Sacks

CHAPTER 7

OPERATIONALIZING TELEHEALTH

KEYWORDS | telehealth, legislation, competency, cost, licensure

The delivery of healthcare services using electronic communication between provider and patient who are not in the same location is known as *telehealth* or *telemedicine* (US Department of Health & Human Services [USDHHS], 2023). Telehealth was slowly expanding prior to 2020 (Barnett et al., 2021) but accelerated rapidly beginning with the COVID-19 pandemic due to the public health emergency necessitating the ability to care for patients without in-person contact. Both patients (Eldaly et al., 2022) and providers (Siraj et al., 2021) found value in the telehealth platform and it became an accepted mode of healthcare delivery beyond the pandemic. Telehealth has similar clinical outcomes as compared with in-person care (Hatef et al., 2023).

APPs and physicians require appropriate training, support, patient feedback, and reimbursement for telehealth to be an effective and sustainable mode of healthcare delivery. Telehealth programs have unique components, and scope of practice and competencies have been incorporated in APRN, PA, and medical education curricula, ensuring successful adoption by future workforce programs (Garber & Gustin, 2022; Noronha et al., 2022). The rapid expansion of telehealth care delivery has forced academic medical institutions to implement clinical training to teach digital health skills to providers across the medical education continuum (Noronha et al., 2022).

Patients in rural communities benefit from telehealth because they are able to see providers from their own homes and do not have to travel the long distances often required for in person visits. It can also be difficult to recruit providers to rural areas, which is another benefit of telehealth (Kichloo et al., 2020). Totten et al. (2022) found that telehealth can improve patient outcomes such as access to and quality of care, provider outcomes such as knowledge and self-efficacy, and payer outcomes such as reduced costs or maintenance of payments to rural providers. Telehealth has been found to be more convenient, providing greater access for many patients. It provides patient and provider flexibility, is more efficient in terms of time and use of office space, and allows for remote work (Hatef et al., 2023).

Telehealth allows patients with non-emergent issues to receive care, reducing volumes in emergency departments. Disadvantages to telehealth include lack of awareness of telehealth services, lack of internet, computers, or other required technology, and the lack of palpable physical examinations. There is also a concern of cybersecurity threats with the protected health information that could possibly be tampered with when providing telehealth care (Kichloo et al., 2020).

THE FINANCIAL IMPACT

A critical step in the revenue cycle is payer enrollment in a health insurance network or government program (i.e., Medicare, Medicaid) as a medical provider. Government regulations and payer policies surrounding the level of reimbursement for telehealth strongly influence an organization's likelihood to implement a telehealth program. When providers are enrolled in a payer system or network, they can bill for services after providing care, and the reimbursement from payers is a primary revenue source for healthcare systems. At the start of the COVID-19 pandemic, when the public health emergency was declared, federal policy changes relaxed regulations surrounding telehealth and expanded reimbursement parity (USDHHS, 2023).

Variability in federal telehealth policy adds to the complexity for organizations wishing to operationalize telehealth. Additionally, many private payers have expressed concerns about overutilization of telehealth services by providers or patients. Reimbursement laws vary by state, and many allow private payers room to interpret telehealth coverage policies in a way that limits utilization or reduces reimbursement (Bajowala et al., 2020).

Governmental payers have simplified many of the coding and billing requirements to make training for providers easier and more consistent with in-person patient encounters. There is a perception that since telehealth may be able to be delivered at a lower cost than in-person care it should be reimbursed at a lower rate. Whether care is provided via telehealth or in person, providers need the support of schedulers, nurses/medical assistants, information systems staff, and billing/compliance experts to deliver high-quality care. There may be additional ongoing costs for equipment and systems necessary to provide telehealth to ensure data is secure and safe. According to the USDHHS (2022), after the public health emergency ends, providers will be required to provide telehealth services through technology vendors that are HIPAA compliant and must enter into HIPAA business associate agreements (USDHHS, 2022). These costs are frequently minimized by payers, legislators, and other non-direct patient care professionals, and parity in payment remains a barrier to widespread adoption.

Patients of various ages and with a wide range of diseases and diagnosis may benefit from telehealth services. Although patient access can be enhanced through telehealth, access to telehealth is not universal for all patients. Technology such as rural internet and broadband access is not homogeneous throughout the United States. Certain underserved populations may not own or have access to the technology, such as a computer, smartphone, or laptop with the reliable data connections necessary to engage with providers via telehealth. Others may have access to the equipment, but it may not be located in a private space conducive to personal medical discussions or behavioral health treatment. Patients may have distrust about the privacy of telehealth or concerns about encroachment of the healthcare system into their personal space. The security of telehealth platforms needs to be constantly reviewed and kept current to assure privacy and cybersecurity safety.

Organizations should develop clear telehealth workflows that align the same resources as available with in-person care delivery. Moreover, the same patient satisfaction experience and evaluation surveys used for in-person patient care visits must be delivered to patients who have telehealth experiences to allow the opportunity to compare the patient's perceived benefit or lack thereof.

THE IOWA EXAMPLE

At University of Iowa Health Care, there was little telehealth uptake prior to the pandemic. An attempt several years prior to contract with a co-branded third party to provide 24/7 on-demand acute primary care to the university students, staff, employees, and surrounding community members was fraught with issues. Utilization was very poor despite significant marketing investments as if the patient population was not ready for virtual care. The third-party information system did not connect to the UI enterprise information system, which caused significant difficulties to coordinate care when the patient needed escalation from telehealth to in-person care. The providers did not have any information about telehealth evaluation, even though the patients expected a seamless transition between care settings. UI providers were also not accustomed to having external contracted providers caring for patients under the UI brand. UI providers were concerned about the quality of external providers and demanded all of the third-party providers be credentialed and privileged through our own systems, adding to the administrative complexity. The result was significant negativity and pessimism regarding the value of the program to the patients and enterprise at large.

COVID-19 IMPACT ON TELEHEALTH

As noted above, telehealth has been available for healthcare delivery but was not widely utilized as provider reimbursement for telehealth services was restrictive. With the COVID-19 pandemic, the federal and state governments eased restrictions and allowed providers to be reimbursed for telehealth visits at the same rates as in person visits, and for both new and established patients (USDHHS, 2023). Historically there have been certain specialties that utilized telehealth, most notably radiologists, psychiatrists, and cardiologists, but regulations and policies have been different from state to state (Kichloo et al., 2020).

As the COVID-19 pandemic unfolded, healthcare organizations began to look toward innovative approaches to manage what was an unprecedented situation, part of which led to the rapid utilization of telehealth. The general focus was providing care while keeping patients out of the hospital and clinics as much as possible to minimize collateral spread of the highly transmittable COVID-19 virus. New methods and protocols were necessary for the care and treatment of patients with COVID-19. Providers, health systems, and public health officials were faced with developing systems and protocols to create a patient care pathway from respiratory symptom development to recovery from disease. New approaches and care innovations using the same symptom algorithm for evaluation of COVID-19 symptoms over the phone or through an online symptom checker allowed for the appropriate next step in treatment, whether admission to the hospital for observation or a telehealth encounter.

University of Iowa Health Care developed a COVID-19 response utilizing telehealth that was particularly well received by patients. The response began by having a group of providers trained in telehealth delivery and ready to evaluate the results of COVID-19 testing. If the patient tested positive and was at risk for complications, providers ensured the patient had access to home monitoring protocols such as an oxygen saturation monitor, blood pressure cuff, and thermometer, and enrolled in a home monitoring program via telemedicine (Bryant et al., 2022). Telehealth proved beneficial for ongoing monitoring of COVID-19 patients by a combination of nursing personnel and providers who contacted the patient daily or every other day to assess their clinical status. Providers used telehealth to monitor and identify patients who had developed worsening symptoms and were then directed to be seen in person for additional treatment. As therapies evolved, this same virtual screening and telehealth system was used to identify patients who would benefit from convalescent plasma, antibody, or Paxlovid therapy. This intensive outpatient virtual treatment resulted in high patient satisfaction, high-quality care, and low morbidities (Bryant et al., 2022).

The University of Iowa Health Care program serves to represent a best practice telehealth program example. The clinical cohort of patients was clearly defined. There was a specific workflow for the way the patients were enrolled and monitored in the program. All of the clinical documentation, laboratory results, medications, and vitals were clearly visible to all healthcare personnel caring for the patient. Most importantly, all team members (physicians, APPs, nurses, laboratory personnel, schedulers, etc.) working within the program had ongoing training on the clinical pathways as well as the technology. Telehealth, although rapidly expanded as a result of the pandemic, has been successfully adopted and continues be an integral model of healthcare delivery that should continue to be evaluated to expand patient access and improve the health and well-being of patients.

The pandemic provided rapid relief from regulations and policies that have been plaguing the use of telehealth in the past. When patients were left with few options to receive care, telehealth was a great relief, and now that providers are able to be reimbursed this is a big step forward (Hoffman, 2020). Hospitals were challenged by masses of patients requiring in-person care while limiting the number of patients and visitors in waiting rooms to prevent spreading the illness, and triaging hospital beds to care for those in greatest need. Having the option of telehealth to care for patients has made a difference in the care patients can receive and the safety of the hospitals, staff, and patients that must be seen in-person (Hoffman, 2020). As the COVID-19 emergency resolved, providers and healthcare organizations may need to adjust practices and resources if the state and federal governments do not continue to reimburse similarly to in-person visits, as telehealth visits may decrease considerably.

APP RESOURCE ALLOCATION

Staffing shortages across healthcare organizations is not a new phenomenon. Organizations expanding telehealth coverage may allocate provider resources to solely telehealth, only in-person care, or a combination of both. Unique to the pandemic, telehealth volumes rose while in-person ambulatory visits declined. Telehealth capacity could not keep up with demand, and there was a significant need to expand to all provider types to care for the large volumes of patients that required evaluation with COVID-19-like symptoms via telehealth, as well as managing patients with positive COVID-19 in their homes.

In the case of University of Iowa Health Care, the response to the constant and continued increase of telehealth patients was first using existing providers, then ultimately hiring dedicated telehealth APPs specific for this patient population at one-year assignments for short-term contracts to care for the COVID-19 telehealth patients safely and efficiently. Due to pandemic conditions, APPs who were affected in the opposite manner and faced with closed clinics and canceled surgeries in an effort to prevent further spread could be reallocated to where patient care demands were high, a testament to the agility of the APP workforce. As patient care volumes increased in the telehealth realm, it would be remiss not to mention that APPs working in intensive care units were equally faced with significant patient volumes, and with extensive acuity.

ONBOARDING, EDUCATION, AND LEGISLATION

The framework and processes to recruit and train multiple APPs for telehealth in a timely and efficient manner requires clear objectives and purpose. These objectives are very similar to any ramp up in staffing and include creating a telehealth APP job description that clearly encompasses the needed technical, clinical, and communication skills; an efficient and thorough interview and hiring process with a specific focus on telehealth; creating a consistent APP onboarding and education process targeting telehealth competencies; and providing resources available to assure APPs are up to date in a rapidly changing environment.

When reviewing the job requirements for telehealth APPs, consider whether license to practice permits the provider to physically work remotely outside the state, as this may vary by state and licensing boards. Technological requirements should be clearly spelled out, and each candidate should be required to provide proof that adequate bandwidth is available at their work location and that HIPAA privacy can be maintained when providing telehealth from any remote location.

Interviewing telehealth provider job candidates using video/digital technology provides an opportunity to evaluate how the applicants navigate both the technological aspects and general communication using a digital platform. While the same general onboarding principles apply to any new APP, onboarding telehealth APPs may vary, based on whether they will be providing telehealth 100% remote, entirely on-site, or a combination.

UNIVERSITY OF IOWA HEALTH CARE: THREE-DAY REMOTE TELEHEALTH PROVIDER ONBOARDING

- Day 1 focused on HR requirements, mandatory healthcare compliances, and EHR training.
- Day 2 required 1:1 meeting with the lead APP to review education material and specific telehealth compliances. Review of workflows, processes, and telehealth visit simulation.
- Day 3 trained with an APP working telehealth to observe and begin independently caring for their own patients under the observation of an experienced telehealth APP.
- Ongoing training was offered if additional skills were needed to understand and perfect the EHR and workflows.

As with any new model of care delivery, it is important to have a method in place for communicating the most recent and appropriate information. Organizations should have communication pathways in place to relay information to remote providers.

COMPETENCY METRICS AND QUALITY

It is most common to identify patients with similar symptoms, diagnoses, and/or care pathways/protocols as ideal candidates for telehealth. Common diagnoses such as diabetes have been shown to have good outcomes with telehealth (Momin et al., 2022). Patient cohorts based upon medication regimen complexity and multidisciplinary teams working closely together, such as APPs and pharmacists, are ideal to support the patients (Bell et al., 2022). Regardless of the way patients enter a telehealth program, the triggers for transitioning to standard in-person care or continuing in the virtual program need to be defined and communicated to all telehealth staff and patients.

Equally important is defining patient populations not well suited for telehealth, such as those patients with complex clinical conditions, those needing physical exams, and for therapeutic care requiring human-to-human touch (Hatef et al., 2023). Providers work together to determine the patient populations eligible for telehealth to assure quality is equitable regardless of the visit type, so that a clearly defined care pathway can be used by schedulers, nurses, and other non-provider groups to support the patient and the providers. Decision-making associated with patient care is complex, and the determination of whether a patient needs to be seen via telehealth or in-person is best left to the provider. Patient preference may influence whether telehealth is appropriate, because some patients perceive telehealth as a barrier and prefer an in-person physical exam or communicate more effectively in person (Hatef et al., 2023). For some medical or surgical specialties, the equipment necessary to examine the patient in a direct-to-patients digital platform does not widely exist. As technology changes, it is likely mobile, robust equipment will become available in this space to support expanding patient populations.

COST CONTAINMENT AND DIGITAL SYSTEMS

A crucial component of a successful telehealth initiative is a robust digital systems architecture. Multiple technologies and systems exist for telehealth, all capturing different aspects of the technology, but none perfectly meets the needs for every organization. Organizations should evaluate the pros and cons and identify the systems that will efficiently meet the needs of the patient populations they serve. Early systems include the hub-and-spoke model, which resembles a wagon wheel where pathways (spokes) shoot out from a central data hub, illustrated in Figure 7.1. This model required patients to go to specific physical satellite locations to use dedicated telehealth equipment to connect to providers physically located at other sites. These systems generally required patients to travel outside their home or community, which tended to be dissatisfying compared to newer systems that can connect directly with patients in their own home, workplace, car, or anywhere with an internet or cellular connectivity.

When referring to telehealth, synchronous audio/video telehealth over a two-way video link using broadband connections first comes to mind. Such a system is a heavy technological lift, and in some circumstances, an asynchronous system (which is known as store-and-forward method) is convenient and provides adequate patient support for high-quality care. These systems require patients to upload data, answer questions, and/or upload photos to a secure site and allows the review of uploaded data and interaction with the providers efficiently and without significant technological maintenance. Dermatology is one specialty group that patients can be well served with a store-and-forward system because photos can be uploaded and reviewed by an APP and, if needed, shared with a dermatologist for consultation to review and develop treatment plans based upon the data.

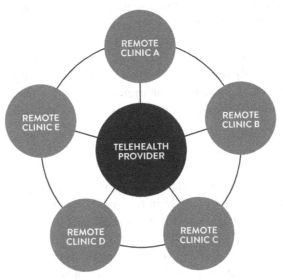

FIGURE 7.1 Telehealth hub and spoke model.

Whatever digital system or structure is chosen must be easily accessible for both patients and providers. The vendors in this space underwent rapid development cycles during the pandemic to improve their system reliability and ease of use. Many EHR vendors now have systems directly integrated into their platforms, including the patient portal, or they have developed relationships with third party vendors to allow deep integration into providers' standard clinical workflows. It is difficult for providers to be well trained on multiple systems for different clinical scenarios, so integration into enterprise systems requires less extensive provider training. Information from telehealth activities must also be freely available to other members of the healthcare team outside telehealth providers so all clinicians caring for the patient have as comprehensive of a picture of the patient's care as if seen in a traditional clinic setting. Deep telehealth integration in multiple circumstances also improves telehealth system reliability.

APP LICENSE TO PRACTICE TELEHEALTH

There are currently no special medical or nursing licensing requirements to provide telehealth; however, many states have issued standards of practice for telehealth that address matters such as prescriptive authority, competency, and scope of practice. Generally, state laws will require that telehealth should be held to the same standard of care as if the service was performed in-person. Providers must be aware of the jurisdiction of the patient, as an APP who provides telehealth to a patient located in another state will be subject to the laws and jurisdiction of the state where the patient is physically located (Iowa Board of Nursing, 2022). Providing patient care across state lines is common when the provider or patient resides close to a bordering state, cares for patients who may reside in warmer climates for the winter months, caring for college students who attend an out-of-state school, or caring for a transient workforce, such as remote workers who have geographically relocated. Multi-state licensing compacts have been considered, but the only true alternative at the present time is for providers to be licensed in multiple states. This adds to the cost and administrative overhead for the program.

SUMMARY

The onslaught of the COVID-19 pandemic brought rapid changes in healthcare delivery, including an unprecedented increase in telehealth, particularly in the ambulatory care setting. Organizations that successfully implemented a robust telehealth program used a number of best practices as outlined within this chapter. Licensing, cybersecurity, HIPAA, and payer policies are some of the issues at the forefront of telehealth implementation. As healthcare organizations transition out of the COVID-19 pandemic, telehealth will continue to be a method of healthcare delivery. Patients have grown accustomed to the convenience and access to healthcare providers, and a large population of rural patients are better served as telehealth offers increased patient access and bypasses rural healthcare provider shortages. Telehealth has proven beneficial for patients, providers, and healthcare organizations and will continue to be an alternative method for care delivery that will continue beyond the pandemic.

REFERENCES

Bajowala, S. S., Milosch, J., & Bansal, C. (2020). Telemedicine pays: Billing and coding update. *Current Allergy & Asthma Reports, 20*(10), 60. https://doi.org/10.1007/s11882-020-00956-y

Barnett, M. L., Huskamp, H. A., Busch, A. B., Uscher-Pines, L., Chaiyachati, K. H., & Mehrotra, A. (2021). Trends in outpatient telemedicine utilization among rural Medicare beneficiaries 2010 to 2019. *JAMA Health Forum, 2*(10), e213282. https://doi.org/10.1001/jamahealthforum.2021.3282

Bell, J. S., Ooi, C. E., Troeung, L., Craik, S., Walton, R., & Martini, A. (2022). Protocol for a pilot and feasibility study of nurse practitioner-pharmacist telehealth collaboration to simplify complex medication regimens. *Research in Social & Administrative Pharmacy, 18*(9), 3687–3693. https://doi.org/10.1016/j.sapharm.2022.03.010

Bryant, A. D., Robinson, T. J., Gutierrez-Perez, J. T., Manning, B. L., Glenn, K., Imborek, K. L., & Kuperman, E. F. (2022, March 11). Outcomes of a home telemonitoring program for SARS-CoV-2 viral infection at a large academic medical center. *Journal of Telemedicine and Telecare.* https://doi.org/10.1177/1357633x221086067

Eldaly, A. S., Maniaci, M. J., Paulson, M. R., Avila, F. R., Torres-Guzman, R. A., Maita, K., Garcia, J. P., & Forte, A. J. (2022, November). Patient satisfaction with telemedicine in acute care setting: A systematic review. *Journal of Clinical and Translational Research, 8*(6), 540–556. https://www.ncbi.nlm.nih.gov/pmc/articles/PMC9741928/

Garber, K., & Gustin, T. (2022, March/April). Telehealth education: Impact on provider experience and adoption. *Nurse Educator, 47*(2), 75–80. https://doi.org/10.1097/nne.0000000000001103

Hatef, E., Wilson, R. F., Hannum, S. M., Zhang, A., Karrazi, H., Weiner, J. P., Davis, S. A., Robinson, K. A. (2023, January). *Use of telehealth during the COVID-19 era: Executive summary.* Agency for Healthcare Research and Quality, 23-EHC005. https://doi.org/10.23970/AHRQEPCSRCOVIDTELEHEALTH

Hoffman, D. A. (2020, June 16). Increasing access to care: Telehealth during COVID-19. *Journal of Law & the Biosciences, 7*(1), Lsaa043. https://doi.org/10.1093/jlb/lsaa043

Iowa Board of Nursing. (2022). *Standards of practice for telehealth.* https://www.legis.iowa.gov/docs/iac/chapter/03-22-2023.655.7.pdf

Kichloo, A., Albosta, M., Dettloff, K., Wani, F., El-Amir, Z., Singh, J., Aljadah, M., Chakinala, R. C., Kanugula, A. K., Solanki, S., & Chugh, S. (2020). Telemedicine, the current COVID-19 pandemic and the future: A narrative review and perspectives moving forward in the USA. *Family Medicine & Community Health, 8*(3), e000530. https://doi.org/10.1136/fmch-2020-000530

Momin, R. P., Kobeissi, M. M., Casarez, R. L., & Khawaja, M. (2022). A nurse practitioner-led telehealth protocol to improve diabetes outcomes in primary care. *Journal of the American Association of Nurse Practitioners, 34*(10), 1167–1173. https://doi.org/10.1097/jxx.0000000000000759

Noronha, C., Lo, M. C., Nikiforova, T., Jones, D., Nandiwada, D. R., Leung, T. I., Smith, J. E., & Lee, W. W. (2022). Telehealth competencies in medical education: New frontiers in faculty development and learner assessments. *Journal of General Internal Medicine, 37*(12), 3168–3173. https://doi.org/10.1007/s11606-022-07564-8

Siraj, A., Salehi, N., & Karim, S. (2021). Refining telemedicine: A plea from healthcare workers during a pandemic. *Cureus, 13*(4), e14664. https://doi.org/10.7759/cureus.14664

Totten, A. M., Womack, D. M., Griffin, J. C., McDonagh, M. S., Davis-O'Reilly, C., Blazina, I., Grusing, S., & Elder, N. (2022). Telehealth-guided provider-to-provider communication to improve rural health: A systematic review. *Journal of Telemedicine & Telecare.* https://doi.org/10.1177/1357633X221139892

US Department of Health and Human Services. (2022). *Power up your telehealth with Telehealth.HHS.gov for patients [Video].* YouTube. https://www.youtube.com/watch?v=p_2cK4obj94

US Department of Health and Human Services. (2023, February 16). *Telehealth policy changes after the COVID-19 public health emergency.* https://telehealth.hhs.gov/providers/policy-changes-during-the-covid-19-public-health-emergency/policy-changes-after-the-covid-19-public-health-emergency

*"Tell me and I forget. Teach me and I remember.
Involve me and I learn."*

—Benjamin Franklin

CHAPTER 8

APRN AND PA STUDENTS

KEYWORDS | students, preceptors, documentation

Educating the next generation of healthcare providers should be part of the mission of every organization regardless of size or structure. Linking clinical practice to didactic education and research completes the tripartite mission, especially at academic health centers where students at every level, whether baccalaureate, graduate, medical students, residents, or fellows are part of the educational purpose. Through clinical experiences with knowledgeable preceptors and a broad opportunity of clinical environments across all sizes of organizations, establishing a pathway to facilitate the education of the future healthcare workforce is pivotal in addressing the shortages facing healthcare organizations.

Clinical practicums are an important element of the APRN and PA educational curriculum (Lofgren et al., 2021; Min et al., 2021). Through clinicals, students apply their didactic knowledge to actual patient care situations to fulfill and complete their education. Clinical placements provide students the opportunity to observe and receive guidance from practicing APPs serving in a formal preceptor role. Alongside their preceptor, students experience routine interactions with patients and other members of the care team, understand the application of the EHR system, apply didactic learning content to practice, and develop clinical skills and confidence in their abilities (McQueen et al., 2018).

CMS: STUDENT DOCUMENTATION REQUIREMENTS

The Centers for Medicare & Medicaid Services (CMS) updated documentation requirements for billing of professional services in 2020. These updated requirements reduce administrative burden as it relates to documentation. Board certified and privileged physicians, physician assistants, and APRNs (including nurse practitioners, clinical nurse specialists, certified nurse-midwives, and certified registered nurse anesthetists) serving as the responsible provider to patients and preceptor to students can review and verify (sign and date) rather than re-documenting notes made in the health record by other healthcare learners such as residents and PA and APRN students. Duplicative documentation has often been seen as a barrier for some providers to take on students, and therefore this change opened up opportunity for a more efficient use of student participation and engagement. As with any change, questions arise surrounding the applicability and legal implications of CMS changes, and therefore communication that includes various scenarios helps alleviate any unwarranted ambiguity for providers questioning taking on students.

AFFILIATION AGREEMENTS

Before any students are placed for clinicals, an affiliation agreement between the school and the organization must be approved and signed by both parties. The *affiliation agreement* is a written agreement used to define the shared responsibilities between both parties: what the school will provide, what the healthcare organization will provide, and details about the requirements for the student and the process. It may take several weeks or months for an affiliation agreement to be completed as it typically is reviewed or revised by the legal department of both the school and the healthcare organization.

Terms of the agreement provide details about the obligations of the school, the organization, and delineates their joint responsibilities. Details include the number of students, the date on which the students are to use the clinical site, the dates of the agreement, and the termination criteria for the agreement.

OBLIGATIONS OF THE SCHOOL

- Provide a designee from the school responsible for the development, maintenance, and supervision of a given number of students enrolled in the program, including clinical experiences and evaluation.

- Assure students maintain health insurance (or an equivalent alternative care plan) prior to the student's commencement sufficient to satisfy minimum standards of coverage established by the organization for all health science students experiencing significant clinical exposures as part of their training.

- Provide an avenue for the preceptor to evaluate the student.

- Submit a physical examination and immunization report satisfying the requirements of the organization for health screening.

- Provide a pathway to promptly report illness and absence to the organization's clinical preceptor.

- Comply with the organization's dress code.

- Comply with the school's plan for student accident or illness while in the organization.

- Be covered by the school's professional legal liability insurance with designated limits agreed upon.

- Designate the maximum number of consecutive training shifts with appropriate time off.

---

continues

continued

- Adhere to both organizations' nondiscrimination requirements.
- Verify that each student has completed the requisite items prior to arrival at the organization.
    - Abuse training
    - Age-related training for patients served
    - Safety and infection control
    - Criminal background check
    - Health screening
    - HIPAA and confidentiality agreement
    - Orientation to organization: mission, governance, improvement
    - Patient safety and medical error reduction compliance
    - Diversity training
    - Patient and staff rights and responsibilities
    - Quality, standards and teamwork
    - Safety and security
    - Harassment prevention
    - Proof of insurance form with copy of insurance card

OBLIGATIONS OF THE ORGANIZATION

- To allow student participation in the patient care programs.
- The organization retains priority for use of the facilities for educational purposes (e.g., conference rooms, simulation labs, etc.). Schools will negotiate with the organization to use the facilities for selected specified education experiences.
- To provide practice areas and observational opportunities within the clinical areas.
- To enable students, under guidance of the school's clinical placement designee and in consultation with appropriate organizational personnel, to select an area of interest for clinical placement.

- The assignment and the quality of care given shall be under the overall supervision of the organization's preceptor and organizational leader, who shall be accountable for all practicums performed by students. Student assignments may be adjusted by the organization to facilitate the provision of appropriate care for patients, taking into account the patients' conditions, skills of the student, and the number of students that can be accommodated at the same time.

- To share the use of available conference areas and instructional materials.

JOINT RESPONSIBILITIES

- The personnel of the organization and the faculty of the school will cooperate in the development of experiences for students and the concurrent and terminal evaluation of the experience.

- Provide an atmosphere conducive to learning.

- Mutual exchange of information, planning and evaluation will take place on a regular basis.

- Opportunity to attend meetings related to the course of study in which the students are involved.

- Either party may require the withdrawal of any student from the clinical areas whose conduct or health may have a detrimental effect on patients or personnel of the organization.

Affiliation agreements further describe the rights of the organization and outline the withdrawal of a school faculty member from the clinical area whose conduct or health may have a detrimental effect on patients or personnel in the organization. The agreement details that students and faculty of the school serve as independent contractors, and assures in writing neither can claim employee benefits, workers' compensation coverage, or payment of taxes. Affiliation agreements include language that neither party is obligated to make payments of any kind to the other party and that services rendered by students covered by the affiliation agreement is educational in nature, and, therefore, the organization or patients will not pay any monetary compensation to students. Affiliation agreements are governed by and construed under the laws of the state in which the student engages in clinical practicum.

Organizations accepting students from multiple schools must track and maintain all the separate affiliation agreements with various schools. This volume of agreements, with rolling expiration dates and number of students each semester, can be administratively challenging to manage. Having organizational resources to oversee, maintain, and assure the student placement process abides with all policies and procedures accordingly underscores the need for ongoing clinical and academic partnerships.

STUDENT PLACEMENT PROCESS

It is important that APP student placement processes and programs are structured in a way to support the organization's overall strategy. Supporting a strong partnership between educational programs and healthcare systems assures having adequate preceptors as a core requirement for a quality clinical experience for students. Often organizations will adopt an exclusive partnership with their preferred educational programs, limiting clinical practicum experiences to schools within the exclusive partnership.

A comprehensive analysis of the perceptions of precepting students in the current healthcare environment noted that there is need for academic and professional ownership of APRN education at every level. (Lofgren et al., 2021). The same study found that hospitals and clinics are not able to keep up with the demand for APRN student placement in clinical practicum sites, resulting in a higher demand than capacity. Organizations are faced with the challenge of having the resources to respond to and accommodate the increasing number of requests for clinical placement, and at the same time assure the students are prepared for clinical practicums from their academic programs. Variability and lack of uniformity in the placement process can result in dissatisfaction from students, schools, faculty, and preceptors (Lofgren et al., 2023). This reinforces the need for strong relationships between the academic APRN and PA programs and healthcare organizations to meet the clinical placement demand of the growing APP programs. Strong academic and clinical partnerships reinforce placement of prepared and experienced students, eliminating strain on preceptors hosting students from multiple programs.

PRECEPTING STUDENTS AS PROFESSIONAL DEVELOPMENT

APPs often have interest in teaching and educating or are interested in informal leadership opportunities. Precepting students can fulfill a desire for professional growth and allow APPs to expand their skills in teaching, instructing, communicating, mentorship, and sharing clinical knowledge and best practices. There are some instances where APP preceptors can obtain professional development credit toward national recertification; continuing education credits; or incentives such as university library access, a state-level tax credit, credit for service in annual performance evaluation, a tuition discount, or personal satisfaction from preparing the next generation of APRNs (Lofgren et al., 2021).

PRECEPTOR TAX INCENTIVES

States have reported a shortage of APP clinical preceptors as one of the challenges to growing a robust workforce of healthcare providers (Carelli, 2019). As a response to the preceptor shortage, states such as Maryland, Georgia, Colorado, South Carolina, and Hawaii offer a state income tax credit for practicing Physician Assistants and Nurse Practitioners who serve as a preceptor for APRN and/or PA students. Each state has their own documentation requirements to qualify for their tax credit program. Georgia pioneered the program in 2014 by offering tax credits to physicians precepting medical students and expanded the program in 2019 to include APPs to benefit the uncompensated community-based preceptors who train healthcare providers (Georgia Preceptor Tax Incentive Program, 2023).

Precepting APP students can be satisfying and support professional development, strengthening overall engagement. Work schedules and clinical demands of the APP need to be considered as precepting a student will likely be in addition to normal clinical work expectations. For APPs compensated based on relative value units (RVUs), clinical efficiency may be impacted for those APPs precepting students (Lofgren et al., 2021).

A strong and stable partnership between schools and preceptors can foster lasting relationships with new graduates, alumni, and current and former preceptors to assist them in finding meaning in the preceptor role and enhance their professional growth (Burt et al., 2021). Other ways to incentivize preceptors are to offer complementary continuing education programs and to allow APPs to network and develop relationships with faculty and academic programs, or in some cases provide adjunct faculty status (Heusinkvelt & Tracy, 2020).

Accepting APP students for clinical practicums may prove advantageous for future recruiting efforts in many organizations. Strong, positive relationships with educational programs and academic professors can translate to a larger network of APP candidates interested in employment at the organization. Students can be a talent pipeline into the organization and serve as a hiring pool to consider for open positions in the future. Many organizations choose to hire or consider former students for open positions, knowing they have had the opportunity to get to know them personally and have been able to observe their skills firsthand. Students ultimately hired as APPs have an advantage of knowing the organization and have a realistic job preview via their practicum experience, thus improving the transition from new graduate into employment.

Meeting the population health needs of the most vulnerable and high-risk patients is a major concern. (Young et al., 2020). Collaborating with community health centers and rural hospitals for placing APRN and PA students for clinical practicums supports the mission of expanding services into these high-risk areas and provides value to the greater community. Students well prepared to serve these rural and underserved patients help improve the health and welfare of these communities and ease the burden on larger healthcare systems.

ESTABLISHING A PRIORITY SYSTEM FOR STUDENT PLACEMENT

Having a priority system for determining which students to accept into clinical placement can support the education mission of the organization, allow professional development for APPs wanting to mentor and precept the next generation of APPs, and support the organization's goal to recruit from a pipeline of highly skilled students. Academic and clinical partnerships have significant value and it is imperative to build these relationships to address the needed economic, market, and generational changes in the healthcare workforce that are affecting our systems and to be more integrated and efficient.

BARRIERS ASSOCIATED WITH APP STUDENT CLINICAL PLACEMENT

Administrative burdens in maintaining affiliation agreements with multiple schools include:

- High demand and low supply of preceptors (especially with high demand areas such as primary care and women's health)

- Varied level of student readiness leaving preceptors to fill in education gaps

- No priority system in selecting schools

- High volume of requests and dealing with multiple schools may create dissatisfaction among departments, making them less likely to accept students and support APPs' precepting

- Administrative burden of tracking and ensuring students adhere to all compliance requirements

---

IDENTIFYING INTERNAL PRECEPTORS

Prior to placing students, each organization should identify the pool of willing preceptors to be sure there are adequate resources. University of Iowa Health Care surveys all APPs three times per year in advance of each academic semester to identify those interested and willing to precept a student. APPs may choose to precept any or all of the academic semesters (spring, summer, fall) and respond to the survey with their name, department, credentials, and the number of hours they are able to precept. To precept a student, APPs are also required to obtain approval from their APP lead or department leadership.

The list of potential preceptors is compiled and provided to the exclusive partnership educational program. The educational program directors match their students with available preceptors on the list specific to the patient populations and clinic experience needed for the curriculum. Once the educational program has matched their students on the list, the committee convenes to review the list and address any concerns or gaps.

The guidelines for student placements are available on the organization's website. This site serves as a means for consistent and current communication for students, schools, prospective students, and other interested parties. The website also hosts a helpful decision tree, as seen in Figure 8.1, to help visually guide students, schools, and prospective students through the clinical placement process.

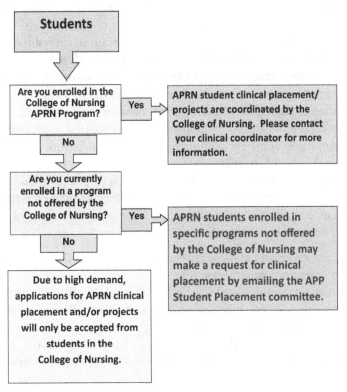

FIGURE 8.1 Clinical placement decision tree.

ACADEMIC PARTNERSHIPS/CLINICAL PRECEPTORS

APPs are a significant part of the workforce, so consideration should be given to building relationships with APRN and PA academic programs. Resources at the organizational level should be attributed accordingly to sustain these relationships to assist with affiliation agreements, background checks, and other documents needed to place students, as well as thoughtful career counseling for staff interested in furthering their education to align with future workforce needs. Connecting the academic education programs and the healthcare organization in care delivery will bridge the gap and strengthen the overall ability to better meet the population health needs of this country (American Association of Colleges of Nursing, 2016). Identification of appropriate preceptors, evaluation and assessment for clinical practicums for APRNs and PAs, and the overall process for student placement for clinical practicum experiences are all essential for success (Amirehsani et al., 2019; Doherty et al., 2019; Hawkins, 2019; Heusinkvelt & Tracy, 2020; Hudak et al., 2019; Min et al., 2021; Roberts et al., 2020).

As APRN and PA programs grow, it is important for healthcare organizations to identify which schools will be a best fit to partner with their organization. A valued and functional relationship with the academic program will include frequent contact with and responsiveness from clinical instructors and regular clinical site visits. Administrative time and resources may be reduced when strong partnerships exist between the healthcare organization and the academic program (Lofgren et al., 2023). Organizations having accommodated students from various schools have the perspective of analyzing the strengths and weaknesses of various academic programs. A strong program meets academic rigors; the students are motivated and high-quality learners; and the school contacts are organized, responsive, and structured so that the paperwork and other behind-the-scenes items are completed promptly and thoroughly. A poor experience with a school, student, or instructor may discourage APPs or organizations from accepting students in the future. Care should be given to selecting those schools who are reputable and whose actions/values are aligned with growing a strong collaboration between school and healthcare organization. A case study detailing an academic clinical partnership can be found in Appendix I.

In a strong academic and clinical partnership, schools will provide concrete course program details and supplemental resources, including learning objectives, well in advance of the student coming on-site to conduct their clinicals. Schools may also provide education to preceptors to enhance the student experience. Providing an annual conference for preceptors to expand their knowledge of current clinical practice issues is one way to support the continual education needs for APPs. Schools may also provide guides, toolkits, and other resources to enhance the experience of both preceptor and student.

STUDENTS FINDING THEIR OWN PRECEPTORS

The practice or necessity of students being required to identify and locate qualified preceptors on their own (without assistance from their educational program) is a process concern from the organization's perspective. Clinical sites and preceptors are in high demand, and organizations are aligning and partnering with specific educational programs to manage and prioritize the number of requests to their providers. Having central oversight ensures affiliation agreements are in place, and the student is in good standing and officially admitted to the APRN or PA program before any contact be made between student and preceptor. From the student's perspective, if unable to find their own preceptors it may delay their program completion date, or a student may resort to paying an outside company costly fees for placement. Many professional organizations and governing programs, such as the National Task Force on Quality Nurse Practitioner Education (2022), are no longer allowing students to find their own preceptors. Likewise, state boards of nursing are also addressing the issue by writing administrative rules. An example of the Iowa Board of Nursing's rules for APRN program preceptorship is provided here:

IBON ADMIN RULES

655—2.16(152) APRN program preceptorship.

2.16(1) A preceptor shall be selected by the nursing program in collaboration with a clinical facility to provide supportive learning experiences consistent with program outcomes.

a. A nursing education program shall not require students to find their own preceptors. The nursing education program and student shall work together to find an appropriate preceptor.

b. The student shall have the majority of preceptorship learning experiences with a preceptor who is an APRN or physician with the same role and population focus for which the student is preparing.

2.16(2) The qualifications of a preceptor shall be appropriate to support the philosophy, mission, and outcomes of the program.

a. The preceptor shall be employed by or maintain a current written agreement with the clinical facility in which a preceptorship experience occurs.

b. The preceptor shall be currently licensed as an advanced registered nurse practitioner or physician according to the laws of the state in which the preceptor practices.

c. The preceptor shall function according to written policies for selection, evaluation and reappointment developed by the program. Written qualifications, developed by the program, shall address educational preparation, experience, and clinical competence.

d. The program shall be responsible for informing the preceptor of the responsibilities of the preceptor, faculty and students.

e. The program shall retain ultimate responsibility for student learning and evaluation.

2.16(3) The program shall inform the board about the preceptorship learning experience process.

a. Written preceptorship agreements shall be reviewed annually by the program.

b. The board may conduct a site visit to settings in which preceptorship experiences occur.

c. The rationale for the ratio of students to preceptors shall be documented by the program.

[ARC 5286C, IAB 11/18/20, effective 12/23/20]

SUMMARY

Having a solid relationship between students, educational programs, and healthcare providers is essential to meet the workforce needs and the educational requirements for APRN and PA education. Given the changing climate in healthcare, a well-prepared group of PAs and APRNs will be necessary to serve the healthcare needs and fill gaps in access to quality care. Organizations should commit both time and resources to educating APP students. Precepting students can be a fulfilling professional development opportunity for current APPs, and having an organized system that values the educational pathways for APPs allows for higher levels of preparation through established relationships with all interested parties and is a key aspect of fulfilling the future workforce with quality APPs.

REFERENCES

American Association of Colleges of Nursing. (2016). *AACN advances nursing's role in interprofessional education.* https://www.aacnnursing.org/our-initiatives/education-practice/teaching-resources/interprofessional-education

Amirehsani, K. A., Kennedy-Malone, L., & Alam, M. T. (2019). Supporting preceptors and strengthening academic-practice partnerships: Preceptors' perceptions. *The Journal for Nurse Practitioners, 15*(8), e151–d156. https://doi.org/10.1016/j.nurpra.2019.04.011

Burt, L., Sparbel, K., & Corbridge, S. (2021). Nurse practitioner preceptor resource needs and perceptions of institutional support. *Journal of the American Association of Nurse Practitioners, 34*(2), 348–356. https://doi.org/10.1097/jxx.0000000000000629

Carelli, K., Gatiba, P., & Thompson, L. (2019). Tax incentives for preceptors of nurse practitioner students in Massachusetts: A potential solution. *Journal of the American Association of Nurse Practitioners, 31*(8), 462–467. https://doi.10.1097/JXX.0000000000000257

Doherty, C. L., Fogg, L., Bigley, M. B., Todd, B., & O'Sullivan, A. L. (2019). Nurse practitioner student clinical placement processes: A national survey of nurse practitioner programs. *Nursing Outlook, 68*(1), 55–61. https://doi.org/10.1016/j.outlook.2019.07.005

Georgia Preceptor Tax Incentive Program. (2023). *Augusta University.* https://www.augusta.edu/ahec/ptip/

Hawkins, M. D. (2019). Barriers to preceptor placement for nurse practitioner students. *Journal of Christian Nursing, 36*(1), 48–53. https://doi.org/10.1097/cnj.0000000000000519

Heusinkvelt, S. E., & Tracy, M. (2020). Improving nurse practitioner and physician assistant preceptor knowledge, self-efficacy, and willingness in a hospital medicine practice: An online experience. *The Journal of Continuing Education in Nursing, 51*(6), 275–279. https://doi.org/10.3928/00220124-20200514-07

Hudak, N. M., Pinheiro, S. O., & Yanamadala, M. (2019). Increasing physician assistant students' team communication skills and confidence throughout clinical training. *The Journal of Physician Assistant Education, 30*(4), 219–222. https://doi.org/10.1097/jpa.0000000000000278

Lofgren, M., Dunn, H., Dirks, M., & Reyes, J. (2021). Perspectives, experiences, and opinions precepting advanced practice registered nurse students. *Nursing Outlook, 69*(5), 913–926. https://doi.org/10.1016/j.outlook.2021.03.018

Lofgren, M., Dunn, H., Gust, C., Worrell, A. M., & Dirks, M. (2023). Advanced practice RN student practicum placements: An academic health center and college of nursing collaboration. *Journal of Nursing Administration,* online ahead of print. doi:https://doi.org/10.1097/nna.0000000000001348

McQueen, K. A., Poole, K., Raynak, A., & McQueen, A. (2018). Preceptorship in a nurse practitioner program: The student perspective. *Nurse Educator, 43*(6), 302–306. https://doi.org/10.1097/nne.0000000000000498

Min, E. A., Bowden, W. P., Gerstner, L. R., & Guthrie, J. R. (2021). Credentials and core clerkships: Who's training our physician assistant students (and does it matter)? *The Journal of Physician Assistant Education, 32*(3), 185–188. https://doi.org/10.1097/jpa.0000000000000366

National Task Force on Quality Nurse Practitioner Education. (2022). *Standards for quality nurse practitioner education. A report of the National Task Force on Quality Nurse Practitioner Education* (6th ed.). https://cdn.ymaws.com/www.nonpf.org/resource/resmgr/ntfstandards/ntfs_final.pdf

Roberts, L. R., Champlin, A., Saunders, J. S. D., Pueschel, R. D., & Huerta, G. M. (2020). Meeting preceptor expectations to facilitate optimal nurse practitioner student clinical rotations. *Journal of the American Association of Nurse Practitioners, 32*(5), 400–407. https://doi.org/10.1097/jxx.0000000000000304

Young, S. G., Gruca, T. S., & Nelson, G. C. (2020). Impact of nonphysician providers on spatial accessibility to primary care in Iowa. *Health Services Research, 55*(3), 476–485. https://doi.org/10.1111/1475-6773.13280

"There are no secrets to success. It is the result of preparation, hard work, and learning from failure."

—Colin Powell

CHAPTER 9

APP BUSINESS PRO FORMA

KEYWORDS | business, staffing models, clinical tracks, pro forma, caseload

A *pro forma* is a standard method to provide the rationale and expected return on investment (ROI) for hiring an APP. Successfully completing a business pro forma for the purpose of hiring an APP into a new or vacant position requires knowledge about the organization's hiring processes, the patient population, the practice location desired, the medical staffing model, and the caseload expectations for the position. Defining these key elements prior to hiring an APP ensures that the position has clear purpose and ensures the pro forma is comprehensive, setting the stage for a successful APP hire.

STANDARDIZED PROCESS FOR HIRING

Having a clear delineation of the necessary skill level is essential for completing the business pro forma. Questions that are helpful to guide practices and attempt to optimize the productivity and functionality of the role include the following:

- How will the role function? Is this for a new APP role or a role to be integrated with existing teams? What are the hours and days of work? Does it include weekends and holidays? Is it inpatient versus outpatient or a hybrid practice model?

- What does the scope of practice involve? Examples include rounding on patients, attending bed huddles, admission and discharge orders, consults, documentation goals, and caseload expectations.

- What are the productivity expectations and timelines to meet expectations? Examples include the number of patients per day or session, the length of time it takes for a patient to be seen, knowing the average census and acuity of the patients to serve, the frequency and timing of when admissions and discharges take place, how many and types of other providers are part of the team, and if there are cross coverage or call expectations.

- How will the APP role align with the organization's other strategic goals? Examples include decreasing length of stay, improving patient satisfaction, increasing nursing and other provider satisfaction, improving continuity of care, and improving patient access.

The pro forma basics should be initiated by the department of human resources or an administrator and vetted by experts for scope of practice, financial analysis, compensation and classification, and senior leadership. For example, from a scope of practice perspective, a centralized office for APPs would provide feedback and approval on the following elements:

- The required/desired board certification and license is appropriate for patient population

- The credentialing date is reasonable and realistic with anticipated date of hire
- There are clear role expectations and rationale for the position, which supports top-of-license practice
- There is an APP lead in place to support this role; if not, an identified person to support the role
- Is the role an APP lead/supervisor position?
- There is a clear reporting structure for the APP role

APP job descriptions should be broad enough not to define every single APP role across an organization but specific enough that it is clear the role requires an APRN or PA license. Each department or service line should have the ability to tailor a section of the job description to the specific needs that align with the pro forma and be included as an attachment. For example, details such as the required board certification for a specific patient population or a desired skill set would be important when matching pro forma to job description.

The pro forma helps an organization quantify a financial rationale for the position. Additionally, having top-of-license work well-defined—including a clear schedule template with details of what type of patients will be cared for by the APP and, conversely, what type of patients are cared for by the physician—helps to calculate an estimated return on investment to an organization. The department should be able to quantify exactly how the APP role is essential to patient care and patient access. This information adds to the role clarity and will be helpful for all team members in understanding the clinical practice model and types of billing potential. Compensation for the APP position should be included in the business analysis. Maintaining market value for APP positions within geographic locations is important for the pro forma and in the hiring process. Both the start date and anticipated privileging and billing dates should be included, reflecting realistic and reasonable timelines. Modification of privileges can take additional months after the initial privileging dates. When department colleagues understand the length of time this takes, as well as the time it takes for modification of privileges that include revenue-generating procedures, it helps to anticipate revenue generating ability of the new APP hire in the first year. The department approver, administrator, APP lead, and any additional supporting roles for the APP position should be included by name on the pro forma.

THE FOUR TRACKS

Quantifying the value of an APP position has its challenges because the role is often underwritten by physicians or bundled in payment models that do not capture APP specific relative value units (RVUs) or is associated with care coordination that requires a provider but are unquantifiable. Certain details relating to how the position will function within a department are important for operations and essential for approval for a pro forma. APPs play unique roles within the healthcare delivery system, and defining the operating model by track is a tangible step in dissecting other critical elements. APP positions can be categorized in the following tracks:

Ambulatory: The ambulatory APP cares for patients in an outpatient-clinic-type setting in both primary and specialty areas. Target APPs for the ambulatory setting usually are board certified as primary care or those with specialty certification. Best practices require the department to define which patients will be seen by the APP independently and which patients need to be evaluated by physicians. Schedule templates may include eight or nine half-day sessions per full-time clinical position. This clinical setting often requires weekend and evening coverage (defined by clinical service area) and should be clearly communicated and addressed in the job requirements. Productivity metrics include defined RVU targets and patient satisfaction scores.

Hospitalist non-intensive care unit: The hospitalist non-ICU service line cares for patients in the inpatient hospital setting or as part of a consult service and may include caring for patients in the skilled or long-term care settings or step-down units. Comprehensive healthcare is provided to patients in these settings with a wide range of complex and comorbid disease conditions across a variety of specialties. Target APPs for this clinical setting are board certified with specialty certification or additional residency or fellowship training that relate to the patient population foci. Patient caseload ranges are often variable from approximately eight to 15 patients based on patient-specific acuity and patient population. Caseload expectations often increase to 16 to 36 patients during the overnight hours or off shifts and again is determined based on the acuity and patient population (Kapu et al., 2016). This clinical setting often requires 24/7 coverage (defined by clinical service area) and should be clearly communicated and addressed in the job requirements. Productivity metrics include, but are not limited to, improved length of stay, improved discharge time, improved complication comorbidity (CC) and major complication comorbidity (MCC) documentation, and improved team communication surrounding the plan of care that is often reflected in improved patient satisfaction scores.

Hospitalist ICU: The hospitalist ICU service line cares for patients in the neonatal intensive care unit (NICU), pediatric intensive care unit (PICU), cardiovascular intensive care unit (CVICU), medical intensive care unit (MICU) and surgical neuro intensive care (SNICU). ICUs provide care to patients with severe or life-threatening illnesses and injuries that require constant care, close supervision from life support equipment, and high-risk medications to ensure stabilization. The hospitalist ICU services require 24/7 coverage schedules. Patient caseload ranges from four to seven patients based on patient specific acuity, and patient population and often caseload expectations may increase to 10 patients overnight or on off shifts (Kapu et al., 2016). Target APPs for this clinical setting should be board certified as acute care or those with specialty certification or additional residency or fellowship training that relate to the patient population foci. Productivity metrics include, but are not limited to, documenting complication comorbidity (CC) and major complication comorbidity (MCC), improved team communication surrounding plan of care, improved patient satisfaction scores, and targeted admission to stabilization times based on specified metrics.

Surgical/procedural: The surgical/procedural service cares for patients in the operating room (OR), cardiac catheterization lab, or infusion suites. The surgical/procedural patient undergoes some aspect of technical or operative procedure. Patient caseload ranges are based on the procedural protocols within the specialty and may require 24/7 coverage (defined by clinical service area) depending on hours of operation. Target APPs for this clinical setting should be board certified as acute care or those with specialty certification that relate to the patient population foci. Depending on the type of procedures, many times APPs may have additional training specific to the procedure (e.g., vein harvesting in a cardiac catheterization lab). Productivity metrics include, but are not limited to, the number and success of procedures completed per shift, procedure completion time, and duration based on available benchmark data.

Appendix J describes in more detail a clinical operating guide for determining best practice examples for each of these tracks. This document summarizes important details when creating APP practice models and can be used as a guide and adopted as needed. Often APPs do not fall into one specific track but instead function in a hybrid model across tracks. The percentage in each track should be noted to help define the number of sessions and patients, panel sizes, or caseload expectation based on the track percentage. This in no way represents an all-inclusive policy or procedure, but rather was developed for department leadership requesting guides for building and establishing practice models that integrate APPs into their designated areas and could support the additional data elements needed for completing the business pro forma.

SCOPE OF PRACTICE AND SCOPE OF EDUCATION

Accurate attribution of the work effort by APPs is vital for workforce planning to project APP and physician staffing needs, determine clinic space, and calculate APP needed support staff (Brooks & Fulton, 2020). Because of the data points included on a business pro forma that require approval from multiple interested parties, assuring top-of-license practice when hiring APPs is a priority. Having a definition of what "top of license" means to an organization helps all team members understand what the goal is when hiring an APP. When the need to perform essential activities is due primarily to lack of adequate support or staffing, often APPs are required to step in; however, this keeps them from practicing to the top of license. The productivity of specific employees is the responsibility of the employee's supervisor (Lucatorto & Walsh-Irwin, 2020). Therefore, assuring all team members recognize the scope of practice and definition of top-of-license practice for APPs is critical to success. Clarity surrounding the definition of top-of-license practice for organizations helps guide the pro forma and the common understanding by everyone involved that APPs are billable providers and should be deployed with the following hiring goals:

- The work requires advanced clinical and cognitive skills

- The work could not be done effectively by someone else with a different set of skills

- The work must utilize the full extent of their education, training, and experience

PAs are educated as medical generalists and often have additional training in the way of residency or fellowships in a specific patient population. APRNs also have transition to practice or specialty residency or fellowships, but NPs are educationally prepared to provide patient care to at least one patient population as defined by nationally recognized role and population foci, called the national APRN Consensus Model. Consideration must be given to the type of APRN or PA based on the patient population to ensure scope of practice equates to scope of education. The APRN Consensus Model describes the four roles of the APRN (CNM, CRNA, CNS, and CNP) with their corresponding population foci (APRN Consensus Work Group & the National Council of State Boards of Nursing APRN Advisory Committee, 2008). It is important to have an understanding of scope of practice and education background when completing the pro forma.

MEDICAL STAFFING MODELS

Organizations are making it a priority to capture their return on investment using value-added metrics, as well as establishing APP-specific onboarding, mentoring, and professional growth and development programs. These programs not only utilize multiple organizational resources but highlight the need for understanding the financial aspects of APPs. This underscores the need to specifically engage and educate APPs in their roles as providers. Tracking APP reimbursement is crucial in today's environment, as well as ensuring APPs have a strong knowledge base of the differences in inpatient versus outpatient billing guidelines (Brooks & Fulton, 2019). According to data from AMGA Consulting's 2020 Medical Group Operations and Finance Survey, over the past four years the median APP-to-physician ratio has increased by an average of 27% across all specialty types (Wagner & Horton, 2022, p. 29). There are many practice models using APPs in the ambulatory setting, in the OR, and on procedural teams, as well as inpatient hospital and ICU settings. APPs can generate revenue functioning independently, as well as augment physicians by delivering preventative care in primary care settings and provide care in medical and surgical settings, thus freeing up physicians to see new patients, referrals, or patients with more complex medical or surgical issues (Wagner & Horton, 2022).

OPTIMIZING MEDICAL STAFFING MODEL

Topics to address when completing a pro forma to assure the medical staffing model is accurately vetted:

- The request should specify whether additional resources are needed to optimize the APP position to work towards a full caseload and to the top of their license and education. This may include additional exam rooms or equipment or additional staffing resources, such as medical assistants or nursing staff.

- The job description should be finalized and included as part of the pro forma. Likewise, other documents that address the anticipated financial growth, the department organizational chart, and any other pertinent documents that support the addition of the position should be included.

- Certain APP positions may be eligible for remote work, such as telemedicine positions or other roles that may not be patient facing. However, very specific guidelines should be in place if remote work is an option.

- APPs across the organization work in various care settings and have diversity in their scope of practice; individual administration and/or documentation efforts need to be evaluated.

- APPs who also take part in research as part of their FTE or function in the role of lead/supervisor for a cohort of other APPs caring for similar patient populations may have a reduced clinical load.

Models of care that highlight the value of adding APPs often focus on quality and cost-avoidance productivity data. For example, Kleinpell and Kapu (2017) have identified several sources of quality measures to enable practice-specific evaluation of NP roles and initiatives. Healthcare is among the most complex of human systems, and coordinating activities and integrating new with old ways of treating patients while delivering high-quality, safe care is challenging (Braithwaite et al., 2020). Physician productivity is a standard measure available for healthcare leaders to use in making decisions and is voluntarily submitted as a component of membership into the Medical Group Management Association and published as national benchmarking data (Lucatorto & Walsh-Irwin, 2020). A significant challenge when trying to apply the same type of business analysis to APPs is the lack of specificity for APRNs and PAs in choosing taxonomy codes and therefore the lack of benchmarking data available. Regardless, organizations should create business pro formas that guide their hiring practices and attempt to optimize the productivity and functionality of the role by asking detailed questions to ensure the medical staffing model is optimized.

CLINICAL FTE

Information on the full-time equivalent (FTE) of the position should be specified so it may be accurately reflected in the job posting and discussed with job applicants. The total FTE for the position should be included in the pro forma, along with the clinical FTE (cFTE). The FTE and cFTE should be equal when there are no administrative or research role requirements as the best practice guidelines within the cFTE should include the time allocated for documentation. FTE should reflect allocated time for non-clinical activities such as research, administration, or teaching.

New FTE positions may have a higher level of scrutiny than backfill positions. This is especially true for unbudgeted positions, which may require a more detailed financial analysis to demonstrate the position is financially favorable to the organization. Situations where the department is not currently meeting budget or is not expected to meet budget with the addition of an APP position should require further explanation with extended long-term return on investment analysis. If the APP position is a replacement position, the exiting employee's name, job code, and departing date should be listed. Often, an APP position may be requested to replace a physician or resident, and having information regarding who was providing the work effort prior is helpful data to reinforce the role should be replaced at the APP level.

The organization may fund APP positions from professional or technical hospital revenues. Each funding source may have their own methods for approving or reviewing position requests. In many cases, it is necessary to review the accounting code as part of the approval process. How the funds flow from the productivity of the APP role should be defined so there is no ambiguity and the revenue can be accounted for in the pro forma.

FULL CASELOAD EXPECTATIONS

All organizations have variable ramp-up cost expectations and metrics. For example, RVU targets for a three-year ramp up for new APPs may be less than replacement APPs. The net patient revenue, expenses, practice overhead, and direct revenue make up the traditional calculations of the pro forma. However, being able to address the financial aspects for an APP pro forma involves understanding the caseload expectations. APPs gain skills and efficiency as they become more experienced, and therefore, the patient load expectations should increase accordingly. Anticipating a ramp-up period allows the organizations to project the ROI given the adequate investment as described throughout this textbook. APPs need to leverage their full potential by increasing caseload and caring for patients that expand their knowledge base. The type of billing model—whether independent RVU billing, partnered with a physician team non-billing, split/shared billing, or a combination—should be described and detailed. Defining the APP's track helps determine the type of billing education needed for the APP to succeed.

Utilizing resources within an organization for the APP pro forma requires coordination of APP expertise and finance expertise to ensure the pro forma has outlined realistic expectations. This team approach assures the checks and balances required for right sizing and setting realistic expectations are outlined for both new and replacement APP positions. The APP hiring pro forma allows everyone to proactively clarify how the position will impact productivity, increase revenue, increase physician productivity, or contribute to cost-avoidance quality improvement metrics. Appendix K is an example of an APP business pro forma that can be adopted and utilized as needed.

SUMMARY

Supporting patient care growth with organizational initiatives that include detailed pro formas ensures the right balance of provider teams to reflect fiscally responsible quality patient care. Pro formas specific to the APP role require collaborative resources from the greater organization because individual departments may be unfamiliar with the APP scope. Accurately defining all aspects of the pro forma described in this chapter sets the stage to support APPs entering the workforce and ensures the APP position has been vetted and scrutinized for content accuracy at every level. APPs are an organizational investment and promote positive patient outcomes, but only when thoughtfully planned to meet the organization's strategic mission.

REFERENCES

APRN Consensus Work Group, & The National Council of State Boards of Nursing APRN Advisory Committee. (2008, July 7). *Consensus model for APRN regulation: Licensure, accreditation, certification & education.* https://ncsbn.org/public-files/Consensus_Model_for_APRN_Regulation_July_2008.pdf

Braithwaite, J., Vincent, C., Garcia-Elorrio, E., Imanaka, Y., Nicklin, W., Sodzi Tettey, S., & Bates, D. W. (2020). Transformational improvement in quality care and health systems: The next decade. *BMC Medicine, 18*(1), 340. https://doi.org/10.1186/s12916-020-01739-y

Brooks, P. B., & Fulton, M. E. (2019). Demonstrating advanced practice provider value: Implementing a new advanced practice provider billing algorithm. *Journal of the American Academy of Physician Associates, 32*(2), 1–10. https://doi.org/10.1097/01.Jaa.0000550293.01522.01

Brooks, P. B., & Fulton, M. E. (2020). Driving high-functioning clinical teams: An advanced practice registered nurse and physician assistant optimization initiative. *Journal of the American Association of Nurse Practitioners, 32*(6), 476–487. https://doi.org/10.1097/jxx.0000000000000415

Kapu, A. N., McComiskey, C. A., Buckler, L., Derkazarian, J., Goda, T., Lofgren, M. A., McIlvennan, C. K., Raaum, J., Selig, P. M., Sicoutris, C., Todd, B., Turner, V., Card, E., & Wells, N. (2016). Advanced practice providers' perceptions of patient workload: Results of a multi-institutional survey. *JONA: The Journal of Nursing Administration, 46*(10), 521–529. https://doi.org/10.1097/NNA.0000000000000396

Kleinpell, R., & Kapu, A. N. (2017, August). Quality measures for nurse practitioner practice evaluation. *Journal of the American Association of Nurse Practitioners, 29*(8), 446–451. https://doi.org/10.1002/2327-6924.12474

Lucatorto, M. A., & Walsh-Irwin, C. (2020). Nurse practitioner productivity measurement: An organizational focus and lessons learned. *Journal of the American Association of Nurse Practitioners, 32*(11), 771–778. https://doi.org/10.1097/jxx.0000000000000538

Wagner, R., & Horton, F. (2022, March/April). The calculus of addition: Three factors to consider before hiring more APCs for your medical group. *AMGA Group Practice Journal,* 28–32. https://www.amga.org/AMGA/media/Consulting/PDFs/CalculusofAddition_ThreeFactors.pdf

"First, do no harm."
—Hippocratic Oath

CHAPTER 10

CREDENTIALING AND PRIVILEGING

KEYWORDS | credentialing, privileging, compliance, competencies, taxonomy, malpractice insurance

The academic rigor of APRN and PA programs prepare APPs to assess the health status of patients and families through histories, physical exams, differential diagnoses, interpretation and ordering of laboratory tests, medication management, and formulation of treatment plans. However, educational pedigrees and clinical competency alone do not provide APPs the ability to see, treat, and bill for services rendered when employed by a healthcare organization. Hospitals and healthcare organizations have internal processes that evaluate providers and ultimately give them permission to practice. Credentialing and privileging is required by The Joint Commission (TJC) and the Centers for Medicare & Medicaid Services (CMS) and integrated as policy into hospital bylaws (CMS, 2020; TJC, 2022b). These requirements are designed to protect the public and ensure quality and safe care. APPs entering clinical practice must undergo the credentialing and privileging process to be approved by the healthcare organization where they are employed to provide care, treat patients, and bill for the services rendered. Credentialing is an extensive process during which an organization performs a substantial amount of background checks, primary source verification, and competency validation, which allows an APP to practice to the top of their license, experience, and education.

Credentialing is the verification process through which a healthcare organization validates the APP's educational background, training, and experience. Privileging is the process by which the organization's governing body grants permission to provide specific aspects of patient care (Hittle, 2010; McMullin & Howie, 2020). When an APP is privileged in hospital or clinical settings, they have met the organization's stringent requirements and have permission to see, touch, treat, consult, and care for patients. It is essential for organizations to understand the importance of accuracy surrounding these processes, and provide the support needed for comprehensive and successful outcomes.

Organizational bylaws describe the privileging process, including structure, membership appointments, terms, and responsibilities of internal reviewers from committees such as APP panels, composed of both APRNs and PAs; medical and surgical panels, composed of physicians; and eventual approval by the organization's governing body. These committees or panels are made up of organizational leaders who collectively approve the definitional statements that describe the scope of practice for an APP within an organization. Membership appointments to these panels or subpanel committees are often inclusive of members who are licensed, experienced, and educated at the same level.

In most healthcare organizations, the credentialing and privileging process is coordinated through a clinical/medical staff office. The credentialing process begins with verification of the APP's education, training, board certification, malpractice claim history, Medicare/Medicaid sanctions, licensure sanctions, and criminal background checks. The clinical/medical staff office then provides their findings to the various panels through a series of review and approvals. At University of Iowa Health Care, the committee review pathway starts with the APRN/PA subpanel that then reports to the medical and surgical credential committees, the organization's clinical system committee or hospital advisory board, and then onto the managed care committee. Specific to APPs, the APRN/PA subpanel is composed of four PAs, four APRNs, one physician who works closely with a PA, one physician who works closely with an APRN, and a chair of the committee. The APRN/PA subpanel is responsible for reviewing the initial privileging applications, any modification of privileges, and review of all affirmations of privileges. The APRN/PA subpanel investigates complaints related to clinical or professional issues, makes recommendations to the professional peer committees, reviews and updates definitional statements, and reviews in-depth scope of practice discussion items. Having an APRN- and PA-specific review committee ensures that documents will be thoroughly evaluated by a peer group familiar with the education, board certification, and licensure needed for safe patient care.

PRACTICE READY

There is a shared responsibility between the organization and the APP to efficiently move through the steps necessary to issue clinical practice privileges. The process requires detailed form completion and documentation and ideally starts immediately after the APP accepts an employment offer. In most cases, the process is time sensitive, and any delays in either completing the application or providing the necessary documents ultimately affect the ability of the APP to provide patient care.

Having all forms and documents readily available and electronically accessible is an important aspect of being practice ready. Missing information, inaccurate information, or delay in completing or providing information will postpone the ability to practice and risks pausing the employment start date. Maintaining a checklist of the required documents will help provide clarity and organization and help make the entire process smooth and efficient:

- Recent professional photo (jpg)

- Copy of all state licenses: PA, RN, and APRN

- Copy of State Controlled Substance Certificate (SCSC)

- Copy of federal Drug Enforcement Administration documents (Note: Fees associated with federal DEA may be waived for state or government employees)

- Copy of ALL diplomas: associates, bachelors, masters, doctorate

- Copy of UPDATED curriculum vitae: Any gap in employment greater than six months requires explanation

- Copy of all board certifications: PA-C, Certified Nurse Practitioner population foci (AGNP acute or primary, FNP, NNP, PNP acute or primary, PMHNP, or WHNP), Certified Registered Nurse Anesthetist, Certified Nurse Midwife, or Clinical Nurse Specialist

- Copy of all certification cards (e.g., Basic Cardiac Life Support, Advanced Cardiac Life Support, Pediatric Advanced Life Support, Neonatal Resuscitation Program, etc.)

- Evidence of required immunizations per organization policy such as COVID-19, TB, and MMR

- Completed universal practitioner credentialing application

- Clinical logs for procedures and clinical rotations

- Names, titles, emails, addresses, and phone numbers of three to four clinical references. It is important to remind the APP to contact the references to confirm accuracy of the contact and request they be responsive in returning all requests in a timely manner. If references aren't notified, it can delay the process if too much time passes from the time of response from a reference in comparison to the initial date of the application.

CREDENTIALING PORTFOLIO

Guiding APPs in maintaining a credentialing portfolio is beneficial for future reaffirmation of privileges and ongoing professional compliance. Suggestions include:

- Encourage APP to be organized with all documents

- Keep contact information from colleges and universities (registrar's office) of how to obtain all documents related to diplomas, transcripts, etc.

- Keep a log of billable procedures and documentation of competencies

- Set up a system for storing information that is confidential and safe but easily accessible

- Update and maintain all board certification, licenses, and other pertinent documents throughout the duration of career

- Always have digital backup

- Maintain an updated list of professional references with current contact information

Communicating the importance of timely gathering and submission of the required documents helps ensure the APP understands their role and accountability in the process. Clearly listing the documents needed and consistently following up until all documents are accounted for assures the organization's due diligence in the best possible timeline to get the APP established to care for patients. Follow-up and clarity around any questions about what is needed should be communicated often because it is easy to overlook or assume the APP understands when, in fact, they may have minimal to no experience with the process.

Advances in technology and systems designed to streamline data collection and form completion for the credentialing process may be available. Many organizations have implemented electronic systems that have eliminated the need for pen and paper form completion and allow for an online application and the ability to upload the appropriate documentation. Web or cloud portals and dashboards allow visibility to the application status for the APP, the clinical/medical staff office, human resources, and other interested parties. Electronic systems may allow for routing of documents to the panels and sub panels, reminders to the applicant when documents are missing, and generally streamlines the application process.

IPPE, OPPE, FPPE, COMPETENCIES

Organizational bylaws also detail the process for validating the performance and competency of privileged providers. This process is known as professional practice evaluation, and metrics were originally defined by the Accreditation Council for Graduate Medical Education and have since been adopted by TJC. These six provider core competencies include patient care, system-based practice, communication, practice-based learning, and professional and medical clinical knowledge (TJC, 2022a). The intent for Ongoing Professional Practice Evaluation (OPPE) is that the organization examines data on performance for all providers with privileges on an ongoing basis, rather than only at the two-year reappointment process (Holley, 2016; TJC, 2022b). Focused Professional Practice Evaluation (FPPE) is used when there is an unsatisfactory OPPE review because of patterns of preventable or unsafe behaviors and practices (Makary, 2011). Organizations have specific policies within their bylaws related to how an FPPE review is started, including who can initiate and the detailed process involved when invoked.

After an APP has been granted privileges and has enrolled in the managed care billing program within the organization, the OPPE requirement to demonstrate and document clinical competency on a defined cycle validates that the APP is practicing safely. Competency is a combination of observable and measurable knowledge, skills, abilities, and personal attributes that constitute an employee's performance assuring the delivery of safe, quality care (Hunt, 2012).

An example of the steps for formal process for competency documentation and evaluation is further defined as follows: 1) initial PPE which applies to new staff members with active privileges, and 2) ongoing professional practice evaluation (OPPE), which applies to APPs assessed every three to six months (Holley, 2016; Hunt, 2012; Makary et al., 2011). Organizational bylaws may permit issuance of initial or provisional privileges to new APPs for a standard period of time (such as six months) with some level of PPE to be completed by a defined proctor for skills and competency to be closely monitored and evaluated during initial employment. Orientation to unit-based practices and procedures is required by TJC and may be implemented concurrently to the PPE processes. Using competency-based orientation templates for APPs that can be adopted for specific departments or divisions based on the six core competencies is a comprehensive approach to meeting this requirement. Appendix L is one example of a template that can be adapted by any organization wanting to adhere to this form of compliance competency.

COMPETENCY ASSESSMENT

To make the assessment of ongoing competency more objective and continuous, TJC suggests using standard mechanisms for collecting data as follows (TJC, 2022b):

- Periodic chart review or record review
- Direct observations or proctoring
- Monitoring of diagnostic and treatment techniques and/or outcomes
- Discussion with other individuals involved in the care of the patient (360 evaluation)
- Simulations
- External peer review

Establishing metrics for OPPE can be challenging as the metrics specifically related to patient care, practice based learning, and medical clinical knowledge reflect the clinical specialty of the APP. Metrics for professionalism, communication, and system-based practice can be universal and completed by all APPs regardless of board certification, patient population, or licensure. One example of a standardized and easily measured metric is in Appendix M. This is an example of a six-question chart review intended to be distributed every four to six months to all APPs. This is a very simple chart review completed by peers that identifies high-level documentation indicators that reflect system-based competency.

APPLICATION EXAMPLES

CREDENTIALING AND PRIVILEGING

It is helpful for organizations to provide specific template examples to help APPs accurately complete their documents. Appendix N provides an example of Iowa's Statewide Universal Practitioner Application (ISUPA) guide for APPs. As noted in the example, the more specific you can be to clearly outline the information needed, the stronger the assurance every APP will fill it out fully understanding what is expected. Information entered on the application is validated and primary source verified to ensure that the information is factual and the APP applying for privileges aligns with who they are; their education, license, and certifications are accurate and up to date; and the experience and past employment are accurate and without gaps in practice. Primary source verification is an important requirement sanctioned by many accreditation bodies, including but not limited to CMS and TJC (National Association of Medical Staff Services [NAMSS], 2023). Primary source verification means the information is verified directly with the original source or an agent of that source. For example, a license itself is verified directly with the state board of nursing or board of physician assistants rather than merely obtaining a photocopy of the license card. Board certification is verified directly with the certifying board, education degrees are verified directly through their academic program, etc. Likewise, references are contacted directly and respond to questions about experience and skills. The credentialing process provides a documented level of assurance that the provider meets all the baseline criteria to be considered for privileging at the organization. The organization relies on the due diligence and accuracy of the credentialing process to grant privileges, and assuring APPs understand what information is being asked of them through specific and detailed examples underscores the information is accurate.

BILLING APPLICATION

There is a separate process for managed care organization credentialing and privileging so APPs can bill for services rendered for the care they provide. APPs are not always knowledgeable about the managed care billing application process, and Appendix O showcases another example of a guide that walks the APP through the document to help them complete the form accurately. APPs may need assistance during this application time frame to ensure the information asked is clearly understood and answered correctly.

NPI AND TAXONOMY CODES

Every provider must apply for a National Provider Identifier (NPI) through CMS. The NPI is a Health Insurance Portability and Accountability Act (HIPAA) Administrative Simplification Standard that mandates a unique identifier for healthcare providers and health plans (Dillon & Hoyson, 2014). Covered healthcare providers and all health plans and healthcare clearinghouses must use the NPIs in the administrative and financial transactions adopted under HIPAA. A provider taxonomy code is chosen when a practitioner applies for an NPI through the National Plan and Provider Enrollment System. One or more provider taxonomy codes (provider type/specialty) must be identified on the NPI application, which defines the healthcare provider type, classification, and area of specialization. The provider can indicate, using the taxonomy code, where they specialize in their medical practice. Although the healthcare taxonomy code set for PAs and APRNs is a less extensive listing than for physicians, up to four taxonomy codes may be specified on the NPI application (NAMSS, 2023).

When providers enroll with a Medicare contractor through the Provider Enrollment, Chain, and Ownership System (PECOS), they must indicate their specialty. Physicians have multiple choices of specialty while APPs can only choose their designation within the PECOS system, either nurse practitioner or physician assistant.

PROVIDER TAXONOMY CODE

A taxonomy code is a unique 10-character code that designates a provider's classification and specialization. This code will be used when applying for an NPI. To become a Medicare provider and file Medicare claims, providers must first enroll in the Medicare program. To enroll, providers must have an NPI. And to get an NPI, the application will need to include the taxonomy code that reflects the classification and specialization. Providers may select more than one code or code description when applying for an NPI but must indicate one of them as the primary code (CMS, 2022).

The National Uniform Claim Committee (NUCC) is presently maintaining the code set. It is used in transactions specified in HIPAA and the NPI application for enumeration. Effective 2001, the NUCC took over the administration of the code set. Ongoing duties, including processing taxonomy code requests and maintenance of the code set, fall under the NUCC Code Subcommittee (NPIdb, 2023; National Uniform Claim Committee, 2023).

Both the APP taxonomy code and the PECOS APP specialty designation options are limited relative to the robust specialty list for physicians. Limited specialty designations have been identified as a barrier to practice. For example, issues have arisen when Medicare Administrative Contractors do not reimburse two evaluation and management (E/M) visits billed by an APP with the same taxonomy or same specialty for the same patient on the same day. To be reimbursed appropriately, the patient would require scheduling the E/M visits on two separate days, which is not in alignment with patient-centered care and is especially unfeasible in rural areas. Given the number and granularity of physician specialties recognized for purposes of Medicare enrollment, and the demand for healthcare providers often filled by APPs, advocating to apply an APP clinical specialty on claims beyond the existing nonspecific CMS specialty codes may optimize reimbursement for the care rendered.

Similarly, when an APP sees a patient as a new patient, and the same patient is seen as a new patient by another APP in a separate specialty within three years, the claim is only reimbursed if submitted as an existing patient, regardless if the APPs are practicing in separate specialties and the patient has separate clinical diagnoses. APRNs and PAs are helping to fill in the gaps for the changing practice of healthcare today, and being able to be adequately and appropriately reimbursed for services provided is essential.

STATE CONTROLLED SUBSTANCE CERTIFICATE AND FEDERAL DEA REGISTRATION

Each provider must comply with their state license requirements for controlled substance certification. In many states, each provider must be registered under both state and federal controlled substances acts. In Iowa, federal registration is with the Drug Enforcement Administration (DEA) and state registration is with the Iowa Board of Pharmacy. Application for state controlled substance certificate can be completed when the practice location is known and the APRN or PA license has been issued. The federal DEA application may be completed after the state controlled substance certificate has been issued. Prior to issuing registration, the DEA will verify the provider's employment with the healthcare organization. Registration fees may be waived by the DEA if employment is with an authorized government organization. Guidelines and timelines for DEA registration may be found at https://www.deadiversion.usdoj.gov/drugreg.

PROFESSIONAL REFERENCES

Professional references are a vital part of the credentialing and privileging process, and APPs should thoughtfully choose which professionals to list as references. References are required to be at the same professional level or above, and may not be friends, family, or other students. Professional references should be clinical faculty, APPs in the same specialty, or physician colleagues who have recent knowledge through observation of the APP's professional abilities. As a professional courtesy, APPs should contact references ahead of the process and verify contact information prior to submission. The way the reference process is managed is key in expediting APP credentialing.

Accurate and ongoing oversight between the department credentialing contact, the APP, and the clinical/medical staff office warrants clear and efficient processes to remove the potential for delays due to missing/incomplete information. The sequencing is important and requires attention to detail as well as ongoing communication with all interested parties. As stated earlier in this chapter, the APP must be issued board certification in order to apply for and be issued a state license, have an active state license in order to obtain state controlled substance certification (SCSC), and hold an SCSC certification in order to apply for DEA registration. Until an APP has completed the credentialing and privileging process, including all internal privileging panels, they are not able to care for patients and therefore are a non-billable provider.

GRANTED AND MODIFIED PRIVILEGES

Privileges are specific to a clinical specialty or patient population, and often are department specific. *Delineation of privileges* is the specific list of privileges for APPs granted to practice within the department, unit, specialty, or patient population, which have been approved by department chairs and organizational leaders. When an APP has a dual appointment with separate clinical site locations within one organizational entity, they generally will need to have privileges specific to the patient population specialty and location at each site. Competencies for privileges were designed to reflect entry into practice and basic foundational skills (Klein, 2008). These are often referred to as core privileges, and as additional specialty or population specific procedures are refined, it is the responsibility of the APP and the organization to ensure expertise and competency to modify or add privileges.

The delineation of privileges is a formal document that indicates the scope of practice for the APP at the organization, and specifies the criteria that must be met to show competency for each privilege. Hickman (2016) noted in an evidence-based review that despite the prevalence of acute care nurse practitioners, there is limited exploration into how they are credentialed or privileged to perform invasive procedures. It has been identified that credentialing and privileging for invasive procedures varies across organizations and typically involves proctored observations by a provider with the same privilege, and the number of proctored observations varies by hospitals and procedure (Hickman, 2016; Jalloh et al., 2016; Klein et al., 2020; Pittman et al., 2018). As PAs and APRNs grow in multiple settings, Halsted's model of "See one, do one, teach one" may be modified by organization-specific guidelines. For example, APPs must observe someone else doing the procedure a specified number of times and have someone competent and privileged in the procedure observe them doing the procedure a specified number of times, both of which are documented and submitted when modification of privileges is requested (Kotsis & Chung, 2013). Reaffirmation of privileges typically occurs every two years (Holley, 2016; Hunt, 2012) and requires verification of competency by the clinical peer group. Appendix P illustrates an example of peer evaluation questions used for reaffirmation of privileges. These documents can be adapted and edited for each organization's specific policies and procedures and used as a template.

The organization's bylaws or policies specify the process for modifying privileges. As noted above, initial privileges are granted upon preliminary credentialing and privileging approval and can be modified accordingly as APPs grow and develop additional skills throughout their practice. All clinical privileges are based upon the APP's training, experience, and demonstrated competence. A document to request modification of privileges is in Appendix Q.

STATE TORT/MALPRACTICE INSURANCE

A State Tort Claims Act provides liability protection for state government employees, without dollar limits, for clinical services rendered in a designated state. The State Tort Claims Act is the equivalent of an occurrence malpractice policy. The Federal Tort Claims Act is federal legislation enacted in 1946 that provides a legal means for compensating individuals who have suffered personal injury, death, or property loss or damage caused by the negligent or wrongful act or omission of an employee of the federal government (University of Iowa Health Care, 2023). When providers engage in moonlighting activity outside of the organization, they are responsible for maintaining their own malpractice coverage with adequate liability limits.

MALPRACTICE INSURANCE

The University of Iowa Hospitals and Clinics (UIHC) is an agency of the state of Iowa, which self-insures the tort liability of the state and its employees under the provisions of the State Tort Claims Act, Chapter 669, Code of Iowa.

Providers under contract as house staff members with the UIHC are covered by Iowa's State Tort Claims Act when they are providing services within the scope of their training during assigned rotations at the University of Iowa Hospitals and Clinics and assigned rotations elsewhere in Iowa (University of Iowa Health Care, 2023).

SUMMARY

APPs have become widely used in organizations across the country to meet the provider demands in nearly all areas of clinical practice. The credentialing and privileging process ensures APPs are practicing safely and competently, protecting themselves, the organization, and, most importantly, the patients. Organizational bylaws specify how providers are verified and authorized to provide care through the credentialing and privileging process. Understanding the importance and value of credentialing and privileging is critical so the organization can safely deliver quality patient care, get reimbursed for services rendered, and avoid the financial impact associated with a poorly orchestrated and unknowledgeable process. Having expertise at every level throughout the process assures efficiency and accuracy, which is paramount to the long-term investment.

REFERENCES

Centers for Medicare & Medicaid Services. (2020, Feb. 21). *State operations manual, rev. 200.* https://www.cms.gov/Regulations-and-Guidance/Guidance/Manuals/downloads/som107ap_a_hospitals.pdf

Centers for Medicare & Medicaid Services. (2022, Nov. 15). *Find your taxonomy code.* https://www.cms.gov/medicare/provider-enrollment-and-certification/find-your-taxonomy-code

Dillon, D., & Hoyson, P. M. (2014). Beginning employment: A guide for the new nurse practitioner. *The Journal for Nurse Practitioners, 10*(1), 55–59. https://doi.org/10.1016/j.nurpra.2013.09.009

Hickman, R. L. (2016). Evidence-based review and discussion points. *American Journal of Critical Care, 25*(4), 362–363. https://doi.org/10.4037/ajcc2016431

Hittle, K. (2010). Understanding certification, licensure, and credentialing: A guide for the new nurse practitioner. *Journal of Pediatric Health Care, 24*(3), 203–206. https://doi.org/10.1016/j.pedhc.2009.09.006

Holley, S. L. (2016). Ongoing professional performance evaluation: Advanced practice registered nurse practice competency assessment. *The Journal of Nurse Practitioners, 12*(2), 67–74. https://doi.org/10.1016/j.nurpra.2015.08.037

Hunt, J. L. (2012). Assessing physician competency: An update on the Joint Commission requirement for ongoing and focused professional practice evaluation. *Advances in Anatomic Pathology, 19*(6), 388–400. https://doi.org/10.1097/PAP.0b013e318273f97e

Jalloh, F., Tadlock, M. D., Cantwell, S., Rausch, T., Aksoy, H., & Frankel, H. (2016). Credentialing and privileging of acute care nurse practitioners to do invasive procedures: A statewide survey. *American Journal of Critical Care, 25*(4), 357–361. https://doi.org/10.4037/ajcc2016118

The Joint Commission. (2022a). *2023 hospital accreditation standards* (1st ed). https://www.jointcommission.org/standards

The Joint Commission. (2022b, Feb. 4). *What are the key elements needed to meet the Ongoing Professional Practice Evaluation (OPPE) requirements?* [FAQs]. https://www.jointcommission.org/standards/standard-faqs/hospital-and-hospital-clinics/medical-staff-ms/000001500/

Klein, T. (2008). Credentialing the nurse practitioner in your workplace: Evaluating scope for safe practice. *Nursing Administration Quarterly, 32*(4), 273–278. https://doi.org/10.1097/01.NAQ.0000336723.18312.3f

Klein, T. A., Kaplan, L., Stanik-Hutt, J., Cote, J., & Brooks, O. (2020). Hiring and credentialing of nurse practitioners as hospitalists: A national workforce analysis. *Journal of Nursing Regulation, 11*(3), 33–43. https://doi.org/10.1016/S2155-8256(20)30132-0

Kotsis, S. V., & Chung, K. C. (2013). Application of the "see one, do one, teach one" concept in surgical training. *Plastic & Reconstructive Surgery, 131*(5), 1194–1201. https://doi.org/10.1097/PRS.0b013e318287a0b3

Makary, M. A., Wick, E., & Freischlag, J. A. (2011, June 20). PPE, OPPE, and FPPE: Complying with the new alphabet soup of credentialing [Editorial]. *Archives of Surgery, 146*(6), 642–644. https://doi.org/10.1001/archsurg.2011.136

McMullen, P. C., & Howie, W. O. (2020). Credentialing and privileging: A primer for nurse practitioners. *The Journal for Nurse Practitioners, 16*(2), 91–95. https://doi.org/10.1016/j.nurpra.2019.10.015

National Association of Medical Staff Services. (2023, January). *Health care provider taxonomy code set, ver. 23.0.* https://taxonomy.nucc.org/

National Uniform Claim Committee. (2023). *Health care provider taxonomy code set.* https://taxonomy.nucc.org/

NPIdb. (2023). *NPI number lookup.* https://npidb.org/

Pittman, P., Leach, B., Everett, C., Han, X., & McElroy, D. (2018). NP and PA privileging in acute care settings: Do scope of practice laws matter? *Medical Care Research & Review, 77*(2), 112–120. https://doi.org/10.1177/1077558718760333

University of Iowa Health Care. (2023). *Malpractice insurance.* https://gme.medicine.uiowa.edu/about/malpractice-insurance#:~:text=The%20State%20Tort%20Claims%20Act%20provides%20the%20house%20staff%20member,no%20tail%20coverage%20is%20required

"If you think compliance is expensive—try non-compliance."
–Former US Deputy Attorney General Paul McNulty

CHAPTER 11

ORGANIZATIONAL COMPLIANCE

KEYWORDS | coding, billing, clinical documentation, compliance, evaluation and management, auditing

Healthcare is evolving at a rapid pace with new techniques, equipment, and methods of providing services to patients. As one of the most highly regulated industries, the rules and regulations that govern it are changing at equally rapid speeds. An effective organizational compliance program is vital to reduce regulatory risk. While the structure of a compliance program may vary widely across the industry, the goal of upholding the organizational value, as well as complying with the myriad of laws and regulations, remains the same. At a basic level, compliance is about prevention, detection, collaboration, and enforcement (Troklus & Vacca, 2016). Simply stated, an effective compliance program helps the organization fulfill its commitment to patients, families, and employees.

Within healthcare, the role of the compliance office is one of oversight spanning multiple areas and topics: policies and procedures, privacy, conflict of interest, auditing and monitoring, and education. Overseeing education and auditing activities specific to coding and billing is one of the many ways the compliance office helps fulfill the organization's commitment to doing the right thing.

EVALUATION AND MANAGEMENT EDUCATION

APPs are a growing workforce and require additional knowledge specific to the regulations surrounding their profession, especially related to coding and billing practices. Education related to evaluation and management of patients should, as a best practice, be provided at the start of employment. Many organizations utilize online/electronic training modules, which can be completed independently and self-paced. Required training for new providers would include the basics of evaluation and management (E/M) coding guidelines, copy/paste best practices, teaching providers rules, and involvement by other members of the healthcare team. Utilizing techniques to increase comprehension (such as embedding "Test Your Knowledge" questions, which require the end user to answer prior to moving on to the next section) not only reinforces the information discussed in that section but also addresses some of the common scenarios within the organization where questions or issues typically arise.

ONGOING EDUCATION

Annual changes to the American Medical Association coding guidelines and the rules embedded in the Medicare Physician Fee Schedule make it necessary for healthcare organizations to provide ongoing education to ensure compliant coding practices. To provide effective education, it is necessary to create material suited to the target audience by utilizing a variety of techniques to provide up-to-date coding and billing information to all relevant parties. In-person, virtual, and online presentations, as well as tip sheets, frequently asked questions, and pocket cards (or the electronic equivalent), are some examples of educational methods.

"TEST YOUR KNOWLEDGE" EXAMPLES FOR AN E/M TRAINING MODULE

Q1. The Office of the Inspector General states that every provider who provides or supervises the provision of services to a patient is responsible for the correct documentation of the services rendered.

  a. True

  b. False

Q2. In cases where evaluation and management (E/M) services are provided, the provider is responsible for assuring that:

  a. A patient's medical record includes appropriate documentation of the applicable key components of the E/M services provided

  b. That documentation adequately reflects the procedure or portion of the services provided

  c. That all documentation is present and accurate

  d. All of the above

Q3. While it is true that a percentage of E/M charges are reviewed and audited by coders for accuracy, for most departments, the vast majority of E/M charges are selected by the provider and released directly for billing. The provider is responsible for the accuracy of the documentation and that the level of service selected is supported by medical necessity in relation to the nature of the presenting problem.

  a. True

  b. False

Answer key

Q1: a. – True

Q2: d. – All of the above

Q3: a. – True

Although much of the material is tailored to a specific request, some topics, such as E/M services as discussed above, support more standardized education. Organizations should develop and implement standardized online education about changes surrounding coding and billing guidelines by utilizing tools available within an organization, allowing providers to complete required education at a time that fits best into their schedule.

Having a set schedule for education ensures that providers stay current on best practices. Providers should complete coding and billing education initially at hire and annually thereafter. For example, after guideline changes went into effect for the Office E/M code set in 2021, the annual coding education may be focused on a summary of those changes as a supplement to any additional education that was provided prior to the rule changes. Annual coding education should reflect real time identified trends. Examples may include:

- Proper documentation of patient risk factors
- Documentation of ordered tests
- Discussion of management with external providers
- Order/review versus independent interpretation
- Review of data from external sources

APPs have become a part of the clinical makeup of most healthcare organizations. As the rules and regulations continue to change specific to coding and billing, it is important to understand how these changes impact not just the physician profession, but how they apply to the APP profession as well. Because there is no crosswalk to easily define how to apply certain rules to APPs, it is important for the compliance office and other groups within the organization to work together to design workflows that minimize burdens while still meeting the regulated requirements. For example, operational leaders and frontline staff may help determine the workflow, but the compliance office will help make sure it meets the regulated requirements.

As a coding and billing education resource for the organization, the compliance office's education team must work collaboratively with key team members to meet the unique needs of each group. It is vital to engage not only executive leadership, but those providers, including APPs, on the receiving end of the educational training and materials. Understanding the training profile of the organization and engaging the clinical workforce/leadership as well as the payer relations and revenue cycle leadership is vital for educational success and overall provider buy-in.

While much of the educational material created by a compliance office can apply to all provider types (e.g., evaluation and management education), there are instances where the material needs to be tailored to specific groups. For example, when the Centers for Medicare & Medicaid Services (CMS) finalized changes related to review and verification of medical record documentation (CMS, 2019), it was necessary to understand not just the rule change but also how that fit in to clinical practice workflow. Education should be provided surrounding how various members of the healthcare team are affected by the implementation of this change and any nuances to consider when implementing changes specific to APPs. To effectively tailor the material to the APP group, it is important to work collaboratively with key members of the APP leadership team. A compliance office's understanding of the regulations coupled with their understanding of APP clinical scope of practice allows for educating to the change and a resource to address questions that arise before, during, and after implementation.

CLINICAL DOCUMENTATION

The Clinical Documentation Improvement (CDI) department works with providers to ensure that clinical documentation accurately reflects patients' severity of illness and intensity of service, resulting in an appropriate expected length of stay (LOS) and diagnosis related group (DRG). In addition, CDI department works closely with compliance to ensure adherence with coding guidelines and regulations. CDI activities are primarily engaged for inpatient and procedural documentation. CDI teams help to translate clinical documentation into hospital coding and billing language through review of patient cases to be sure the most accurate diagnoses, including complexity and severity of disease, are being assigned. CDI teams function as part of specialty teams and often take a role in huddles, rounds, and education with providers. They reach out to providers with questions to ensure that all documentation is accurate, clear, and consistent. CDI teams work hard to partner with providers and bridge the gap between providers and the office of compliance team.

Here are some CDI responsibilities:

- The primary purpose of CDI is concurrent review of the healthcare record to increase the accuracy, clarity, and specificity of provider documentation.

- CDI teams bridge the gap between the providers and hospital coders to clarify at-risk documentation prior to claim submission.

- Responsible for concurrent reviews of healthcare records to help ensure accuracy, clarity, and specificity of provider documentation.

- Collaborate extensively with providers, coding staff, healthcare administration, and other patient caregivers to improve accuracy and completeness of documentation.

- Ensure accurate capture, documentation, and report of conditions considered to be hospital acquired conditions and patient safety metrics.

- When provider documentation is illegible, incomplete, imprecise, inconsistent, conflicting, or unreliable the CDI team communicates with the provider to obtain the necessary information and clarify the healthcare record.

- Provide data and other documentation-related metrics to service teams and healthcare administration.

CDI QUERY EXAMPLE

Dear APP,

The below listed diagnosis is noted in the anesthesia note. The diagnosis isn't currently documented in the assessment and plan. Please clarify in the discharge summary or progress notes the clinical relevance/validity of the conditions identified:

- Heart failure

If you agree that the diagnosis is valid, please specify the type and acuity of heart failure in your progress notes:

1. TYPE:
   - ❏ Diastolic
   - ❏ Systolic
   - ❏ Other (please specify) _____
   - ❏ Clinically unable to determine
   - ❏ Unknown

2. ACUITY:
   - ❏ Chronic
   - ❏ Other (please specify) _____
   - ❏ Clinically unable to determine
   - ❏ Unknown

Clinical Indicators: - Anesthesia: CHF

Last OSH Echo EF 65% DDG1 LVSF WNL

Cont. ARB, CCB, not on diuretic

Medications: Amlodipine 5mg po daily, HCTZ 25mg po daily, losartan 50mg po daily

By submitting this query, we are seeking further clarification of documentation to accurately reflect all conditions that you are monitoring, evaluating, treating or that extend the hospitalization or utilize additional resources of care. Please utilize your independent clinical judgment when addressing the question(s) above.

Thank you, CDI Team

APP/PHYSICIAN CLINICAL PARTNERSHIP PRACTICES

The rules continually evolve when capturing clinical practice when physician and APPs are practicing collaboratively, for example split shared and incident to rules. This is an area where partnership between the compliance office and APP leadership is necessary to ensure understanding of the clinical practice happening in real time and accurate implementation of changes. It is important to include a variety of clinical settings from inpatient, observational units to ambulatory outpatient and community-based clinics. Many physicians and APPs practice in both hospital-based and clinic-based settings, and because the rules can vary based on clinical setting, it is vital to understand the collaborative or independent nature of the physician and APP relationship and also the specifics of each clinical setting. Open communication between the compliance office and physician and APP leadership teams helps them understand the educational materials needed for the different provider types based on the roles they serve. Likewise, it is important to be able to provide profession-specific education addressing additional educational materials for related concepts.

AUDITING

Coding and billing require ongoing collaboration between the compliance office and APPs beyond one time education. According to the US Sentencing Guidelines, "the organization shall take reasonable steps to ensure that the organization's compliance and ethics program is followed, including monitoring and auditing" (US Sentencing Commission, 2021, §8B2.1(5)A). An organization can conduct auditing and monitoring activities in a variety of ways, such as new provider and risk-based audits. These methods of auditing are used to monitor the effectiveness of education as well as assessing the organization's compliance with rules and regulations. Auditing a variety of topics using various methods of data analysis helps to ensure identification of potential areas of risk for the organization. Although the topics can vary from evaluation and management service to procedures, providing feedback to the appropriate provider group is imperative. To do this, provider-coded claims and coder-coded claims are not typically intermingled within an audit and therefore take thoughtful review. This helps to ensure the feedback provided is relevant to the provider(s) receiving the information and the person(s) best able to mitigate the potential risk identified through the audit.

While the audit scope will change for each audit topic, the risk-based audit process remains relatively stable. First, the audit topic is identified through an annual risk assessment process as well as review of regulatory changes and monitoring of internal trends. Once the audit topic is selected, data analysis is used to identify population scope. For example, the population scope of an audit could be determined to be providers that bill 99205/99215 a minimum number of times in a calendar year. Providers that bill below the set minimum would be considered out of scope for the audit. Next the audit scope is defined to ensure consistent review across the entire audit population. Examples include correct level of service and modifier assignment, compliance with attestation rules, and use of templates.

After providers are identified and the audit scope is outlined, a sample of claims is reviewed for all elements. After all claims have been audited, a preliminary letter summarizing the findings is sent to the audited provider, coding group, and department administrator(s) outlining the findings and recommendations, focusing on clinical language rather than coding language. Summaries include a description of the audit topic and scope, detailed explanations of errors and other findings, and next steps. In the case of provider audits, if a provider falls below the passing threshold set for each audit, a meeting is requested to review results. These meetings serve to not only provide focused education to the provider on the errors identified, but a clinical perspective to auditing staff to better understand what is being conveyed in the clinical documentation which could change the final audit results. Once the results are finalized, the audit will either be considered complete based on a satisfactory score or may be moved in to one of two follow-up processes: 1) a three-month data analysis to determine the impact of the audit/educational session and potential next steps or 2) further review in accordance with organizational policy to determine if there are any additional federal repayment obligations.

EXAMPLE OF AUDIT FINDINGS

The Compliance Office has completed a claim review of E/M coding and documentation.

Background:

We are primarily reviewing whether documentation supports the level of service for the charges submitted (we look at coder-assigned codes separately). However, we also provide feedback on other areas such as: teaching guidelines and required signatures/statements and observations about contradictory statements and copy/paste.

Findings:

Over coded Claims: 2

MRN: 1 DOS: x/x/xx CPT code originally billed: 99204, FS CPT code recommended: 99203, FS

Explanation: This new patient presented to clinic for evaluation of iliac aneurysm. External records from {***} were reviewed and duplex imaging was ordered. The scan revealed {***}. Decision was made to follow up in two years for duplex surveillance. Based on the status of the patient and the documented medical decision-making, this is best supported by CPT code 99203, FS.

MRN: 2 DOS: x/x/xx CPT code originally billed: 99204, FS CPT code recommended: 99203, FS

Explanation: This new patient presented to clinic for evaluation of lower extremity swelling and possible AV fistula. External records from {***} were reviewed and duplex imaging was ordered. Venous duplex showed {***} with no indication for intervention and decision was made to follow up as needed. Based on the status of the patient and the documented medical decision-making, this is best supported by CPT code 99203, FS.

Claims with other findings: 1

MRN: 3 DOS: x/x/xx CPT code originally billed: 99204, FS CPT code recommended: 99214, FS

Explanation: The patient was previously seen on x/x/xx by you, which was within the three-year time period; therefore, this should have been coded as an established patient. The system should be set up to catch this type of error from occurring; this is not your error and feedback has been passed along.

Next Steps:

We do not feel a meeting is needed at this time. However, if you need any assistance regarding this review or any other billing/documentation related issues, we are happy to help. Please know that our review efforts are ongoing and there is always potential for future reviews to occur.

NEW PROVIDER AUDITS

All new providers who perform evaluation and management services should have a documentation audit conducted, typically within the first six months of their clinical service. This audit follows the above- outlined audit process with a retrospective review of 10 evaluation and management services with the following purpose:

- Opportunity to evaluate and address areas of concern
- Audit/educate on best practice vs. minimum standard required
- Relationship building: an introduction to the compliance auditing and educational activities of the organization and providing a key resource for future questions or compliance concerns

RISK-BASED AUDITING

In addition to new provider audits, organizations should implement an ongoing risk-based audit process. Unlike the new provider audit process, where a provider would only be audited once, a provider could be audited many times under the risk-based audit process as the topics change. Risk-based audit topics are determined in a variety of ways. An annual compliance auditing and monitoring plan will lay out some of the key areas of focus, such as major coding changes or hot topics from the Office of the Inspector General. Additional topics may be identified based on internal trends or external reports such as the CMS Comparative Billing Reports. Once an audit topic is identified, one of a variety of methods is used to review data and identify providers to be audited. Although not an all-inclusive list, here are some ways to review data to identify providers for a given audit topic:

- **Benchmark data:** Providers are identified when they exceed benchmark data for a given set of codes.

- **wRVU data:** Providers are identified based on billing a high volume of wRVUs per day.

- **Primary procedure:** Providers are identified based on the primary procedure billed to determine potential outliers related to billing additional procedures during the same operative session to the primary procedure.

- **Modifier data:** Providers are identified based on high usage of a modifier such as -25 or -59.

RISK-BASED AUDIT: SPLIT/SHARED

There are many factors to take into consideration when understanding how to bill for services performed by APPs, especially when looking at the collaborative or independent relationship with physicians. Three main scenarios exist for billing services performed by APPs: 1) independent billing under their own national provider identifier (NPI); 2) billing incident-to services under the physician's NPI; and 3) split/shared services. Split/shared services have been an area of focus for CMS over the past few years with recent changes in the Medicare Physician Fee Schedule. Based on these recent regulatory changes, as well as posted settlements involving physician and APP billing relationships, it is important to continue to perform ongoing risk audit work on instances where APPs services are billed under a physician's NPI number. Although APPs are always included for risk-based audit topics where the APP service is billed under their own NPI, the scope of additional audits should focus on services billed under a physician NPI but performed either in part (split/shared) or fully (incident-to) by an APP. To effectively perform the audit and provide valuable feedback, it is necessary to understand the clinical workflow. Factors to consider include whether APPs work their own schedule, clinical reasons a physician may see a patient jointly with an APP rather than the APP seeing the patient on their own, understanding the documentation workflow, and knowing who makes the charge selection. Understanding this allows feedback to be tailored based on how providers practice. Taking the responsibility of communicating feedback to the APP helps to positively impact the relationship between the compliance office and the providers as well as improve the likelihood the feedback is implemented. Figure 11.1 shows a split/shared audit finding.

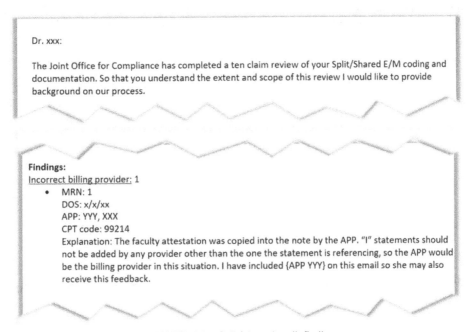

FIGURE 11.1   Split/shared audit finding.

SUMMARY

Although not all new projects or issues rise to the level of a compliance issue, it is important that all members of the organization feel comfortable engaging with the compliance office. By maintaining collaborative relationships across the organization, the compliance office can keep the lines of communication open and be viewed as an ally in the overall mission of the organization. Healthcare organizations and patient care practices are complex in today's healthcare arena, but the overall strategic plans across organizations are most successful when utilizing the rich resources by working together.

REFERENCES

Centers for Medicare & Medicaid Services. (2019). 42 CFR (Code of Federal Regulations) Parts 403, 409, 410, 411, 414, 415, 416, 418, 424, 425, 489, and 498. *Federal Register, 84*(221), 62568–63563. https://www.govinfo.gov/content/pkg/FR-2019-11-15/pdf/2019-24086.pdf

Troklus, D., & Vacca, S. (2016). *Compliance 101* (4th ed.). Health Care Compliance Association.

United States Sentencing Commission. (2021). Effective compliance and ethics program. *Guidelines manual,* §8B2.1(5)A. https://www.ussc.gov/sites/default/files/pdf/guidelines-manual/2021/CHAPTER_8.pdf

"In any given moment we have two options; to step forward into growth or to step back into safety."

–Abraham Maslow

CHAPTER 12

PROFESSIONAL DEVELOPMENT

KEYWORDS | training, development, leadership, recognition, retreat, conference, learning, committee

Creating a workplace environment that supports and encourages ongoing professional development has been linked to job satisfaction, engagement, and perceived positive impact on clinical practice (Mlambo et al., 2021). Professional development for clinical staff includes a variety of activities and strategic learning opportunities that encompass more than just keeping skills and competencies up to date. *Professional development* means embracing the approach of a lifelong learner, seeking out ways to improve personally and professionally, adding to the depth and scope of technical knowledge, identifying areas of improvement, setting goals, and taking action towards achieving those goals. Many organizations offer an array of professional development opportunities intended to help APPs progress professionally through technical clinical skills, advanced knowledge, leadership opportunities, and personal growth.

Professional development opportunities can be offered at the department/unit level, at the organizational level, or through participation in professional organizations. Clinical departments develop their APPs professionally through subject matter expertise, a collaborative learning environment, and promoting top-of-license practice and efficiency (Hilty et al., 2019). At the organizational level, professional development may occur through collaboration across services; exposure to broader concepts; embracing diversity, equity, and inclusion; and adapting to a variety of clinical disciplines. At the national level, professional organizations provide best practices, guidelines, and exposure to new directions and methods with a broader perspective (Hilty et al., 2019).

EXAMPLES OF PROFESSIONAL DEVELOPMENT OPPORTUNITIES

- Relevant CME/CEU offerings

- Providing opportunities for APPs to present information learned at a conference or course to their work group or team

- Subscribing to listservs and newsletters for learning opportunities and events hosted by professional organizations

---

LEADERSHIP PATHWAY DEVELOPMENT

Strong leadership within a healthcare organization can be linked to increased job satisfaction, positive well-being, lower burnout rates, and improvement in patient outcomes and quality care (Cummings et al., 2021). It is important that organizations invest in and prioritize growing and developing leadership skills through targeted training that sets the stage for APPs who are seeking additional pathways that go beyond their clinical education. Leadership skills can include topics such as recruiting, hiring, onboarding, retention, engagement, facilitating performance, coaching, and documentation.

Providing training and education relating to leadership skills helps develop consistent practices and education within the organization, strengthens supervisory skills, and promotes reliable, equitable employment practices. If an organization fails to support the development and growth of APPs, they may alienate this rapidly growing group of healthcare providers (Kapu & Jones, 2016).

Providing ongoing training to grow skills and knowledge helps prepare APPs interested in leadership pathways to be well-rounded and effective future leaders within the organization. Leadership continuity is a strategic approach that includes succession planning. Identifying APPs who aspire to hold leadership positions and providing specialized leadership skills training helps train experienced APPs to transition from clinical practice to leadership (Bugos et al., 2023). University of Iowa Health Care offers an Executive Leadership Academy for high potential emerging leaders, including APPs, where training is provided on the healthcare system, quality/process improvement, project management, finance, marketing, and professional relationships. This program and others similar to it are designed to prepare the next generation of APRN and PA leaders to optimize team care and operationalize strategic and effective clinical models.

There are a variety of ways that organizations can engage their APPs in leadership and professional development. Recorded webinars that may be viewed on demand, are an approach used by University of Iowa Health Care to provide advanced education on a variety of topics. For example, a Revenue Cycle Bootcamp for APPs was created and recorded in webinar format. Other recorded webinar educational topics include the credentialing and privileging process, conflict of interest disclosures for APPs, and social media for APPs. Organizations with multiple work locations and 24/7 work environments may find that the recorded webinar format increases the reach of educational programs.

As was introduced in Chapter 1, having an infrastructure through an enterprise leadership group that complements nursing, medical, and other existing infrastructures can provide resources related to APP leadership development through some of the following activities:

- **APP lead meetings:** Bringing together a cohort of APP leads on a regular basis to discuss issues, share knowledge, and be kept current on pertinent organizational matters

- **1:1 mentorship with APP director:** Individual meetings to guide, mentor, and discuss issues related to their role and assimilation within the organization

- **Communication conduit with APP lead cohort:** Advance knowledge of issues, policies, and organizational practices that impact APPs

- **Organizational committee opportunities:** Broader understanding of how committees impact APPs within the organization

- **Networking opportunities:** Enhance collegial relationships and offer networking support

- **Resource direction for operational issues:** Access to leadership to discuss/brainstorm topics pertaining to APPs

- **Formal APP lead orientation:** Summary of pertinent topics and introduction to the leadership role within the organization

LEADERSHIP COMPETENCIES

The American Nurses Association (ANA) has developed a model which defines and identifies competencies for leaders. ANA describes *competency* as an "expected level of performance that results from an integration of knowledge, skills, abilities, and judgment" and categorizes leadership competency into three distinct groups: leading yourself, others, and the organization (ANA, 2018, p. 3). ANA describes competencies for leading others as being an effective communicator, encouraging the development of the team while leveraging diversity and unique talents, and being a collaborative leader who will address issues and problems directly. Being part of a team includes aligning with and supporting organizational strategy, understanding change and project management, being decisive, and using business acumen while problem-solving. Using a strategic perspective is important to understand the viewpoint and the organizational geography and culture. Self-awareness is key, and APP leaders should take time for self-examination and reflection to know and understand their own strengths and weaknesses and actively work towards personal improvement. ANA (2018) describes leaders as motivated, adaptable, and fostering an environment of trust, credibility, and integrity.

LEAD ORIENTATION

Informal training through retreats, seminars, webinars, and burst formats are accessible methods for providing education. A formal training program may also be appropriate for leaders who are new to their role or need a refresher on leadership skills and topics. University of Iowa Health Care has embraced the utilization of APP leads as informal and influential leaders within a clinical department and offers a half day APP lead orientation to introduce new leads into the role and provide information and resources. Curricula for the training was developed with input from existing APP leads, finance, HR, and department and physician leaders on topics that would be pertinent to a new APP lead. Here are some of the topics covered in this course:

- APP central office staff, function, mission
- Organizational charts
- APP steering committee oversight
- Roster of APP leads
- Shared governance
- Support for APP leads, role expectations
- Training resources
- Leader mindset
- Time tracking and attendance
- Organizational strategic plan, policies, bylaws
- Intranet resources
- Committees
- Practice models
- Productivity
- Top of license
- Business pro forma
- Recruitment
- Onboarding new APPs
- Credentialing and privileging
- Employee engagement
- Employee recognition
- Professional development
- Labor relations
- Performance evaluations
- Magnet
- OPPE/IPPE
- Student clinical placement
- Informatics

- Incident reporting
- Professionalism
- Recommended reading

APP REWARDS AND RECOGNITION

With healthcare organizations facing staffing shortages, turnover, burnout, and compassion fatigue, efforts to improve the employment experience through creating a culture of recognition becomes a critical initiative (American Association of Critical-Care Nurses [AACN], 2005). The AACN recommends having a system in place that includes formal recognition for APPs for their contributions and the value they bring to the work of the organization. Promoting organizational, individual, and team employee recognition and appreciation can increase satisfaction and mitigate burnout (Kapu et al., 2021). A culture of recognition utilizes best practices for day-to-day and large-scale recognition and encouragement of APPs. Organizational leaders need to coach, guide, and encourage APPs to take individual initiative in achieving broad departmental or organizational goals. Recognizing APPs for their unique contributions includes giving credit for an APP's ideas and work, formally and informally. A humble leader will share credit, acknowledging the contributions and success of others ahead of recognition or attention for themselves (Kalina, 2020).

Professionalism is a core competency and reflects a set of behaviors that can and should be practiced and learned. This includes behaviors that demonstrate respect for others, integrity, being accountable, and conflict resolution skills. In healthcare, professionalism may be measured through patient satisfaction scores, feedback by APRN and PA students, being a highly requested provider, and being available and willing to be a positive resource for colleagues. These are characteristics that should be recognized and rewarded because these attributes are essential for future APP leaders.

Informal recognition is equally important, and intention should be given to recognize employees who are also champions in their roles but don't interact as often with leadership. Some employees may be quieter, more introverted, or may not be comfortable bringing their accomplishments forward to their leaders. In these situations, leaders should seek out their accomplishments so that they can be appropriately recognized.

A leader can create a culture of gratitude within their team by encouraging, recognizing, and thanking exemplary APPs. It is human nature to feel valued when efforts are acknowledged and appreciated from their leaders, peers, and other interested parties. Encouraging team members to speak up for each other helps reinforce the culture of gratitude. Time can be made for this at staff meetings or in daily huddles. Providing timely feedback and follow-up as soon as possible after a positive event, achievement, or interaction is important. Describing the actual behavior being recognized and who benefited from the positive work behaviors (patients, team dynamics, leadership, etc.) will reinforce continued behaviors, and APPs, like all professionals, should be recognized for their contributions.

INFORMAL RECOGNITION EXAMPLES

Individual appreciation:

- Take time one-on-one just to thank them; don't discuss any other issue
- Send a handwritten thank you note in the mail or leave it on their desk
- Send a thank you email to the APP and cc other pertinent leaders
- Take an APP to coffee or lunch
- Bring in a favorite treat for an APP as a thank you

Praise APPs in front of other staff and/or their leaders:

- Regularly acknowledge good performance during staff meetings
- Create a bulletin board where APPs and other staff can post kudos for others
- Create lighthearted awards: social director award, early bird award, clean desk award, etc.
- Know and celebrate your employees' work anniversary
- Have a "traveling trophy" or token mascot in the work group that can be passed along and re-gifted to someone who goes above and beyond
- Establish a place to display memos, posters, and photos recognizing the APP team efforts
- Submit an article highlighting the accomplishments of the team or feature an APP on the organization's social media.

When developing a formal recognition program, consider whether similar programs already exist within the organization that can be adapted accordingly for APPs. A recognition program should have clearly defined outcomes and expectations, assigned oversight, and funding should be secured in advance. The recognition program details should be clear, including application or nomination process and how the recognition will be communicated, the timeline, and who is eligible. Organizations may develop a formal clinical award program to recognize clinical excellence among members of the healthcare team. An Advanced Practice Provider of the Year Award is one example that would recognize an APP who most embodies those aspects of a truly great patient service provider, including technical skill, humanism to patients and families, collaboration with colleagues, and advocacy. A clear nomination process should be determined including the program deadlines, nomination method, and criteria for award selection.

TAKE TEN LEADERSHIP SERIES

While APP leads benefit from ongoing professional development training, lack of time is often a constraint for attending. University of Iowa Health Care resolved this constraint by providing a 10-minute "burst" training via a "Take Ten Leadership Series" at regularly scheduled APP lead meetings. A shorter training format may be optimal because the effectiveness of leadership development is not driven by program length or mode of delivery, but rather targeted approaches to improve leadership (Cummings et al., 2021).

SAMPLE TAKE TEN TRAINING TOPICS

- Interviewing Best Practices
- Mentoring Toolkit
- Generations at Work
- Turnover Statistics
- Job Descriptions
- Resilience for Leaders
- Job Postings
- Credentialing and Privileging Resources
- Using OneNote
- Performance Evaluations
- Employee Engagement
- Setting Performance Goals
- Creating Hiring Pipelines

LEADERSHIP TRAINING—TAKE TEN FORMAT

- 10-Minute Leadership Training during regular scheduled meetings

- Introduce a topic

- High-level overview with contacts at the end to reach out individually if more information is requested

- Review current practice/guidelines

- Roundtable discussion following: "Tips and Tricks"

COMMITTEE & PROJECT INVOLVEMENT

Serving on a committee, whether at the department, organization, state, or national level, allows APPs to gain a more strategic perspective and a broader view of their profession and the organization, grow collaborative relationships, network, and represent their profession in long-term planning and strategies. When contemplating a committee appointment, consideration should be given to appointing APPs who are engaged, experienced, have a desire to grow and expand their leadership skills, and bring a level of diversity to the committee. Those serving on committees are expected to be actively engaged and demonstrate these behaviors:

- Regular attendance and engagement

- Carry out committee assignments

- Represent and be a professional voice for APPs

- Regularly summarize committee activities to the APP director

- Brief report-out at monthly APP lead meetings

Each member of the APP team should be aware of their job expectations and understand how their work aligns with the strategic goals for the department, unit, and the organization, which can help guide direction for becoming engaged and active participants on committees or projects at every level.

Leaders and APPs should work together to establish relevant professional development goals that go above and beyond regular job duties, such as projects and committees that would allow them to contribute their skills in a more meaningful way. Professional development activities should be aligned with organizational strategic goals, such as participation in a process improvement project. Optimally, goals should develop the employee while moving the organization forward.

SAMPLE LIST OF INTERNAL COMMITTEES FOR ADVANCED PRACTICE PROVIDERS

- APP (APRN/PA) steering committee or council
- APRN/PA managed care billing subpanel
- APRN/PA credentialing and privileging subpanel
- APRN/PA student placement committee
- Peer review professional committee
- Peer review medical committee
- Peer review surgical committee
- Nurse leadership council
- CME advisory committee
- Clinical systems committee
- Clinical staff affairs subcommittee
- Provider well-being working group
- APP leadership symposium committee
- Provider coding & documentation advisory committee
- Clinical revenue cycle governance committee
- Clinical documentation improvement committee
- Pediatric advocacy committee

VALUE-ADDED LEARNING ACTIVITIES

Overall, an engaged and satisfied employee will view the organization's values positively, recommend the organization as a good place to work, and be able to see themselves working at the organization in the future (Kang et al., 2020). Other indicators of engagement and satisfaction are opportunities for professional development and the ability to learn and grow in their field. Table 12.1 provides a list of activities that enhance the professional value and experience of the APP. Not every APP will want to explore every area, but for those who are interested in learning more, gaining some experience, and exploring their interests, a guide to value-added professional work activities may be helpful. The categories of value-added work activities are research, precepting, scholarly publishing, mentoring, leadership, education, committees/policy/service, and quality improvement. An academic medical center with a tripartite mission of education, patient care, and research is an ideal setting for offering an array of activities for APPs wishing to grow professionally. Participation in these activities benefit the APP by providing valuable experience and a breadth of knowledge. Departments may wish to encourage and incentivize those APPs who seek out and participate in additional value-added activities (see Table 12.1).

TABLE 12.1 VALUE-ADDED LEARNING ACTIVITIES

AREA OF INTEREST	STRATEGIC PILLAR ASSIGNMENT	ACTIVITIES	EVIDENCE/ DOCUMENTATION
Research	Research & Discovery	■ Conduct a literature search on a topic of interest, then write a summary and present to your work group ■ Present evidence-based practice poster or presentation at local, state, or national conference ■ Participate in formal research project outside of regular work duties through data collection, literature review, or other areas ■ Submit an IRB research proposal ■ Lead or co-lead a research study and disseminate findings	Documentation of participation or attestation from leadership
Precepting	Student Success	■ Consistently precept APP or medical students in your department ■ Provide unit-based continuing education for ongoing learners ■ Create and implement training, workflows, education materials for areas of practice ■ Mentor DNP project to its completion ■ Present at local, state, or national conference related to APP students	Documentation demonstrating precepting/educator role, project oversight

continues

TABLE 12.1 VALUE-ADDED LEARNING ACTIVITIES (CONT.)

AREA OF INTEREST	STRATEGIC PILLAR ASSIGNMENT	ACTIVITIES	EVIDENCE/ DOCUMENTATION
Scholarly Publishing	Research & Discovery	■ If previously published, mentor an APP student or peer towards scholarly publishing ■ Serve as a co-investigator or research coordinator on a research study, or grant proposal submission outside of regular work duties ■ Publish in a professional journal or author a book chapter ■ Peer review for a professional journal	Copies of published materials, submissions, attestation of peer review or mentorship
Mentoring	DEI & Collaboration	■ Meet your department grand round presentation attendance recommendations ■ Precept, train, or onboard other APPs within department ■ Lead and implement activities to promote teamwork, collaboration, and engagement within your workgroup ■ Serve as a formal mentor for APPs within your workgroup	Attestation or documentation from department leadership verifying participation
Leadership	DEI & Collaboration	■ Executive Leadership Academy ■ Clinical Leadership Development Academy (CLDA) ■ Serve as a presenter and planning committee member for APP Leadership Symposium ■ Obtain Health Systems Leadership Certificate through the College of Nursing ■ Obtain MHA or MBA through accredited program ■ Serve in a leadership role within your professional organization	Certificate of completion or written verification of role from organization

Education	Student Success	■ Lead journal club or other department collaborative learning opportunities ■ Provide an uncompensated (unpaid) lecture at nursing or PA school or present at a symposium or conference (unpaid) ■ Volunteer in community activities (e.g., free medical clinic, school guest speaker, etc.) ■ Develop a presentation or poster for local, state, or national conference	Documentation of lecture, training, education, journal leadership, poster submission
Commit-tees Policy Service	Engagement	■ Serve as an interdisciplinary resource within area of practice ■ Actively participate in organizational committee; provide regular updates to APP Director ■ Join your professional organization(s) and attend meetings ■ Become knowledgeable about local, state, national policy and issues; share this knowledge within your team ■ Participate in community organization that is healthcare-related	Verification from committee chair, education provided, community service participation
Quality Improvement	Patient Care	■ Participate in QI initiatives in your area of practice ■ Identify and lead process improvement efforts within area of practice ■ Attend Lean Improvement Model for Health Care training ■ Become a subject matter expert on the processes and systems that support quality in your work area and provide education within your workgroup	Overview of QI project role and outcome, documentation of education provided

LEADERSHIP RETREAT AND SYMPOSIUM

The cohort of APP leads is strengthened as trust is grown and camaraderie develops. The impact of mentoring and an openness to sharing ideas and experiences relies on the group of APP leads having a trusting, collegial relationship. Bringing together APP leads informally to grow and strengthen these relationships builds on professional unity.

Holding leadership retreats off-site, in an informal environment where a facilitator can guide the group through collaborative games, drills, and exercises, further promotes a culture of teamwork. Coordinating a meal following a half day filled with activities is a successful approach in bringing together the cohort and providing fun, lighthearted activities as a respite from the otherwise high stress and demanding rigors of their day-to-day role. Retreats should be held at regular intervals with thoughtful planning, clear goals, input from the team, and support from leadership to allow participants to step away from daily responsibilities to attend.

A convenient and accessible way to offer professional development on a large scale is to provide a seminar, retreat, or symposium with didactic course offerings and education centered around topics of interest. One example is to host a leadership symposium for APPs seeking to grow and enhance their leadership skills and operational knowledge. A day-long symposium provides a series of educational presentations to enhance participants' leadership knowledge, skills, and abilities, which are critical in today's changing academic healthcare environment. Attendees of the symposium are presented with information regarding the business, legal, and financial decisions that will better equip APPs with the tools required to analyze, plan, and implement solutions to the challenges they face. To offset any costs associated with hosting a symposium, an organization may charge a nominal fee to attend. Offering CEU/CME credit will further support the professional development need for APPs.

EXAMPLES OF LEADERSHIP SYMPOSIUM TOPICS

- Discuss effective elements of organizational change.

- Review APP bylaws and their relationship to state and national agencies.

- Review communication basics, coaching philosophy and techniques, and discuss constructive feedback techniques to improve work relationships.

- Discuss billing, coding, and revenue cycles and their relationship to APP billing and documentation; describe the process to capture, collect, and manage patient service revenue.

- Determine how administrative and clinical functions contribute to the success of the organization.

- Establish a pro forma that can translate to an operating budget for each department.

- Explore concepts of hiring and team building to promote success within healthcare; explore best practices for recruiting and retaining staff and leaders in APP roles.

- Explain the steps for APP credentialing, privileging, and ongoing professional practice evaluation as well as their impact on APP practice; discuss professional development opportunities for leadership.

- Identify metrics that equate to productivity and value from APP contribution.

- Review organizational structure, including APP leadership.

- Gain awareness of your communication style and its impact on others, and learn techniques for communicating effectively with coworkers who have different styles.

- Discuss strategies for advocating with policymakers regarding issues.

- Identify proactive behaviors for burnout recognition and treatment.

- Identify barriers to help-seeking behaviors among healthcare professionals.

- Learn about comprehensive approaches healthcare enterprises are taking to address the sustained stressors of the industry.

- Review change management strategies deployed at the start of COVID-19.

- Describe the purpose and process of publishing.

- Identify strategies for effective precepting and teaching in the clinical setting.

- Explore strategies for team engagement for career development.

SUMMARY

Organizations will benefit by creating a workplace environment that supports and encourages ongoing professional development by offering a selection of opportunities intended to help APPs progress through technical clinical skills, advanced knowledge, leadership opportunities, and personal growth. There are many ways organizational leaders can support, grow, and develop APPs and can impact the profession within the organization. APPs serve as mentors, inspire professional growth, and encourage others to become involved in organizational initiatives (Kapu & Dubree, 2021). APPs deserve to be recognized for the work they contribute not only in the clinical arena but also as leaders within the organization alongside their physician and nursing colleagues.

REFERENCES

American Association of Critical-Care Nurses. (2005). AACN standards for establishing and sustaining healthy work environments: A journey to excellence. *American Journal of Critical Care, 14*(3), 187–197. https://doi.org/10.4037/ajcc2005.14.3.187

American Nurses Association. (2018, July). *Competency model.* https://www.nursingworld.org/~4a0a2e/globalassets/docs/ce/177626-ana-leadership-booklet-new-final.pdf

Bugos, K., Mansour, S., Stringer, M.A., & Kuriakose, C. (2023). Highlighting an advanced practice fellowship for leadership transition. *Journal of Nursing Administration, 53*(3), 181–182. https://doi.org/10.1097/NNA.0000000000001265

Cummings, G. G., Lee, S., Tate, K., Penconek, T., Micaroni, S. P. M., Paananen, T., & Chatterjee, G. E. (2021). The essentials of nursing leadership: A systematic review of factors and educational interventions influencing nursing leadership. *International Journal of Nursing Studies, 115*(103842). https://doi.org/10.1016/j.ijnurstu.2020.103842

Hilty, D. M., Liu, H. Y., Stubbe, D., & Teshima, J. (2019). Defining professional development in medicine, psychiatry, and allied fields. *Psychiatric Clinics of North America, 42*(3), 337–356. https://doi.org/10.1016/j.psc.2019.04.001

Kalina, P. (2020). "Humble, hungry and smart?" A cautionary tale for inclusive healthcare leaders. *The International Journal of Health Planning & Management, 35*(5), 1267–1269. https://doi.org/10.1002/hpm.2990

Kang, J. Y., Lee, M. K., Fairchild, E. M., Caubet, S. L., Peters, D. E., Beliles, G. R., & Matti, L. K. (2020). Relationships among organizational values, employee engagement, and patient satisfaction in an academic medical center. *Mayo Clinic Proceedings: Innovations, Quality, & Outcomes, 4*(1), 8–20. https://doi.org/10.1016/j.mayocpiqo.2019.08.001

Kapu, A. N., Borg Card, E., Jackson, H., Kleinpell, R., Kendall, J., Lupear, B. K., LeBar, K., Dietrich, M. S., Araya, W. A., Delle, J., Payne, K., Ford, J., & Dubree, M. (2021). Assessing and addressing practitioner burnout: Results from an advanced practice registered nurse health and well-being study. *Journal of the American Association of Nurse Practitioners, 33*(1), 38–48. https://doi.org/10.1097/jxx.0000000000000324

Kapu, A., & Dubree, M. (2021). Today's advanced practice leader: Value contribution to healthcare systems and delivery of accessible, high-quality patient care. *JONA: The Journal of Nursing Administration, 51*(4), 179–181. https://doi.org/10.1097/nna.0000000000000994

Kapu, A. N., & Jones, P. (2016). APRN transformational leadership. *Nursing Management, 47*(2), 19–22. https://doi.org/10.1097/01.NUMA.0000479443.75643.2b

Mlambo, M., Silén, C., & McGrath, C. (2021). Lifelong learning and nurses' continuing professional development, a metasynthesis of the literature. *BMC Nursing, 20*(1), 62. https://doi.org/10.1186/s12912-021-00579-2

"A leader takes people where they want to go. A great leader takes people where they don't necessarily want to go, but ought to be."

—Rosalynn Carter

CHAPTER 13

MENTORING

KEYWORDS | mentor, leadership, peer mentoring

A formal mentoring program occurs when an organization dedicates structure, time, and resources towards pairing an APP with a peer to provide professional support and guidance. In academic medicine, physician leaders have traditionally used mentoring to help develop and build successful academic careers (Seehusen et al., 2021). Whether a peer mentoring program or a multidisciplinary mentorship, a formal mentoring program provides an established series of predetermined topics designed to decrease role-transition stress, increase satisfaction, and provide professional support (Moss & Jackson, 2019). Furthermore, developing a professional support system for new APPs will decrease frustration, feelings of isolation, and positively impact patient safety and positive patient outcomes (Horner, 2017). There is considerable literature addressing the benefits of a formal mentoring program for APPs in role transition, job satisfaction, and retention (Moss & Jackson, 2019). Kapu et al. (2021) found that having a support system and mentor improved the symptoms of APP burnout. Mentoring has been shown to improve job satisfaction by providing connections with colleagues, growing a sense of belonging and community within the work group, decreasing isolation and frustrations during the first year, and increasing retention of highly qualified APPs (Horner, 2017). As organizations struggle with healthcare employee burnout, one solution may lie in mentorship among care providers as an effective way to contribute to a satisfactory work/life balance and overall wellness (Osman & Gottlieb, 2018). There are professional and personal benefits associated with mentorship for both the mentor and mentee, including personal fulfilment in giving back, renewed interest in their career, and a stronger feeling of empowerment as a professional (Burgess et al., 2018). Multidisciplinary/interprofessional mentorship among groups of varying healthcare disciplines help to promote and strengthen collaborative team-based care (Henry-Noel et al., 2019). Additional benefits include:

- Building and expanding professional network
- Promoting professional learning and development
- Practicing coaching and giving/receiving constructive feedback
- Support for identifying and working towards goals
- Learning about coaching and effective meeting management skills
- Growing a mutually beneficial relationship

It is important to make a distinction between the role of preceptor and mentor. Although both require similar skills, they serve a different purpose in supporting an APP's transition into clinical practice (Moss & Jackson, 2019). A clinical preceptor is a physician or peer APP who facilitates the steps towards clinical competency, providing procedural opportunity, training, and didactic content for a specified period. The end goal from the preceptor perspective is satisfaction that the APP demonstrates top-of-license practice. Mentoring occurs when an experienced member of the healthcare team (mentor) is assigned to an APP (mentee) to provide professional guidance in adjusting to their role and assist with assimilating to the organization and department. Mentoring is focused on helping adapt to the work environment and navigate role expectations, rather than teaching technical clinical competency.

Organizational support is crucial for success and often starts with an internal champion or mentoring committee to provide oversight, develop the program, and address barriers (Moss & Jackson, 2019). Whether developing an organization-wide program or implementing a mentoring toolkit, it is helpful to have a designated person or persons (committee) who ensure consistency and provide a standard curriculum and general program oversight. Having a designated person or committee also affords the opportunity to:

- Serve as the point of contact if there are any issues, dilemmas, or concerns about the program, mentee, or mentors

- Solicit feedback from participants throughout the program

- Provide training, guidance, and communicate all aspects of the program to team members

TRAINING

Mentoring plays an important role in guiding the transition to practice for new APPs. Mentor relationships have been linked with improved role transition and may positively influence self-confidence (Anglin et al., 2021). A peer mentor helps their partner strategize and increase self-awareness in areas such as job performance, working relationships, and personal satisfaction with work. An effective peer mentor listens, gathers information, provides honest and constructive feedback, creates a vision for change, and motivates an individual to action. APPs entering clinical practice rely on experienced colleagues to teach, guide, shape, and support the newest graduates through mentoring (Moss & Jackson, 2019). Professional organizations have recognized the importance of mentoring within the profession as it is an expectation of the American Association of Colleges of Nursing (AACN) that mentoring future generations of NPs is the responsibility of current advanced practice nurses (AACN, 2006).

Mentoring participants should be in good standing, having completed their orientation and onboarding, and have the appropriate level of support through the process. An ideal mentee candidate should be early in their role, yet far enough along that they understand or have observed some of the organizational culture and norms and have a solid sense of the expectations of their clinical orientation.

APPs may be eager to start their mentoring relationships but may also have hesitations about the process if they are unfamiliar with or new to a mentoring program. A best practice for implementation of a formalized program would include time and resources for participant training (Moss & Jackson, 2019). The effectiveness of a program relies on both the mentor and mentee having clear understanding about expectations and outcomes, what the program and their participation entails, and how it is different from a preceptor or supervisor role (Stoeger et al., 2021).

MENTORING PROGRAM IMPLEMENTATION STEPS

- Identify and name desired outcomes from mentoring program
- Determine ROI (return on investment) and success metrics
- Develop program guide and curriculum based on desired outcomes
- Develop communication plan
- Communicate program details and select participants
- Train mentors and mentees
- Check in with mentors/mentees throughout the program
- Survey attendees post-program to obtain feedback
- Make any necessary adjustments to the program

THE MENTOR ROLE

The mentor is responsible for providing new APPs with a solid foundation for independent or collaborative practice, improving integration into the department and the organization, and assisting with the new APP's professional growth (Barker & Kelley, 2020; Higgins & Newby, 2020; Jackson, 2020). The mentor attributes are as follows:

- Experienced APP or member of the multidisciplinary healthcare team
- Provides information, advice, support, and encouragement
- Guides by example through their expertise and experience
- Helps to grow the new APP's professional network
- Trusted advisor and champion

MENTOR RESPONSIBILITIES AND EXPECTATIONS

- Be available to your mentee.

- Reach out to welcome them to the program.

- Introduce yourself.

- Schedule your first and subsequent meetings.

- Make time and the commitment to regularly connect with your mentee both during and outside of your scheduled meetings.

- Share your expectations, professional goals, and career interests.

- Build trust. Lead by example. Foster a supportive environment.

- Keep confidence. Be sensitive to information that your mentee may share privately.

MENTEE RESPONSIBILITIES AND EXPECTATIONS

- Be open to receive information, advice, support, and encouragement.

- Be responsive to the expertise and experience of mentor.

- Be willing to grow professional network.

- Demonstrate willingness to assume responsibility for your own professional growth.

The mentor and mentee can each expect growth and evolution of their professional relationship through the mentoring program (Eller et al., 2014). At first the interpersonal interaction may be formal and cautious as both begin to get to know each other. Over time, as the two continue to meet, the relationship strengthens and trust grows, a key aspect of a beneficial partnership (Eller et al., 2014). Appendix R provides examples of professional correspondence between APPs involved in the mentor program and can be edited accordingly to be more personal and aligned with each organization's program goals.

In some instances, the mentoring partners do not evolve, grow, and strengthen, "and the result is a decline in the mentoring relationship. Generally, this occurs when there is a lack of time invested by one or both individuals, a mispairing, or if there is a breach of trust (Ocobock et al., 2022). It is difficult to grow a trusting relationship when the mentoring partners fail to develop rapport or demonstrate mutual respect. If a breakdown in trust occurs (e.g., one partner breaking issues of confidentiality), the mentoring partnership may need to conclude. The individuals with program oversight should periodically touch base with the participants to ensure the program is on track and the relationship is growing as expected. A contact individual should be identified for the participants to provide concerns and feedback should this become necessary through the course of the program.

MENTORING AGREEMENTS

Establishing an agreement to outline key expectations for a mutually beneficial relationship reinforces commitment to the program and to each other and positively impacts program success. An agreement addresses which organization policies and protocols apply and defines the boundaries or limits of confidentiality. Trust builds when both parties commit to keeping their conversations between themselves, yet each organization should be clear about the situations when confidentiality cannot be offered or expected. Organizations may have their own protocols for when information should be reported to appropriate leadership or pertinent agencies. Examples of these situations might include when there is immediate risk or harm to self or others, research misconduct, criminal activity, or serious violations of policies. Additionally, all professionals must be aware of mandatory reporting laws within their state.

CURRICULUM

A program guide with established curricula provides a structured roadmap for meeting sessions, each with a theme, discussion topic, resources, and homework. The topics and curricula should be designed to support organizational initiatives, ensure conversations are professionally focused, and provide themes and topics beneficial to participants and to the organization. The focus on the program, and in most cases the reason the APPs choose to participate, is to build relationships. Having the questions, themes, and resources established in advance reduces the administrative burden for mentors and allows them to focus entirely on the relationship.

Themes should be specific enough to keep the conversation focused, but not too specific to prevent a free- flowing, interactive conversation. Themes should build upon each other, starting with getting to know more about each other, setting goals and discussing career paths, and, as the relationship grows, include more personal topics such as work/life balance.

PROGRAM GUIDE

Time should be dedicated within the first few sessions of the program for the participants to become more acquainted with each other. Although many times the APPs have worked together and may have a relationship as coworkers, these first sessions will help transition their relationship from colleagues to mentor/mentee. General icebreaker questions may be provided for this session. It's also important for both parties to have a clear understanding of the mentoring expectations by discussing with each other what they hope to accomplish during the sessions and defining what a successful relationship looks like so that both have realistic and well-aligned expectations. This can be revisited throughout the program to ensure that expectations are being met and make any necessary adjustments to bring things back on course. Appendix S is an example of a complete mentor guide that can be edited and adjusted to align with an organization's objectives for an APP mentorship program.

COMMUNICATION

Clear and consistent communication is a key factor for success and occurs in phases throughout the development of a mentoring program. The basis and return on investment should be defined and communicated to operational leaders. Having templates and guides brings consistency and provides structure for the program. Utilizing consistent messaging ensures a system of accountability for all constituents. Program committees and leaders should periodically check in with participants to discuss any issues with the mentoring participants.

SURVEYS

Each organization will have a process for evaluating the quality of the mentoring program. Ongoing evaluation is key for understanding when the desired outcomes are reached, as well as for making changes and adjustments to the programs to become more effective over time (Stoeger et al.,2021). Evaluation methods may include a pre- and post-participation survey to determine the participants' satisfaction and a method for capturing the program outcomes such as long-term engagement surveys and separate turnover/retention statistics. If skill advancement is part of the mentoring goals, the supervisor may provide feedback on observable changes in technical skills, assessment skills, and interpersonal skills. The methods and data collected will help determine ongoing improvements for the program to align with the intended and expected outcomes.

SUMMARY

Organizations that establish a formal mentoring program with a set curriculum and allow for a supportive professional relationship to evolve between participants will facilitate engaged APPs. This chapter outlines the elements of a formal peer mentoring program that can be used as an example and edited accordingly. As noted from the literature throughout the chapter, having a mentorship program demonstrates the professional support for new APPs that facilitates overall engagement and a feeling of belonging to the organization, which ultimately impacts patient safety, positive patient outcomes, and overall job satisfaction.

REFERENCES

American Association of Colleges of Nursing. (2006, October). *The essentials of doctoral education for advanced nursing practice.* https://www.aacnnursing.org/Portals/42/Publications/DNPEssentials.pdf

Anglin, L., Sanchez, M., Butterfield, R., Rana, R., Everett, C. M., & Morgan, P. (2021). Emerging practices in onboarding programs for PAs: Strategies for onboarding. *JAAPA: Journal of the American Academy of Physician Associates, 34*(1), 32–38. https://doi.org/10.1097/01.JAA.0000723932.21395.74

Barker, E., & Kelley, P. W. (2020). Mentoring: A vital link in nurse practitioner development. *Journal of the American Association of Nurse Practitioners, 32*(9), 621–625. https://doi.org/10.1097/jxx.0000000000000417

Burgess, A., van Diggele, C., & Mellis, C. (2018). Mentorship in the health professions: A review. *The Clinical Teacher, 15*(3), 197–202. https://doi.org/10.1111/tct.12756

Eller, L. S., Lev, E. L., & Feurer, A. (2014, May). Key components of an effective mentoring relationship: A qualitative study. *Nurse Education Today, 34*(5), 815–820. https://doi.org/10.1016/j.nedt.2013.07.020

Henry-Noel, N., Bishop, M., Gwede, C. K., Petkova, E., & Szumacher, E. (2019). Mentorship in medicine and other health professions. *Journal of Cancer Education, 34*(4), 629–637. https://doi.org/10.1007/s13187-018-1360-6

Higgins, K., & Newby, O. (2020). DNP student mentorship: Empowering students and nurse practitioner organizations. *Nurse Practitioner, 45*(4), 42–47. https://doi.org/10.1097/01.NPR.0000657320.35417.d2

Horner, D. K. (2017). Mentoring: Positively influencing job satisfaction and retention of new hire nurse practitioners. *Plastic Surgical Nursing, 37*(1), 7–22. https://doi.org/10.1097/psn.0000000000000169

Jackson, D. C. (2020, April). Evaluation of a mentor's training program for nurse practitioners. *The Journal for Nurse Practitioners, 16*(4), 286–289. https://doi.org/10.1016/j.nurpra.2019.12.006

Kapu, A. N., Card, E. B., Jackson, H., Kleinpell, R., Kendall, J., Lupear, B. K., & Dubree, M. (2021). Assessing and addressing practitioner burnout: Results from an advanced practice registered nurse health and well-being study. *Journal of the American Association of Nurse Practitioners, 33*(1), 38–48. https://doi.org/10.1097/JXX.0000000000000324

Moss, C., & Jackson, J. (2019). Mentoring new graduate nurse practitioners. *Neonatal Network, 38*(3), 151–159. https://doi.org/10.1891/0730-0832.38.3.151

Ocobock, C., Niclou, A., Loewen, T., Arslanian, K., Gibson, R., & Valeggia, C. (2022). Demystifying mentorship: Tips for successfully navigating the mentor-mentee journey. *American Journal of Human Biology, 34*(S1), e23690. https://doi.org/10.1002/ajhb.23690

Osman, N. Y., & Gottlieb, B. (2018). Mentoring across differences. *MedEdPORTAL, 14*(10743). https://doi.org/10.15766/mep_2374-8265.10743

Seehusen, D. A., Rogers, T. S., Al Achkar, M., & Chang, T. (2021). Coaching, mentoring, and sponsoring as career development tools. *Family Medicine, 53*(3), 175–180. https://journals.stfm.org/familymedicine/2021/march/seehusen-2020-0341/

Stoeger, H., Balestrini, D. P., & Ziegler, A. (2021). Key issues in professionalizing mentoring practices. *Annals of the New York Academy of Sciences, 1483*(1), 5–18. https://doi.org/10.1111/nyas.14537

"Empowering those around you to be heard and valued makes the difference between a leader who simply instructs and one who inspires."

—Adena Friedman, Nasdaq CEO

CHAPTER 14

METRICS THAT MATTER

KEYWORDS | productivity metrics, documentation, patient satisfaction, RVU, bundled payment

APPs provide a high degree of value and contribute to improvements in patient access, patient safety and quality, physician productivity, patient throughput, continuity of care, and length of stay (Moote et al., 2011). Identifying and measuring APP value and productivity helps to demonstrate their return on investment, yet most healthcare organizations report difficulty in tracking these metrics (Moote et al., 2011). Productivity is often aligned and measured with revenue-generating activities such as relative value units [RVUs], yet this measurement alone does not account for the value of services provided by APPs that enhance patient care (Winter et al., 2020). When analyzing output from APPs, both value and productivity must be considered.

Capturing value and productivity from the work that APPs perform can be challenging. Organizations utilize APPs in multiple specialties and locations and often have various practice models. Although this speaks to the versatility of the APP role and their advanced skill set, it makes it challenging to develop standard productivity metrics to capture return on investment. Creatively capturing APP value and productivity requires innovative and thoughtful approaches to separate the work performed by APPs from the work performed by other members of the healthcare team. Well-defined role expectations provide clarity and focus for the APP, especially when RVU attribution or other direct cause-and-effect relationships are not possible to demonstrate productivity.

Understanding the expectations surrounding practice models, caseload expectations, scope of practice, communication, teamwork, and non-clinical responsibilities is important for projecting potential metrics that demonstrate effectiveness of the APP. This chapter will provide examples of analyzing APP productivity and value in a variety of settings and practice models. This may be challenging, particularly for APPs who practice in inpatient or procedural settings or do not see patients independently, generating RVUs; however, organizations must continue to strive to establish metrics that can be evaluated and (at the very least) described so all team members understand APP role expectations.

APP inpatient productivity metrics that are supported in the literature include increasing patient throughput, improving patient safety and quality, reducing length of stay, improving patient satisfaction, and improving continuity of care (Aiken et al., 2021; Kapu et al., 2014; Kleinpell et al., 2008; Kuriakose et al., 2022; Liego et al., 2014; Moote et al., 2011). Other examples that have significant potential to demonstrate APP value include increasing physician productivity and improving complication or comorbidity (CC) and major complication or comorbidity (MCC) documentation.

VALUE METRICS

- Improve access for patients
- Increase physician productivity
- Reduce length of stay [LOS]
    - Assist with patient throughput
- Improve patient satisfaction
    - Continuity and communication
- Improve documentation

RVU ATTRIBUTION FOR BUNDLED PAYMENTS

Some specialties practice with a bundled payment structure, which can be exceptionally challenging to portray the return on investment for APPs. In a specialty service where APPs may see a variety of patient types requiring pre- and post-op encounters, the RVU attribution varies within that specialty. RVU attribution is a method used by government programs and private insurance companies to determine how much to pay for services rendered, with RVU payments higher for performing complicated medical care procedures or treating complex patients. Payer mix influences RVUs: workers' compensation cases are typically at a higher RVU rate and Medicare/Medicaid at a lower rate for the same services.

A department with bundled services, where APPs see pre- and post-op patients (with no RVUs), may have low overall RVUs. Measuring only collections does not give the full picture of the value of APPs seeing pre- and post-op patients, which ultimately frees up surgeons' time for OR and other activities. Figure 14.1 demonstrates only collections and salary and is a flawed and potentially misleading method of calculating APP productivity, because it does not include the value added by an APP providing non-RVU (bundled) services.

A more effective method calculates the total output generated by the APP, including APP split/shared (direct) encounters, indirect RVUs (patients seen independently by an APP), and an estimate of the output for non-RVU generating pre-/post-op encounters. Figure 14.2 details this method. This analysis begins by calculating the average RVU generated among all APPs within the specialty ($89.71 in the example). Next, the total output is calculated by adding the APP's share of the direct (split/shared) RVUs, the indirect RVUs, and number of pre-/post-op encounters. The total output is multiplied by the average RVU to determine an estimated dollar output.

Team	Collections From RVU Generating Activities	Salary	Net Collections (Collections-Salary)	
APP 1	$ 55,817	$ 100,000	(44,183)	
APP 2	$ 38,689	$ 100,000	(61,311)	Incomplete
APP 3	$ 67,258	$ 100,000	(32,742)	analysis as non-
APP 4	$ 11,104	$ 100,000	(88,896)	RVU generating
APP 5	$ 146,319	$ 100,000	46,319	activities (such as
APP 6	$ 98,355	$ 100,000	(1,645)	pre-op/post-op
APP 7	$ 89,375	$ 100,000	(10,625)	bundled visits)
APP 8	$ 74,921	$ 100,000	(25,079)	are missing from
APP 9	$ 109,024	$ 100,000	9,024	this analysis
APP 10	$ 66,126	$ 100,000	(33,874)	
Average	$ 75,699	$ 100,000	(24,301)	

FIGURE 14.1 Analyzing collections only.

To capture the APP portion of the split/shared encounters (direct RVUs), the organization estimated a 60/40 split between physician/APP and applied the 40% portion to APPs. Each organization can determine what split/shared percentage is a best estimate.

Additionally, for simplicity purposes, the pre-/post-op encounters were assigned a 1.0 RVU. The organization may use a factor other than 1.0 as appropriate.

This method provides a more accurate measure of the overall output an APP provides within the department. Multiplying the RVU output by the average RVU for the APP team determines the total output in dollars, which can then be compared to the APP salary expenses to determine the net contribution.

Although these are "pseudo RVUs," attributed in the example as output, the intention is to provide quantifiable data that demonstrates the non-RVU-generating encounters when APPs see patients in the pre- and post-op setting. This demonstrates the value of APPs using revenue modeling that could easily be translated to increase physician productivity and value to the organization.

Estimate APP portion
of Split/Shared
(example: 40% of total
↓

| Team | $/RVU | Estimating Output | | | | | $ Output Output * $89.71 | Salary | Net Output (Output-Salary) |
		Direct RVUs Split/Shared (APP Share)	Indirect RVUs	# Encounters pre-op	# Encounters post-op	Total Output			
APP 1	$ 61.34	32	1060	129	289	1510	$ 135,462	$ 100,000	$ 35,462
APP 2	$ 62.77	33	1062	98	206	1399	$ 125,504	$ 100,000	$ 25,504
APP 3	$ 82.58	20	501	646	239	1406	$ 126,132	$ 100,000	$ 26,132
APP 4	$ 49.09	72	454	200	375	1101	$ 98,771	$ 100,000	$ (1,229)
APP 5	$ 126.25	244	984	224	153	1605	$ 143,985	$ 100,000	$ 43,985
APP 6	$ 69.13	88	740	176	59	1063	$ 95,362	$ 100,000	$ (4,638)
APP 7	$ 84.98	14	699	352	78	1143	$ 102,539	$ 100,000	$ 2,539
APP 8	$ 74.29	91	610	823	99	1623	$ 145,599	$ 100,000	$ 45,599
APP 9	$ 193.34	143	508	240	179	1070	$ 95,990	$ 100,000	$ (4,010)
APP 10	$ 93.31	435	398	815	124	1772	$ 158,966	$ 100,000	$ 58,966
Average	$ 89.71	117	702	370	180	1369	$ 122,831	$ 100,000	$ 22,831

↑
Average
RVU

Each pre/post op
encounter = 1 output

FIGURE 14.2 Estimating APP output.

IMPACT ON PATIENT SATISFACTION

The Press Ganey Medical Practice survey is the most commonly used survey for outpatient satisfaction in the US (Presson et al., 2017). Increasingly, healthcare organizations are initiating communication skills training for practicing healthcare providers, recognizing the link between effective communication and patient satisfaction and outcomes (Pedersen et al., 2021). Patient satisfaction and experience is another measurement that can demonstrate when APPs contribute positively to the aggregate patient satisfaction scores.

Both the APP and physician, through their communication with patients, can promote a sense of mutual respect and trust that will then carry over to the patient's perception of a confident team. Using similar terminology when referencing APPs is an important concept to familiarize patients to view APPs as providers. For example, using terms such as "physicians" instead of "providers" and not specifically mentioning the APP title can be confusing to the patient completing the survey and may make it difficult to attribute the data to the APP. As with many of these examples, the goal is not to compare APPs to physicians, but rather to demonstrate APP contributions using a variety of metrics.

IMPROVING DOCUMENTATION AND LENGTH OF STAY

Historically it has been challenging to measure and quantify APP productivity on the inpatient services. APPs are frequently utilized on inpatient units in a hospitalist role to strategically address the bulleted issues in the following list (Anen & McElroy, 2017; Gilliland et al., 2016; Kleinpell et al., 2019). These examples demonstrate how APPs can be impactful in the inpatient setting and accentuate the work effort required resulting from APP productivity when they are functioning in unique, but top-of-license roles:

- Assuring accurate documentation in compliance with International Classification of Diseases (ICD) codes

- Decreasing length of stay and improving patient throughput

- Increasing physician productivity

- Attending inpatient huddles for patient continuity, assisting with patient admissions and timely discharges

- Performing procedures

- Evaluating test results

- Communicating changes in plans of care to healthcare team and family members

- Making appropriate referrals and follow up on consults

- Following/developing clinical practice guidelines in specialty areas

Increasingly, the literature has supported inpatient APP metrics surrounding cost avoidance (Kapu et al., 2014), which are challenging to attribute specifically to individuals or teams of APPs. Developing dashboards that allow for the ongoing evaluation of metrics such as expected length of stay compared to actual length of stay, discharge times, etc., allow the ability to capture the impact of APPs. This would be valuable when comparing models of APPs utilized in inpatient units with inpatient units where there are no APPs. Once metrics are identified that demonstrate the value and impact of APPs on inpatient units, the greater the opportunity to replicate the model of care in other areas.

- Clinical units, one staffed with APPs and one without, to compare the difference in length of stay per organizational goals and metrics

- Clinical units with the exact same patient types, diagnosis, clinical composition—one staffed with APPs and one without—to demonstrate cause and effect

COMORBIDITY AND MAJOR COMORBIDITY DOCUMENTATION CAPTURE

Role expectations for an inpatient APP may include management of patients, facilitating and expediting patient discharges, and management of inpatient care bundles. Another example of measuring inpatient productivity related to providing continuity of care and improved overall documentation is the rate of documenting CC and MCC.

The Centers for Medicare & Medicaid Services (CMS) classifies inpatient discharges by Diagnosis Related Group (DRG) and adjusts payments based on the weighting factors assigned to each DRG which considers the level of resources needed to care for patient treatment within that DRG (CMS, 2023). Medicare/Medicaid reimbursement rates are higher for patients with DRG indicating CC/MCC. Tracking the rate at which a CC/MCC is present in provider documentation allows for a comparison of the CC/MCC capture rate among providers over time and may demonstrate when APPs' involvement with documentation results in higher reimbursement.

Figure 14.3 shows a summary of the CC/MCC capture rate in an inpatient unit at University of Iowa Health Care from May 2016 through March 2018. Notice that over time there were periodic dips in the capture rate. Further analysis determined that the dips aligned with the only APP in the unit having time off work (vacation, etc.). Given the unique staffing model where there is only one APP on this inpatient unit, it was observed that when the APP was absent, there were considerable coinciding differences in CC/MCC DRG documentation. For example:

- When the APP is absent 10 or more business days in a month, the CC/MCC capture rate was 65.0%.

- When the APP is absent nine or fewer business days in a month, the CC/MCC capture rate is 78.2%.

- The estimated difference in Medicare reimbursement for a single DRG group (329–331) alone based upon this 13% difference is approximately $140,000 (based on 2017 data).

This analysis illustrates that when demonstrating the productivity of APPs, there may be opportunities to look at work output comparisons when the APPs are not present relative to the value of when they are present. In this case:

- This DRG group reflects only a fraction of the care the service provides.

- If the APP were not functioning in this role, the additional documentation analysis described above would not be done; therefore, the CC/MCC capture rate would be much lower than 65%.

- Thus, the total reimbursement increase by employing an APP to conduct documentation review is likely multiples of this number.

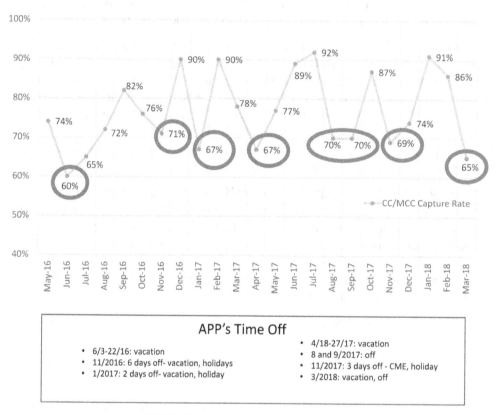

FIGURE 14.3   Department CC/MCC capture rate.

To continue with the analysis and quantify the financial impact of having an inpatient APP functioning in this role, a Medicare Dollar Opportunity benchmark is applied. A Medicare Dollar Opportunity indicates potential for reimbursement for CC/MCC capture rate at the 75th percentile based on the University of Iowa Health Care benchmarking group (Vizient, 2023). Figure 14.4 assigns the Medicare Dollar Opportunity gained by having the APP capturing CC/MCC, and the lost opportunity due to the absence of the APP and the significant dollar opportunities that could have been billed.

Again, these examples may not be easily obtained and require work effort, but this example opens the discussion for operational leaders and APPs to be creative and think of ways to capture the productivity and value of APPs by identifying and analyzing quality metrics comparing time periods when APPs are absent as well as present from inpatient units.

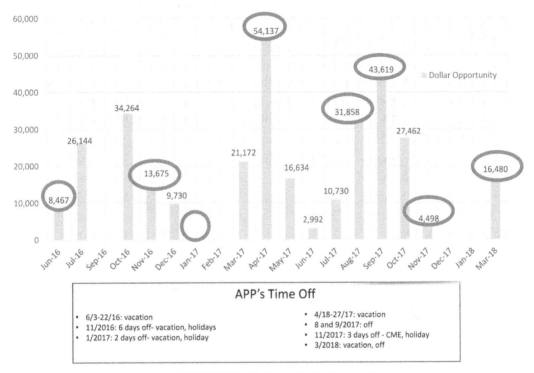

FIGURE 14.4   Medicare Dollar Opportunity.

ELECTRONIC HEALTH RECORD TOUCHES

In clinical situations, APPs may serve in hybrid roles in both outpatient and inpatient services, making it difficult to capture the impact of APP productivity. The daily activities and role expectations of an inpatient/outpatient hybrid APP may include first call for general inpatients and emergency department consults, inpatient rounding, patient exams, progress notes, order placement, discharge planning, discharges, communication with consulting teams (both for primary patients and consults), multidisciplinary bed huddles, procedures, family care conferences, add-on outpatient clinic patients, and assistance with nurse coordinator triage/outpatient phone calls and orders.

Due to the varied functions of the hybrid role, productivity is unable to be captured using RVUs. One way to measure value in this instance would be perform an EHR audit. University of Iowa Health Care performed this analysis over a one-week time frame for one hybrid APP, which showed that the APP had over 5,000 hits or touches to the EHR, all determined to be top-of-license activities.

There is no benchmark data to demonstrate the "normal" number of times per week an average provider was in the EHR; thus the APP's EHR touches were compared to the EHR touches by other providers for that same week.

Figure 14.5 demonstrates the comparison of touches in the EHR for the same week and indicates the APP EHR touch volume is twice the number of the physician resident and fellow and 5–10 times the amount of the faculty physician. This demonstrates APP touches in the EHR are a value add because it frees up time for physicians, ultimately increasing their productivity.

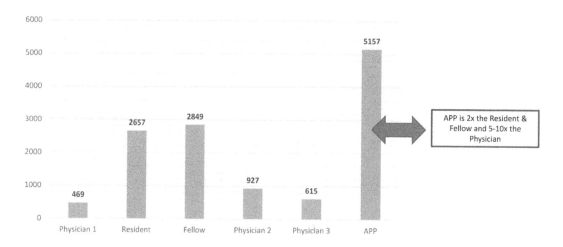

Definition of Audit Trail
any orders/labs/notes/media/reports/diagnosis/documents/flowsheets reviewed, orders made/reconciled, problem list accessed/changed, notes written/pended/signed, and In Basket requests viewed/responded to

FIGURE 14.5   EHR touches in one week.

Comparing the number of RVUs for the same week between the physicians and the APP demonstrates that although the APP was doing 5–10 times the touches in the EHR, they were also receiving 100–250 times less RVU attributions as in Figure 14.6, again demonstrating significantly increased physician productivity because of the APP.

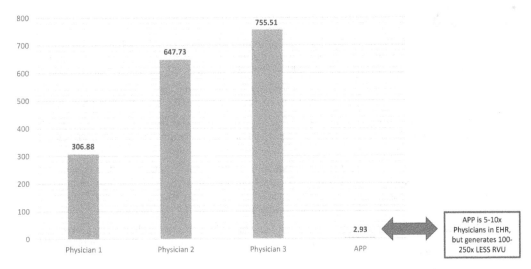

Same Physicians and APP (Resident and Fellow removed, non RVU generating)

FIGURE 14.6   Work RVUs generated.

SUMMARY

Organizational leaders should develop the role expectations and productivity metrics to quantify the return on investment for APPs as part of the care team. The metrics will vary based on the clinical setting. For example, ambulatory metrics are typically centered around improving patient access with a clearly defined patient panel and schedule template, and a work schedule geared towards optimizing an APP's patient-facing time. This is a simpler metric to quantify, but the value-added work of APPs in other settings is also valuable, just more challenging to quantify.

Capturing APP productivity in the inpatient units has been challenging and may include analyzing the work that would not be done if APPs were not present, as was illustrated in the CC/MCC capture rate example. It is imperative for leaders to continue to approach ideas and metrics with an open mind and think nontraditionally on how to capture productivity by billable APP providers that don't have a direct cause-and-effect relationship. The versatility in the ways APPs function in the healthcare system is a key value to the role and is essential to high-quality care. Striving to attribute the productivity of APPs in all areas of healthcare requires creative analysis.

REFERENCES

Aiken, L. H., Sloane, D. M., Brom, H. M., Todd, B. A., Barnes, H., Cimiotti, J. P., Cunningham, R. S., & McHugh, M. D. (2021). Value of nurse practitioner inpatient hospital staffing. *Medical Care, 59*(10), 857–863. https://doi.org/10.1097/mlr.0000000000001628

Anen, T., & McElroy, D. (2017). The evolution of the new provider team: Driving cultural change through data. *Nursing Administration Quarterly, 41*(1), 4–10. https://doi.org/10.1097/naq.0000000000000202

Centers for Medicare & Medicaid Services. (2023, April 10). *MS-DRG classifications and software.* https://www.cms.gov/medicare/medicare-fee-for-service-payment/acuteinpatientpps/ms-drg-classifications-and-software

Gilliland, J., Donnellan, A., Justice, L., Moake, L., Mauney, J., Steadman, P., Drajpuch, D., Tucker, D., Storey, J., Roth, S. J., Koch, J., Checchia, P., Cooper, D. S., & Staveski, S. L. (2016). Establishment of pediatric cardiac intensive care advanced practice provider services. *World Journal for Pediatric & Congenital Heart Surgery, 7*(1), 72–80. https://doi.org/10.1177/2150135115611356

Kapu, A. N., Kleinpell, R., & Pilon, B. (2014). Quality and financial impact of adding nurse practitioners to inpatient care teams. *JONA: Journal of Nursing Administration, 44*(2), 87–96. https://doi.org/10.1097/nna.0000000000000031

Kleinpell, R. M., Ely, E. W., & Grabenkort, R. (2008). Nurse practitioners and physician assistants in the intensive care unit: An evidence-based review. *Critical Care Medicine, 36*(10), 2888–2897. https://doi.org/10.1097/CCM.0b013e318186ba8c

Kleinpell, R. M., Grabenkort, W. R., Kapu, A. N., Constantine, R., & Sicoutris, C. (2019). Nurse practitioners and physician assistants in acute and critical care: A concise review of the literature and data 2008–2018. *Critical Care Medicine, 47*(10), 1442–1449. https://doi.org/10.1097/ccm.0000000000003925

Kuriakose, C., Stringer, M., Ziegler, A., Hsieh, C., Atashroo, M., Hendershott, J., Tippett, V., Shah, D., Cianfichi, L., Katznelson, L., & Mahoney, M. (2022). Optimizing care teams by leveraging advanced practice providers through strategic workforce planning. *JONA: Journal of Nursing Administration, 52*(9), 474–478. https://doi.org/10.1097/nna.0000000000001185

Liego, M., Loomis, J., Van Leuven, K., & Dragoo, S. (2014). Improving outcomes through the proper implementation of acute care nurse practitioners. *JONA: Journal of Nursing Administration, 44*(1), 47–50. https://doi.org/10.1097/nna.0000000000000020

Moote, M., Krsek, C., Kleinpell, R., & Todd, B. (2011). Physician assistant and nurse practitioner utilization in academic medical centers. *American Journal of Medical Quality, 26*(6), 452–460. https://doi.org/10.1177/1062860611402984

Pedersen, K., Brennan, T. M. H., Nance, A. D., & Rosenbaum, M. E. (2021). Individualized coaching in health system-wide provider communication training. *Patient Education & Counseling, 104*(10), 2400–2405. https://doi.org/10.1016/j.pec.2021.06.023

Presson, A. P., Zhang, C., Abtahi, A. M., Kean, J., Hung, M., & Tyser, A. R. (2017). Psychometric properties of the Press Ganey® Outpatient Medical Practice Survey. *Health and Quality of Life Outcomes, 15*, 32. https://doi.org/10.1186/s12955-017-0610-3

Vizient. (2023). *Vizient clinical data base user manual.* https://www.vizientinc.com/what-we-do/operations-and-quality/clinical-data-base

Winter, S., Chan, G., Kuriakose, C., Duderstadt, K., Spetz, J., Hsieh, D., Platon, C., & Chapman, S. (2020). Measurement of nonbillable service activities by nurse practitioners, physician assistants, and clinical nurse specialists in ambulatory specialty care. *Journal of the American Association of Nurse Practitioners, 33*(3), 211–219. https://doi.org/10.1097/JXX.0000000000000439

"Alone we can do so little; together we can do so much."
–Helen Keller

CHAPTER 15

TEAM-BASED CARE

KEYWORDS | teams, value, policy, revenue

Numerous factors contribute to the complexity of healthcare delivery, including multiple constituencies often with divergent priorities and incentives. Patients want access to providers who listen to their needs and provide excellent outcomes. Providers want to curate their patient populations and to have decision-making autonomy and a pool of competent resources. Staff want to be treated equitably and respectfully with enough coworkers to manage the workload. Administrators want to have a positive budget or bottom line to keep the enterprise afloat. Payers want low utilization and high-quality outcomes. Accreditation bodies want adherence to process metrics. It's challenging to align efforts towards a common organizational vision and a team-based approach. Despite these individual challenges and desires, it is imperative for health systems to develop innovative care delivery models that will make a significant impact as we move into the future.

Other industries, such as manufacturing, have seen tremendous efficiency gains over the past century. There is voluminous literature on the benefits of process improvements, such as organizing and optimizing product design, assembly, and packaging to increase throughput without significantly increasing expense. This has been successful in part because disparate groups have been able to align and work collaboratively to a clearly articulated goal. The value of standard work and continual process improvement have been mainstays of the mark toward high efficiency and reliability. The challenge for healthcare is patients cannot be viewed as products on an assembly line, and providers/staff cannot be viewed as interchangeable workers along the production line. The goal cannot be defined as how quickly a patient encounter can be completed at rock bottom cost. Quality and safety cannot be lost or sacrificed, even with efforts to standardize processes to gain efficiencies.

Team composition will by necessity vary by specialty and setting. The traditional nurse and physician as a team has been expanded greatly with the addition of APPs. In some circumstances, physicians have limited understanding of the scope of practice of APPs and only support APP work to be performed similar to traditional nursing roles. Medical and nursing assistants entered healthcare systems many years ago, but depending on the clinical specialty, other disciplines may also be well suited to support the team. Paramedics may be helpful not only in emergency rooms and urgent cares, but infusion centers can also frequently benefit from their training and expertise. In the orthopedic world, published reports have focused on carefully matching the needs of the provider with the skills of team members (Milewski et al., 2022). If the desire is to improve productivity with the EHR, using scribes or medical assistants serving in their designated roles based on their education background is more beneficial and fiscally responsible than using APPs for activities that are not top of license. Cast room assistants or athletic trainers may be even more beneficial if ambulatory throughput for individual providers is an issue. Primary care has seen benefit in team-based care both in fee-for-service access metrics but also in the transition to value-based ones (Teisberg et al., 2020). These interventions have been well documented to improve provider well-being while at the same time improving access and even staff engagement (American Medical Association, 2023). These team structures lead to employees feeling more positive about their work, with higher job satisfaction and less turnover (Brooks & Fulton, 2020).

HEALTH MANAGEMENT AND POLICY

Health management and policy guides the direction of organizations to ensure the implementation of programs such as improving accessibility to services, overall health conditions for designated populations, provider well-being, patient satisfaction, and lowering healthcare costs. The Institute for Healthcare Improvement created the Quadruple Aim to summarize the key challenges identified in the US healthcare system. These four aims specifically included better outcomes, improved provider experience, lower costs, and improved patient experience (Bachynsky, 2020). Health policy promoting reimbursement for team-based care is vital to improving outcomes and has significant impact that shape interprofessional collaboration for optimal use of the skills of all health professionals working together as a team to deliver comprehensive, integrated care. Healthcare systems that support team-based care, as part of the Team Strategies and Tools to Enhance Performance and Patient Safety (TeamSTEPPS) model or a version of their own organizational integrated teams, support a culture where interprofessional care delivery is the expected standard. Patient care models should integrate policies that support optimal healthcare delivery.

REVENUE CYCLE MANAGEMENT

Providers, including APPs, influence the revenue cycle process through their activities that contribute to the charge capture, management, and timely collection of patient service revenue. Historically, revenue cycle has not been part of a team-based approach. As healthcare organizations evolve to a more collaborative model, opportunities exist for revenue cycle leaders to be engaged and part of the team. Revenue cycle/provider collaboration can bring optimization through fee-for-service and quality/value metrics benefiting the entire organization. The complexity of payer reimbursement continues to grow and evolve, accentuating the need for APPs to partner with the revenue cycle team in ensuring they have a full grasp on how their role can assist in the efficiency of the process. Because each step in the revenue cycle is dependent on a previous step, it is vital for the staff and providers to recognize the significant impact they have on each other, the organization, and ultimately on the patients. Ensuring scheduling templates are in place and accurate; open and clear communication between the providers, the

Clinical Documentation Improvement team, and the coders; and adequate training and education on documentation techniques all help to streamline the revenue cycle process. Providers are the most knowledgeable about the care rendered for patients, which in turn is reflected in their documentation so that the organization can bill accurately. The coding team understands payer regulations and coding guidelines, will code based on what the provider documented, and will in turn expect billing to best reflect the performed services. Working as a team, provider and revenue cycle can support each other with training and communication to ensure documentation and coding are appropriate and timely, leading to an efficient and effective outcome.

VALUE THROUGH CONTINUOUS WORKPLACE IMPROVEMENT

Process improvement principles can be applied in healthcare. Historically, the process was optimized for the physician's needs. While the physician continues to be the most expensive resource in the process, that does not justify their needs being met above all others. The real focus should be diverted to the patient's needs and the process improvement principles based on the evidence that demonstrates positive patient outcomes. It is important to engage all staff involved in patient care in order to provide a great patient experience. In this way, patient care ends up being less about a process and more about a group of individuals with different training, experience, and strengths meshing to accomplish improved patient outcomes, which is the essence of team-based care.

One of the keys to a high-functioning healthcare team is clear delineation of various team member roles and responsibilities. Regulatory pressures from payers, accreditation bodies, and other regulatory groups over time have led to incremental adjustments to how care is delivered, but in most enterprises, healthcare delivery processes have not been intentionally organized and planned. This has in part led to tremendous variation in delivery across and within organizations. It is like a sports team that has not created a playbook and just begins every day with some general rules about how to play the game, not cohesively working together, leading to poor outcomes.

As has been discussed in other contexts, there are many considerations when adding APPs to a clinical team. The APP should not be considered a physician extender to follow alongside the physician. Instead, the specific roles and responsibilities within the larger team should be clearly defined, and each member of the team should optimize top-of-license practice. These roles should be matched to the level of education and training of the team member with a mind also toward scope of practice. While all team members may sometimes perform functions generally considered below their license, as a necessary means to make the team flexible, it should not be the norm. Physicians may occasionally need to take vital signs or review a medication list, but if team members are routinely required to perform tasks that are not at the top of their license, engagement in the team and in the enterprise will erode. It is also clear that all providers need to prioritize leadership and advocacy for the team in order to provide an environment of trust, which benefits all involved, including the patient (Guevara et al., 2020; Reddy et al., 2022).

In a team environment, process improvement toward standard work and value stream mapping can be recast in the structure of collective clinical care improvements. This does not reduce the importance of individual accountability, but it does provide a platform to support all team members into a system of process and outcome improvements. Patient satisfaction improvements have been an ongoing challenge to delivery systems. Responsibility for its improvement tends to be placed upon specific disciplines (especially physicians and nurses). Comprehensive multidisciplinary inpatient teams including APP members have been shown to improve patient satisfaction, particularly compared to those with single teams (Will et al., 2019). This may be a result of diversity in approach to patients and improved patient access and also may be equally considered to be an application of process improvement with clearly defined roles and responsibilities instead of historical single disciplinary teams. While patient satisfaction is forefront in multiple organizations, objectives such as inpatient quality and length of stay indices are also likely to show improvement given the right team makeup.

TEAM PROFESSIONAL DEVELOPMENT

Healthcare teams include highly skilled individuals who know their job and have been put together for the benefit of patient care. It may be believed that once healthcare teams are established and deployed they will continue to function at high levels without ongoing team building. Similar to sports teams that regularly practice honing their skills as a team for the game, healthcare providers and staff need time together outside the stressful environment of care delivery to connect, grow trust, and develop rapport. Structured team building activities and communication strategies such as TeamSTEPPS are essential for the sustainability for high functioning teams (Agency for Healthcare Research and Quality, 2017). TeamSTEPPS is a healthcare quality curriculum that allows organizations to improve communication and teamwork skills among healthcare professionals, which has been shown to benefit the work of the team (Buljac-Samardzic et al., 2020). Organizations must integrate such programs to sustain high levels of team functioning in years to come.

IMPLEMENTING TEAM-BASED CARE AT UNIVERSITY OF IOWA HEALTH CARE

Development of a culture of team-based care and process improvement takes time even with the support of and resources from enterprise executive leaders. A sense of urgency exists in healthcare to fix systemic issues to provide higher levels of service to a larger and more diverse patient population. However, providers and staff are prone to fall back into safe, comfortable roles unless there is ongoing support to encourage change. At University of Iowa Health Care (UIHC), family medicine clinics had high patient satisfaction but were struggling with poor staff engagement, provider burnout, lack of accountability, and low clinical volumes. There were no urgent care sites to support patients' needs for care not acute enough for the emergency room, but also difficult to be accommodated in a primary care clinic already filled with scheduled patients. Provider burnout scores were some of the highest in the organization. Change was necessary.

Providers had the philosophy that adding more nurses and physicians was the answer to improvements. Through reviews of national initiatives, such as the American Medical Association Steps Forward, it has been clear that just adding staff to a challenged system was unlikely to provide the desired result. Consequently, leadership started down the pathway of reimagining the primary care system as well as the work within individual clinics. UIHC opened their first ever urgent care site, which outperformed the pro forma expectations. Provider and staff models for urgent care were developed in collaboration with clinical leadership. This approach increased collaboration and inclusivity and reduced care silos and the perception of "us versus them." It forced all the leaders to work together as a team to support different levels of care. The focus has been on what level of care is most appropriate for the patient, and staffing models were developed based on collaboration, avoiding conflict over what number of providers are needed and in what complement. APPs have been critical to the success as they are a constant presence that unites teams together across areas and are seen as trusted partners and independent providers in the care of patients.

Coordinating care across sites was not enough as all providers were struggling to keep up with EHR issues, patient satisfaction, quality metrics, volume expectations, etc. The outdated staffing model of a physician and nurse was falling short. Leadership assembled a core team of nurses and a project manager as a clinical transformation team. The team was trained with the most up-to-date evidence to reimagine work in the outpatient setting. The AMA Steps Forward curriculum, as well as others, were defined as best practice, and TeamSTEPPS outlined an underlying strategy. The team developed a model whereby each 1.0 clinical full-time equivalent (FTE) primary care provider would be supported by:

- 2.0 FTE medical assistants trained for scribing, chart prep, pending orders, health maintenance, and scheduling
- 0.5 FTE RN focused on patient triage, patient education, and care coordination

This strategy has been refined to add productivity metrics that clarify that adult primary care providers meet a 10 patient per four hour session volume to support the staffing model. The providers in the model have increased their patient throughput by 30%, offsetting the expenses of the additional staff. What is even more important is that there have been improvements in staff engagement with lower medical assistant turnover in those clinics, less provider pajama time (taking work home) by the providers, and improved preventive health metrics, all while maintaining high patient satisfaction. The clinical transformation team continues to work closely with those providers who for a variety of reasons have not been able to meet the volume targets associated within the model. A low volume model was subsequently developed with a 1.0 FTE medical assistant and 0.25 FTE RN supporting the provider.

Leadership and support to the team has been crucial in these transitions. Our experience has been that as the model evolves, the entire team begins to see the benefit. Variability exists among teams to fully embrace the volumes; however, the overall workflow burden for the provider is reduced very soon after implementation.

SUMMARY

Team-based care has become a critical approach within healthcare delivery systems with outcomes that are beneficial across multiple dimensions. Demonstrating clear patient outcomes related to team-based care is imperative to positively influence successful healthcare delivery models. Through the impact of outcomes-driven research, development of new interprofessional training programs, team-based clinical practice guidelines, and health policy promoting reimbursement for team care, the overall patient experience can be transformed (Will et al., 2019).

REFERENCES

Agency for Healthcare Research and Quality. (2017, April). *About TeamSTEPPS®*. https://www.ahrq.gov/teamstepps/about-teamstepps/index.html

American Medical Association. (2023, April 18). *Practice innovation strategies: Physician burnout*. AMA Steps Forward. https://www.ama-assn.org/practice-management/ama-steps-forward/practice-innovation-strategies-physician-burnout

Bachynsky, N. (2020). Implications for policy: The Triple Aim, Quadruple Aim, and interprofessional collaboration. *Nursing Forum, 55*(1), 54–64. https://doi.org/10.1111/nuf.12382

Brooks, P. B., & Fulton, M. E. (2020). Driving high-functioning clinical teams: An advanced practice registered nurse and PA optimization initiative. *JAAPA, 33*(6), 1–12. https://doi.org/10.1097/01.Jaa.0000662400.04961.45

Buljac-Samardzic, M., Doekhie, K. D., & van Wingaarden, J. D. H. (2020). Interventions to improve team effectiveness within health care: A systematic review of the past decade. *Human Resources for Health, 18*(2). https://doi.org/10.1186/s12960-019-0411-3

Guevara, R. S., Montoya, J., Carmody-Bubb, M., & Wheeler, C. (2020). Physician leadership style predicts advanced practice provider job satisfaction. *Leadership in Health Services, 33*(1), 56–72. https://doi.org/10.1108/LHS-06-2019-0032

Milewski, M. D., Coene, R., Flynn, J. M., Imrie, M. N., Annabell, L., Shore, B. J., Dekis, J. C., & Sink, E. L. (2022). Better patient care through physician extenders and advanced practice providers. *Journal of Pediatric Orthopedics, 42*(Suppl 1), S18–S24. https://doi.org/10.1097/bpo.0000000000002125

Reddy, S., Todsen, J., & Lee, Y. S. (2022). Physician leadership and advocacy for team-based care. *AMA Journal of Ethics, 24*(9), E853–E859. https://doi.org/10.1001/amajethics.2022.853

Teisberg, E., Wallace, S., & O'Hara, S. (2020). Defining and implementing value-based health care: A strategic framework. *Academic Medicine, 95*(5), 682–685. https://doi.org/10.1097/acm.0000000000003122

Will, K. K., Johnson, M. L., & Lamb, G. (2019). Team-based care and patient satisfaction in the hospital setting: A systematic review. *Journal of Patient-Centered Research and Review, 6*(2), 158–171. https://doi.org/10.17294/2330-0698.1695

"Access to care is now viewed as a primary key to optimizing the value chain within healthcare delivery systems. Absent a concerted, coordinated effort to manage capacity, optimize schedules, prioritize call handling for patients and referring providers, and coordinate transitions of care in the enterprise, the value chain can fracture."

—Woodcock, 2015

CHAPTER 16

PATIENT ACCESS CENTER

KEYWORDS | people, customer service, team-based, collaboration, processes, technology, access, workflows

The Department of Health and Human Services (DHHS) has identified a goal to reduce the proportion of people who can't get medical care when they need it by the year 2030 (USDHHS, 2020). Growth in the APP workforce is a key strategy in increasing patient access to quality healthcare. The value of utilizing a patient access center to support the access and scheduling needs of the patients is crucial to meeting this goal. This includes scheduling to optimize patient access and requires understanding the workflows, processes, capacity, and patient profile for providers. *Patient profiles* include the specific patient populations and scope of practice defined for both APPs and physicians. The access center is part of an optimized healthcare system that includes all people, processes, and technology working in concert to support the ideal patient experience and access to care.

THEME-BASED DEFINITIONS HELP DRIVE A COMMON MODEL

People: Organizational alignment and support; diversity, equity, and inclusion in daily practices and in human resource activities; customer service behaviors; team-focused practices; leadership; mentoring; personal and group accountability; collaboration; relationships; productivity; quality; and closed loop communication

Processes: Standardization of practices across departments; efficient avenues of demand input; external health record collection processes, policies, procedures, and protocols; triage; closed-loop communication for handoffs; escalations; local systems to support staff resilience and engagement

Technology: EHR development for access workflows, automation whenever and wherever possible, health information exchange portals, patient and provider portals, web-based referral and appointment sites, scheduling templates, capacity management and data analytics, workforce management, and telephone systems to support necessary call center technology and patient communication methods

---

COORDINATING PATIENT FLOW

The core business operation of the patient access center is answering calls and scheduling appointments, anchored in strong customer service with a solid understanding of the downstream implications of operational decisions. The access center serves as the first impression to callers, ensuring optimal productivity and satisfaction for the providers, the clinic workflows, the organization's staff, and the community. This is only possible through appropriate training so that decisions are based on a comprehensive understanding of overall relevant operations at every level, from the very first contact.

To have a high-functioning, successful access center, it is essential to have core standard workflows that allow for differentiation between specialties and provider type. This involves policies, procedures, and guidelines surrounding the core business principles of the access center. Examples include standard workflows with the scheduling processes, workflows in the EHR, appointment requests, referral workflows, ownership and accountability, and standards for performance management and productivity. The access center operations should be standardized, and must operate in a centralized function, allowing room for reasonable variances in the operations supporting the individual clinics, departments, physicians, and APPs. Department scheduling guidelines serve as the detailed directions for scheduling and delineate between physician and APP providers. Examples of content in a departmental scheduling guideline for the access center include:

- Provider profiles

- Escalation protocols for patient acuity or urgent needs

- Triage practices

- Outside records requirements

- Specialized "advanced scheduling" directions

These guidelines should be built into the EHR system to promote automation of the system tools as much as possible using guided scheduling, questionnaires, or decision trees. Robust automation leads to decreased dependency on written scheduling guidelines, reduction in scheduling errors, increased efficiencies of scale in cross-coverage, and ultimately will open the door for patient-directed scheduling via a patient EHR portal.

The access specialist, or scheduler, has a key role in patient throughput, the patient experience continuum, and ensuring the plan of care for visits is executed. Patient access is integrated throughout the patient experience with the healthcare system starting from a new patient call to schedule an appointment, to complex routing between healthcare departments and organizations, to shared electronic referral requests for specialty services.

The access specialist manages each one of the inputs and schedules the visits, following workflows developed in the system, as well as following specialty specific guidelines developed by the departments for the following types of scheduling:

- All visit types, all specialties, across all sites of practice

- Incoming referrals

- Telehealth and in-person visits

- Primary care and subspecialties

- Cadence-based procedure and diagnostic testing

Figure 16.1 shows incoming pathways for an appointment, and Figure 16.2 illustrates incoming pathways for a referral appointment.

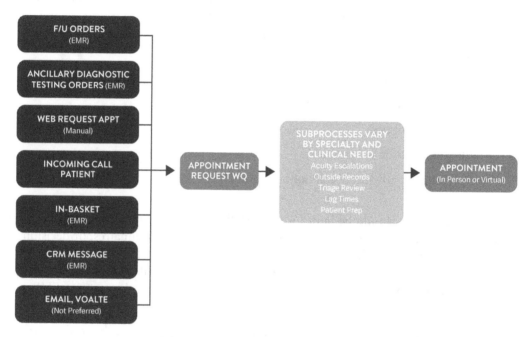

FIGURE 16.1   Incoming pathways for appointment.

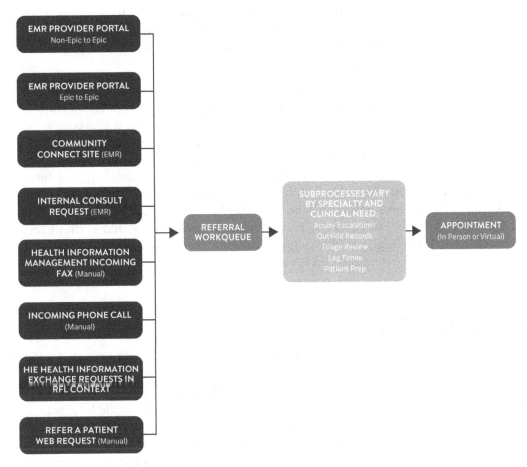

FIGURE 16.2   Incoming pathways for referral appointment.

PATIENT ACCESS COLLABORATIVE

A critical tool for successful operations is defining, measuring, setting goals, and monitoring performance metrics. Networking with national contacts and benchmark organizations is essential in determining targets for goals, as well as ensures the organization is keeping up to date on new operational processes and automations in the access environment. Networking with other sites and benchmarking against others is an element necessary for success, longevity, and outcomes for an access center. One example of an informative and helpful benchmarking group is the Patient Access Collaborative. This group was founded in 2011 by Elizabeth Woodcock and provides an avenue for academic health systems and children's hospitals across the country to join in sharing ideas and data to improve patient access. This group currently represents a collaboration of approximately 100 healthcare organizations, which equate to one of every five outpatient visits across the nation (Woodcock, 2022).

As processes have evolved and technology has advanced, call center capabilities have developed into much more sophisticated operations using new tools and entry points through automation and integration with the EHR. A patient access center (PAC) supports the entire organization, taking on access and scheduling tasks that can be accomplished off-site so the on-site teams can focus on patient care and the customer experience, while the patient is present in the clinical setting. Scheduling guidelines are regularly evaluated and updated with changes including provider types and skill level. This is especially important for the APP role, because they are educated either as generalists or by patient population rather than clinical specialty, and as they gain experience and knowledge, are able to take additional types of patients. A centralized PAC can offer a 24/7 operational team that serves as an access point for both patients and providers.

ROLE CLARIFICATION

The PAC is structured in designated teams of staff trained to be experts in specific areas. The value of a centralized operation should not minimize the importance of efficiencies of scale and cross-training of staff across specialty areas. Each scheduling team may include a designated "lead" who serves as the content expert for the local team and is accountable to ensure the department or clinic-specific scheduling guidelines are regularly updated, and communicate physician and APP practice changes with the team. The lead role would report to and is supported by a patient access coordinator and manager team, which are accountable for a defined set of clinics within the access center. The scope of coverage for the coordinator and manager are similar, but the daily tasks may vary between roles. Key performance qualities necessary for an access coordinator or manager include collaboration, accountability, forward-thinking perspectives, patient access champion mentality, and adaptability to change, while always serving as a patient advocate. Appendices T and U show a job family career ladder and detail role responsibilities and a division of duties.

A centralized PAC is a vital 24/7 service that, without appropriate staffing, would become a barrier for patients receiving care, providers' productivity, and clinical operations. A PAC manager's daily responsibilities are split between managing scheduling teams, collaborating with clinic counterparts, and project work. Managing the scheduling teams includes ensuring staff training and development, daily and monthly monitoring of individual and team performance against established benchmarks, corrective coaching for staff who are underperforming, and providing performance management when warranted.

Operations managers should work collaboratively with clinic counterparts to identify and review potentially inefficient practices or procedures. The PAC manager role has a large emphasis on communication and collaboration as they consult with colleagues to develop optimizations to increase patient access and improve efficiency. The managers are responsible for leading projects focused on employee engagement, PAC initiatives, and enterprise-level projects aligned with the overarching strategic plan to enhance growth.

Most inputs for an access center are received by phone; however, as EHR systems and customer expectations have evolved, the way patients access healthcare is in a constant state of change with an emphasis on more automated pathways being developed such as chat bots, texting, EHR portals, and potentially artificial intelligence.

Consideration should be given to the staffing mix to balance the customer service and efficiency with ensuring the center is not overstaffed. Call centers have historically used a calculation tool called the ErlangC, which is now widely used in healthcare access centers for identifying the full-time equivalent (FTE) staffing needs. This tool is a calculation-based formula that is built on the work of Agner Krarup Erlang, a Danish mathematician and leader in queueing theory in the early 1900s. The ErlangC formula ultimately provides a way to calculate the number of staff resources needed for a defined period of time based on a set of assumptions for the service level goals (Call Centre Helper, 2023). This calculation can provide critical details to operate the access center, including the probability a call waits to be answered, taking into consideration the traffic intensity in the time frame and the number of staff resources available. An example of the Erlang calculator is shown in Figure 16.3.

Type parameters in the boxes below.

The left hand box calculates the number of agents needed to reach a required service level. Use the right hand box if you want to see statistics for the number of agents that you have.

Call Centre Helper Erlang Calculator Version 6.0

This calculator only works up to 600 Agents. For higher volumes please use the online version
https://www.callcentrehelper.com/tools/erlang-calculator/

Calculate the number of agents required to reach an agreed service level:

Incoming calls	400	calls
in a period of	30	minutes
Average Handling Time	257	seconds
Required service level	80.0%	
Probability of target answer time		
Target answer time	20	seconds
Max Occupancy	85.0%	
Shrinkage	30%	

Number of Agents required   #NAME?

Average Handling Time = Average Call Duration + Average time spent in After Call Work (ACW - also known as Wrap-Up time)

Traffic Intensity   57.1   Erlangs

Calculate probability of calls being answered or waiting:

Incoming calls	400	calls
in a period of	30	minutes
Average Handling Time	257	seconds
Target answer time	20	seconds
Number of agents	97	
Traffic Intensity (Erlang)	57.11	

Probability a call waits   #NAME?
Erlang-C Formula

Probability call is answered
in target time (Service Level)   #NAME?

(NB Shrinkage is not included in this calculation, set it to 0%)

Next Page >>

FIGURE 16.3   Erlang calculator.
© Call Centre Helper Erlang Calculator, 2017 (https://www.callcentrehelper.com)

Capacity management is collecting and analyzing the data that drive patient access in today's complex healthcare environment. This practice, and the tools within a capacity management approach, are increasingly driving decision-making.

Data analytics helps us understand how the access center is performing as a key entry point in a patients' care journey. Operational decisions should be data driven and reflect what an access center is not doing, should be doing, or where there can be opportunity to optimize performance on behalf of the physician and APP providers and patients. There are several groupings of key performance indicators (KPIs):

1. Call center metrics:

   a.   Service level (% of time calls are answered at goal)

b. Average speed of answer

c. Abandoned calls

d. Average handle time

2. Staff and HR metrics:

a. Turnover

b. Quality assurance

c. Productivity

d. Staff engagement metrics

3. Access metrics:

a. New patient lag times

b. % of patients seen in defined days (7, 10, or 14 are standard)

c. Schedule and physician and APP utilization (fill rate)

d. Time left on the table

e. Next 3rd available

f. Non-arrival (no-show and late cancellations)

g. Encounters per hour

h. Enterprise-driven cancellations

Capacity management includes not only metrics of supply and demand but also data-driven practices, including physician and APP schedule template build and maintenance. The focus for building scheduling templates should include both how the end user places patients on a schedule and how the template is constructed and maintained in the EHR system. Before engaging with physicians and APPs for a template build, the organization should determine what the most critical rules or guidelines are for ease of use, maximized fill rates based on demand, and standards of practice for how the overall system workflows should function. To improve how the templates function within the system, documentation and education of the guiding principles should occur with each clinical group prior to engaging in build. Other items that may also come into play are the support systems available for the physicians and APPs in the clinic area, such as support staff and room availability.

Template review should be based on the following:

1. Adherence to enterprise scheduling principles

2. Lean approach to build

3. Use of scheduling system tools, focusing on automation

4. Increase in volumes to meet strategic growth plans

5. Increased and simplified access for patients

6. Improve ease of scheduling for end users

Specific templates for APPs should be aligned with the practice model established for the department to best support strategic growth and top-of-license practices. One example includes four primary practice models:

1. APP independently treats new and established patients based on department guidelines

2. APP only treats established patients based on department guidelines

3. APP treats new patients for evaluation, determines if they need to be seen by a surgeon, and manages post-op continuation of care

4. A mixed-hybrid practice model

APP practice models should be established based on state practice laws and organizational bylaws that support the APP to top-of-license practice. Clear guidelines for the access center to operate from are essential in getting the patients seen in a timely manner. Here is a list of scheduling strategies:

- Developing pathways to care with APPs working in partnership with specialists to get patients seen early and integrated into the system without delay

- Allowing APPs to see new patient self-referrals and referrals from non-specialists

- Focusing on the patient experience by allowing first call resolution as often as possible

- Avoiding non-essential handoffs for triage review of patients and EHR review prior to scheduling whenever possible

- Leveraging system tools such as decision trees and patient self-scheduling whenever possible

- Developing clear and concise guidelines for the scheduling team

- Developing patient facing scripting surrounding knowledge about the APP as part of the healthcare team to aid in scheduling discussions and confidence in scheduling with APPs

- Decompressing physician schedules to onboard more complex cases for those physicians

- Open and straightforward templates that enable ease of scheduling and maximized patient access

QUALITY AND SCRIPTING

Quality assurance is a core business function, and in patient access it is measured by patient engagement and satisfaction. It is essential to measure and understand the level of customer service being provided to patients, and what patients experience as they engage with the organization through the patient access center. Measuring key conversation points and focusing on customer service and scheduling accuracy provides a consistently high level of service to patients. Access center calls should be recorded, with a set number of randomized calls evaluated on a periodic basis. Key items in the evaluation include the quality of customer service and the accuracy of the completed scheduling in the EHR. Appendix V provides a sample quality scoring matrix. The organization should also provide scripting prompts for the team. Examples of scripting templates can be found in Appendices W–Z.

Ongoing training and review of quality performance metrics can help address trends related to staff performance. Just-in-time training modules may be used to address emerging issues or local trends with the goal of reversing these before they become habitual or to address an emerging situation. Ad hoc training may be administered for system enhancements such as an upgrade to the EHR or other key technology platforms that require unique training development.

A well-trained, engaged, and quality customer-service-driven access team is a strong organizational asset. To enhance staff retention and limit preventable turnover, consider retention strategies such as engagement surveys; stay interviews; quarterly town hall meetings; remote/hybrid work arrangements; an active staff engagement committee; and increased communication via huddles, debriefs, communication boards throughout the physical site, weekly updates, and a staff-focused monthly newsletter.

Figure 16.4 shows the essential elements of a high-functioning access center.

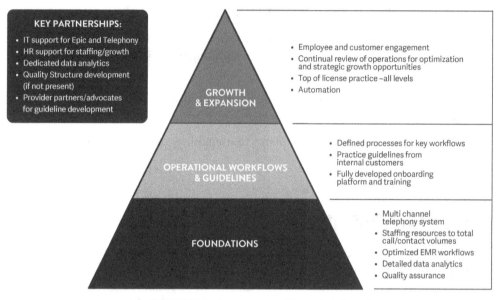

KEY PARTNERSHIPS:

- IT support for Epic and Telephony
- HR support for staffing/growth
- Dedicated data analytics
- Quality Structure development (if not present)
- Provider partners/advocates for guideline development

GROWTH & EXPANSION

- Employee and customer engagement
- Continual review of operations for optimization and strategic growth opportunities
- Top of license practice –all levels
- Automation

OPERATIONAL WORKFLOWS & GUIDELINES

- Defined processes for key workflows
- Practice guidelines from internal customers
- Fully developed onboarding platform and training

FOUNDATIONS

- Multi channel telephony system
- Staffing resources to total call/contact volumes
- Optimized EMR workflows
- Detailed data analytics
- Quality assurance

FIGURE 16.4 Access center hierarchy of needs.

SUMMARY

A patient access center is a complex system, responsible for the first introduction to an organization's healthcare delivery system. A high-functioning access center makes a significant difference and impacts patient access, customers served, and all team members from staff to providers. As the APP workforce continues to grow, patient access centers will integrate the role into the systems for provider optimization. When an access center has organizational support, a solid foundation, and the right staff and leaders to develop processes and technology, it can make a crucial difference in the healthcare delivery system and the potential for future growth of the organization.

REFERENCES

Call Centre Helper. (2023). *Erlang calculation – An introduction.* https://www.callcentrehelper.com/an-introduction-to-erlang-calculations-79806.htm

US Department of Health & Human Services. (2020). *Reduce the proportion of people who can't get medical care when they need it — AHS04.* https://health.gov/healthypeople/objectives-and-data/browse-objectives/health-care-access-and-quality/reduce-proportion-people-who-cant-get-medical-care-when-they-need-it-ahs-04

Woodcock, E. W. (2015). Patient access: Best practices in the ambulatory enterprise. *Group Practice Journal, July/August,* 36–40. https://www.amga.org/performance-improvement/publications/group-practice-journal/archives

Woodcock, E. W. (2022). *Patient access collaborative.* https://www.patientaccesscollaborative.org/

"The road to success is always under construction."
—Lily Tomlin

CHAPTER 17

ORGANIZATIONAL INITIATIVES

KEYWORDS | project management, quality, teams

As APPs continue to span the healthcare industry in essentially every arena, and as healthcare systems strive to capitalize on top-of-license practice, productivity, and excellent patient outcomes, strategic organizational initiatives are paramount to the success of implementing APP projects across organizations. Systemic change occurs when the healthcare system works together to prioritize fully integrating APPs at every level of the organization. Change management can be complex, and using internal project management to support the organization and interested parties is an effective utilization of key resources (Lavoie-Tremblay et al., 2017).

PROJECT MANAGEMENT AND ADMINISTRATIVE OVERSIGHT

Project management involves applying tools and techniques to guide the project work to deliver specific objectives and outcomes (Project Management Institute, 2021). A project manager may be assigned to lead the project team and will plan, manage, control, evaluate, and communicate the project functional group's efforts, from its objective ideation to closing. A project manager serves as a neutral coordinator, an important component of project success in healthcare organizations undergoing transformation (Lavoie-Tremblay et al., 2017). Using organizational resources already in existence to facilitate and collaborate with APP leaders can achieve scheduled targets, scope, and cost (Salapatas, 2000).

THE PROJECT MANAGEMENT INSTITUTE PROJECT FUNCTIONS

- Overseeing and coordinating project work
- Presenting objectives and feedback to interested parties
- Facilitating and supporting the project team through change
- Performing work and contributing insights to the project
- Applying expertise and providing resources and direction
- Maintaining governance of the project

(Project Management Institute, 2021).

The two leading causes of project failure are insufficient involvement of collaborators and infrequent communication with sponsors (Serrador, 2009). To remedy this, project managers develop relationships built on trust and open communication for effective partner management. As with multiple disciplines, APP expertise may be variable or absent within projects. Including APP subject matter experts on the project team will strengthen the knowledge needed to contribute to the project's success. Understanding the commitment to a project and the relationships between different team members as the project progresses is key for successful project implementation (Miller & Oliver, 2015). A designated project manager can gather information from key partners and disseminate it across the teams to prevent duplicate efforts, scope creep, misallocation, and missing milestones, and keep the project focused on important goals and aligned with the organization's overall strategy.

EXAMPLES OF VALUE-ADDED APP PROJECTS

- Improving efficiency, productivity, responsiveness, or effectiveness of patient care, including improving patient access and decreasing length of stay

- Implementing changes needed to transition the organization towards top-of-license practice for APPs

- Creating new and existing services involving APPs, including optimizing practice, throughput, and expanding to underserved areas

---

Using an electronic or cloud-based platform to manage data and track the project status provides a method for clear communication among all project team members. Multiple projects may run concurrently, and consideration should be given to crossover impact and ensuring that project teams are communicating the status of any interrelated objectives.

Feedback and project status should be shared consistently among the project sponsors and team members. Using a cloud-based interface as a shared workplace brings collaboration and communication solutions into a focused workspace available to multiple vested parties. The project team and APP leadership should know where to find project information, have the appropriate access, and know how to use the platform. A shared workspace allows and creates transparent workflows while opening communication and assisting in keeping all partners engaged. The ideal platform achieves an improved ability to collaborate through sharing live videos, instant messaging, and real-time documentation. Many APP projects are large in scale and include multiple departments across a geographical environment and can be much more successful using these platforms.

APPs, like all providers, are primary partners in the implementation and maintenance of projects, successful change implementation, and a culture dedicated to continuous process improvement. APPs and physicians, nurses, and administrative leaders view and respond to problem-solving differently and rely on the expertise of each colleague for a successful project.

MANAGEMENT OF MULTIPLE SITES

There are several tools that should be used to support management of multiple locations where APPs practice. Standardization, dependable communication tools, cross-training, and consistent cultural expectations all support strong management of APP practice regardless of geographical distance between sites. Training, accountability, resource availability, and performance improvement positively impact the operations and outcomes of healthcare. When you focus on managing the process, you will in turn manage the results (Lewis, 2022).

Creating standardized environments across multiple locations improves efficiencies and reduces risk of error as well as improves quality and cost efficiency (Lewis, 2022). Standardization across practice sites (particularly sites of the same specialty or clinic setting such as urgent care or quick cares) allows APPs to optimize the ability to work in various sites without compromising efficiency. Standard processes allow the ability to utilize members of the healthcare team in multiple locations as patient care demands change. Providing the appropriate resources and support is imperative, including standard staffing models, patient flow processes, patient information and instructions, supply and medication vendors. Standardization provides seamless patient care regardless of assignment locations, which helps with clinical practice productivity and promotes the availability of a practice-ready workforce.

The multi-site practice setting is vulnerable to several elements that can significantly impact operations. Environmental factors such as inclement weather, safety factors, and economic factors such as supply chain issues can impact the ability to provide care to patients. Creating strong communication tools across locations ensures a support system at every level.

Daily huddles where APP providers and organizational leadership across locations communicate either in person or virtually about agenda items such as number of patients in the day, staffing concerns, and any patient safety concerns will provide timely communication with everyone. For efficiency, huddles are short, less than five minutes, and set for a recurring time of day.

Huddles should have a mechanism to report any identified concerns to staff. Communication tools that can supplement the huddle can be as simple as a whiteboard, or more sophisticated platforms such as within the EHR or electronic communication board. As with any visible communication board, consideration should be given to adhere to HIPAA and other patient-secured information policies. APPs, like all members of the healthcare team, should be kept abreast of all policies and communication expectations within the various practice locations.

Establishing a separate huddle time for the APP leads and administrative leadership for each location ensures clear communication about anticipated issues and allows for leaders from multiple sites to support each other to foster trusting relationships. Without the designated time to connect on a regular basis, miscommunications or assumptions can occur. The same huddle topics are relevant in a leadership huddle as team huddles: patient volume, staffing concerns, operational concerns, and patient safety concerns.

The challenges of a multi-site setting can be negated with cross-training of support staff for the APPs. This allows opportunity to work in various supportive roles where traditional medical or nursing assistants might be resource-challenged and staffed by paramedics or other healthcare team members that expand their primary scope and flex into alternate roles as needed. Through cross-training, a practice location is able to shift work effort to provide the flexibility to adjust with staffing variances. Cross-training within a single location as well as across multiple locations provides an added flexibility to ensure daily operation needs can be met. An example of tasks that may be easily shifted include patient intake, vitals, and phlebotomy. Radiology technicians can be trained within their scope to support the clinical setting with phlebotomy or patient intake, or medical assistants may be trained to support reception and scheduling. All support the APP to be highly productive and allow for top-of-license practice.

Creating a consistent, positive team-based culture across locations helps get all members on the same mental model regardless of geographic location. This includes setting consistent expectations and, most important, leading not only by example but with respect for all professionals. Training on cultural values should occur during the onboarding process with a sustainability strategy, including annual retraining. Setting a consistent team culture allows leaders and staff to move between locations and supports the practice at every level in employee engagement and satisfaction. Leadership rounding can also help create a culture in which staff feel empowered to identify and address issues during the routinely designated rounding time. Employee engagement is a foundational component to workplace outcome. APPs will feel invested when leadership openly receives feedback and recommendations and allows involvement with change implementation. Understanding culture enables APPs to work synergistically (Menaker & Wampfler, 2022).

Regular, purposeful leadership rounding emphasizes a positive, open, and inclusive work environment. APP leads and practice site administrators should have dedicated time to touch base with staff, observe patient flow, and listen to all APP providers, support staff, and patients to ensure that real-time practice concerns are being addressed. The wide range of inclusive leaders allows for everyone to understand each other's role and identity. Leaders in various roles (provider, administrator, nursing, support staff) tend to focus on different aspects of the practice. Creating a leadership rotation at different sites allows the group of leaders to identify different successes and challenges within each location. Identified items, action plans, and accountable owners should be discussed as leadership groups follow up with issues for closed-loop communication.

FINANCIAL IMPACTS USING APP TEAMS

Healthcare systems can realize financial gains through the effective use and deployment of APPs. With recurrent pressure from the Centers for Medicare & Medicaid Services (CMS) and private insurance for providers to be fiscally responsible with healthcare services, organizations must always seek ways to gain efficiencies and deliver safe and quality care. When organizations optimize an APP's skill set and capabilities through top-of-license practice, there can be measured improvements to documentation and billing, reductions to length of stay and readmissions, improvements to patient appointment access, and a more cost-effective provider option for established outpatient visits and pre/post-surgical care.

APPs who are skilled in documentation and billing demonstrate a comprehensive understanding of Medicare and other insurance billing regulations and reimbursement policies. This includes having the knowledge to understand the differences between inpatient and outpatient documentation and billing, so the APP knows how the care they render to patients is reflected in accurate and concise documentation based on time spent with the patient and the patient's clinical severity. Having this understanding between the relationship of care provided and comprehensive documentation leads to optimal billing and payment.

As noted in previous chapters, APPs are an effective option in both the inpatient and outpatient settings, providing substantial quality and financial value. Many healthcare provider groups have patient appointment wait times that extend many months due to physician shortage, overextended panels, and limited clinic staffing. APPs are clinically exemplar and can care for specific patient types, reducing patient appointment wait times and ultimately increasing patient throughput, volume, and net revenue.

APPs who are employed by surgical practice groups provide pre- and post-op care to surgical patients, resulting in high-quality care and improved overall efficiency. Most surgical procedures provide reimbursement through a global or bundled payment that includes a pre-determined number of pre-op and post-op outpatient visits. These outpatient visits are not reimbursed on their own but rather are included in the global payment, which makes it advantageous to have an APP render the visits in lieu of the surgeon. This frees up time during a surgeon's schedule to see new patients and schedule time in the operating room.

The use of APPs within a healthcare system is a more cost-effective option to render care to designated patient populations within their scope and clinical expertise while overall sustaining and improving quality and patient safety. Although Medicare, Medicaid, and many third-party insurance companies reimburse less for an APP visit, the salary differential outweighs the reimbursement reduction. However, there are situations where CMS does not recognize the specialty practices of APPs, and the reimbursement requires significant clarification and appeal. An example of this is a patient living in a rural state who has multiple comorbidities requiring multiple specialties and receives care provided by two very separate clinical expert APPs, in different departments and specialties, despite the APPs having the same license and taxonomy code. It may be advantageous to the patient to travel on the same day and cluster the appointments but administratively burdensome to appeal the claim when it is denied for reasons stated above. As APPs continue to grow in number and impact the provider shortage in this country, it is a best practice to encourage organizations to collect outcome data based on reimbursement barriers and encourage the expansion of taxonomy codes for APRNs and PAs who practice in specialty areas.

LEADING CLINIC RENOVATIONS

Healthcare is consistently growing and changing in response to improvements in the way care is delivered. The increasing transition from the inpatient to the outpatient setting has drawn new focus on construction and renovation design. Space design can provide significant positive or negative impacts to a practice. When considering development, whether renovation or new construction, there should be significant engagement and collaboration with architecture, engineering, and construction management partners early to develop a space program that meets regulatory requirements, patient population needs, practice efficiencies, and growth planning. Likewise, APP providers should also have input; they have much to offer in the way workflow should be constructed because they are the ones providing care.

The Facility Guidelines Institute (FGI) provides concepts and recommendations in the space design for the delivery of healthcare. The guidelines are updated every four years and used by states to regulate health and residential care facility design and construction and are used as a basis for state-written codes. The guidelines for space construction or renovation ensure the design conforms to regulatory requirements. However, it should be noted that although the guidelines address certain details of construction and engineering that are important for facility design and construction, they are neither intended to be all-inclusive nor used to the exclusion of other guidance or codes, such as local and model codes, or expert frontline input (FGI, 2023).

The Joint Commission is a nonprofit accreditation body of US healthcare organizations and programs and used as a condition of participation for Medicaid and Medicare reimbursement. From a facilities perspective, The Joint Commission expects organizations to assess building design and construction based on local, state, and federal regulations and codes. Typically, the controlling authority is the state health department licensing entity, but when these entities are silent on a particular design requirement, The Joint Commission recognizes FGI as the prevailing authority in the Environment of Care chapter (The Joint Commission, 2023).

Aside from regulatory requirements, there are several other considerations during the design phase of a renovation or new construction project. This includes functional and efficient staff workspace, location of centralized services such as supplies and medications, security considerations such as barriers between the waiting area and the clinical space, and enhancing the patient experience using aesthetics and on-stage/off-stage design. Again, input from APPs in renovations facilitates successful adaption and engagement.

The current trend in the healthcare industry is to create multi-specialty space that provides convenience to the patient with related services. For example, an urgent care practice regularly seeing a significant volume of musculoskeletal injuries may consider co-locating with an orthopedic practice. Housing inter-related services creates a space that a patient can rely on for some continuum of care. Having specialty-trained APPs can further enhance the efficiency of the clinical locations and requires specific onboarding and methodical planning. Additionally, ancillary retail services serving healthcare industry within the same space provides a "one stop shop" environment. Expanding on the example above, a multi-specialty urgent care and orthopedic location may consider adding retail space for braces, splints, and other durable medical items.

The design phase of renovation or new construction is an important phase and should not be taken lightly. Leaders in every area of the practice should be involved in the design to ensure functionality for the users of the space. Creating a solid, confident design is vital to a successful project and will ultimately provide cost savings by eliminating modifications agreed upon in the construction contract. In the construction industry, variations to the design that occur during the construction phase are called *change orders*. Change orders usually occur when there is variation in the scope of the project, an issue with material quantities, or design errors. Research indicates that change orders on construction projects average 10%–15% of the contract value of the project, and change in plans by the project owners is the main source of change orders (Desai et al., 2015). For this reason and many others, involving APPs can eliminate change orders on simple processes such as handwashing stations and supplies. Including those who will work in the space every day will ensure functional and efficient design elements.

QUALITY HEALTHCARE

Healthcare *quality,* as defined by the Institute of Medicine (IOM), is "the degree to which health care services for individuals and populations increase the likelihood of desired health outcomes and are consistent with current professional knowledge" (IOM Committee to Design a Strategy for Quality Review and Assurance in Medicare, 1990, p. 21). For healthcare services to impact health outcomes at a population level, the health system must intervene upstream with a focus on patient-centered prevention, early identification of disease, and management of chronic conditions.

Primary care is uniquely situated to drive quality in this manner. APPs serving in the role of primary care providers (PCPs) serve as a de facto access point to the organization, providing continuity and coordination of care over a person's life span. Patients with established relationships with a PCP have been found to have improved outcomes as compared to patients who do not, and some research suggests that the deeper that relationship, as defined by the number of PCP visits in a year, the better the outcomes (Hostetter et al., 2020). A recognition of the role of the PCP in driving health outcomes for populations has resulted in a demand for primary care services that currently outweighs workforce capacity, and that deficit continues to expand as the population ages.

APPs are a consistently reliable solution to deficits in primary care when functioning independently to care for their own panel of patients. Both independent and team-based models using APPs can stretch capacity to provide care to patients and improve the quality of care. Models where APPs practice independently in states with full practice authority and organizations that support specialty models (e.g., APP-physician co-management) have been shown to improve patient adherence to recommended care guidelines and favorably impact clinical outcomes (Norful et al., 2018). APPs and physicians practicing in any organization, whether independently or collaboratively, share in the responsibility and accountability of all patient care, including patient visits, medication management, diagnostic work-up, patient education, and patient follow-up. This also includes care coordination, documentation, and communication with patients and families. Healthcare delivery today requires top-of-license practice to be able to address the significant population health needs and quality patient care that is expected and desired. Effective models must focus on shared responsibility and distribution of resources, as well as effective communication, mutual trust and respect, and a shared philosophy of care (Norful et al., 2018). As part of any healthcare delivery model, APPs impact healthcare quality while also addressing a primary care shortage.

SUMMARY

This chapter details how organizations address unique initiatives due to continuous changes surrounding healthcare. Keeping abreast of these changes requires resourceful, methodical, and strategic continuous planning. APPs are a common denominator in the equation of healthcare today to meet the demands and challenges organizations are facing. Utilizing resources within a healthcare system or organization, using guiding principles to engage all team members, and promoting inclusive environments support those unique and challenging projects where APPs are instrumental in the success.

REFERENCES

Desai, J. N., Pitroda, J., & Bhavasar, J. J. (2015). A review on change order and assessing causes affecting change order in construction. *International Journal of Multidisciplinary Academic Research, 2*(12), 152–162. https://www.researchgate.net/publication/281823301_A_REVIEW_ON_CHANGE_ORDER_AND_ASSESSINGCAUSES_AFFECTING_CHANGE_ORDER_IN_CONSTRUCTION

Facility Guidelines Institute. (2023). *Uses of the guidelines.* https://fgiguidelines.org/guidelines/uses-of-the-guidelines/

Hostetter, J., Schwarz, N., Klug, M., Wynne, J., & Basson, M. D. (2020). Primary care visits increase utilization of evidence-based preventative health measures. *BMC Family Practice, 21*(1), 151. https://doi.org/10.1186/s12875-020-01216-8

Institute of Medicine Committee to Design a Strategy for Quality Review and Assurance in Medicare. (1990). *Medicare: A strategy for quality assurance* (Vol. 1; K. N. Lohr, Ed.). National Academies Press.

The Joint Commission. (2023). *Design criteria – Facility Guidelines Institute (FGI).* https://www.jointcommission.org/standards/standard-faqs/ambulatory/environment-of-care-ec/000001273/

Lavoie-Tremblay, M., Aubry, M., Cyr, G., Richer, M. C., Fortin-Verreault, J. F., Fortin, C., Marchionni, C. (2017). Innovation in health service management: Adoption of project management offices to support major health care transformation. *Journal of Nursing Management, 25*(8), 657–665. https://doi.org/10.1111/jonm.12505

Lewis, O. (2022, September 21). *Enhancing practice operations through process standardization.* Medical Group Management Association. https://www.mgma.com/practice-resources/operations-management/enhancing-practice-operations-through-process-stan

Menaker, R., & Wampfler, E. (2022, June 23). *Shaping a culture: implications for leaders.* Medical Group Management Association. https://www.mgma.com/practice-resources/human-resources/shaping-a-culture-implications-for-leaders

Miller, D., & Oliver, M. (2015, January 1). *Engaging stakeholders for project success.* PMI White Paper. https://www.pmi.org/learning/library/engaging-stakeholders-project-success-11199

Norful, A. A., de Jacq, K., Carlino, R., & Poghosyan, L. (2018). Nurse practitioner–physician comanagement: A theoretical model to alleviate primary care strain. *The Annals of Family Medicine, 16*(3), 250–256. https://doi.org/10.1370/afm.2230

Project Management Institute. (2021). *A guide to the project management body of knowledge (PMBOK® Guide) and the standard for project management* (7th ed.). Project Management Academy.

Salapatas, J. N. (2000). *Best practices – The nine elements to success* [Presentation]. PMI Annual Seminars & Symposium, Houston, TX.

Serrador, P. (2009). *Stakeholder management: Keeping your stakeholders thoroughly happy* [Presentation]. PMI Global Congress, Orlando, FL.

> *"Healthcare can be challenging, but it is important to never lose sight of the passion when we first chose our professions. Those emotions are the fuel that feeds us and gets us through the tough times and is without a doubt why the world is a better place."*
>
> —Maria Lofgren

CHAPTER 18

LOOKING TO THE FUTURE

KEYWORDS | diversity, equity, inclusion, future leadership, collaboration, AI (artificial intelligence)

Changes in healthcare have not only affected hospitals, clinics, and patients but also many of the professions that have been icons in our healthcare systems for decades. Issues that surround our healthcare systems are vast and multifactorial, and changing at what seems to be a rapid speed. It is almost impossible to capture everything our healthcare systems are facing. Issues range from organizational and system structural changes, processes and practices, resources and personnel, adaptation to new patient records and billing systems, use of information technology and artificial intelligence, best practice approaches to improve health and achieve optimal healthcare outcomes, all while trying to minimize costs, maintain patient safety, and assure the well-being of everyone involved (Grunberg et al., 2023). Leading change in healthcare requires significant collaboration. Information available surrounding research on artificial intelligence (AI) promises innovative approaches to many aspects that support the management of healthcare (Chen et al., 2022). It is daunting to try and anticipate the way this innovative technology will change healthcare delivery as we move into the future.

The APRN and PA professions are evolving as positive forces in contributing to bridging healthcare gaps. The *U.S. News and World Report* showcases these professions as top tiered (Ingram, 2023). Today, healthcare organizations are recognizing APPs as a group of certified and state-licensed healthcare professionals who are essential to operations. Healthcare organizations are under tight scrutiny, and capturing ways to improve systems, identify high productivity and efficient processes, and operationalize APPs at the top of their license is essential for future success.

Legislation plays an important role in our healthcare delivery and cannot be overlooked when evaluating the future. The legislative impact on new innovations such as AI is unknown. Many APRN and PA professional organizations, as well as healthcare organizations, are engaging with legislators to influence the Centers for Medicare & Medicaid Services about specialty practice from an APP scope to resolve reimbursement barriers. The success of APPs has been acknowledged by researchers and healthcare providers alike, and their role has become critical in medical subspecialties and intensive care units, including primary care, where APPs play an essential role in addressing the primary care shortage (Corley, 2017). In today's healthcare environment, all professions are counting on each other, including APPs, to work together to provide improved access for patients, engage as a team for healthcare continuity, and provide value-centered care that results in excellent outcomes.

APRN and PA legislation governing state practices is frequently changing, and it is imperative that organizations are cognizant of the issues that surround the ability, or lack thereof, to provide care to patients, and become educated about the roles of the APP and how these roles can add value. It is essential to continue to move forward and track APP contributions into meaningful and understandable data so as new technology and innovations are introduced, all providers and disciplines are part of the matrix.

Information that is published and shared will benefit not only the APP professions and the organizations who employ them but, most importantly, the patients they care for.

State and federal entities and healthcare organizations should support practice to the full extent of education and training by removing barriers such as regulatory, public, and private payment limitations; restrictive policies and practices; and other legal, professional, and commercial barriers (National Academies of Sciences, Engineering, & Medicine [NASEM], 2021). The elimination of these barriers will improve healthcare access, quality, and value.

DIVERSITY, EQUITY, AND INCLUSION

As the APP workforce continues to increase, and as healthcare services provided by APPs expand, consideration should be given to integrating diversity, equity, and inclusion (DEI) practices and education. The recruitment, retention, and leadership advancement of healthcare providers who are underrepresented is a priority to ensure excellence in patient care, research, and health equity (Davenport et al., 2022). Likewise, DEI efforts include recruiting and retaining a diverse workforce in all professions and building employment pipelines for those underrepresented in healthcare. A diverse healthcare workforce is critical to reducing healthcare disparity and improving patient outcomes (Rosenkranz et al., 2021). DEI efforts supported by leadership, and leaders demonstrating inclusive behaviors, improves both job performance and collaboration (Bourke & Titus, 2019). Organizations are encouraged to name commitment towards diversity as part of their mission and describe their organizational vision as providing an equitable, inclusive, and innovative environment (Stanford, 2020). Looking to the future, DEI may provide opportunities in improving patient outcomes and enhancing the work environment.

The literature shows that providing appropriate care for diverse patient populations requires healthcare workforces to have awareness and ongoing education in matters related to cultural differences and general diversity (Young & Guo, 2020). Just as APPs are required to stay up to date on clinical skills and procedures to best serve their patients, education and training on DEI matters as part of healthcare delivery should be treated similarly (Marcelin et al., 2019). No one profession or group will achieve the health equity needed in this nation without all health professions, working within and across disciplines, aspiring to advance the culture. Working across sectors with steadfast vigilance will be a necessary ingredient not only in understanding but also in taking real action to achieve health equity (NASEM, 2021).

Significant financial resources are spent treating illness, and yet the US under-invests in promoting health and preventing disease in comparison to any other resource-rich country, and still has consistently worse health outcomes (NASEM, 2021). The COVID-19 pandemic revealed many inequities surrounding poverty, racism, and discrimination that shed light on the biases in healthcare and forced a conversation around how physicians, APPs, nurses, and all healthcare industry professions are valued. The COVID-19 pandemic has caused an unprecedented wave of resignations in healthcare workers, with high turnover rates causing difficulty in staffing and impacting the quality of care delivered to patients. Poon et al. (2022) and Kleinpell et al. (2021) examined the effects of the pandemic on APRN barriers to practice with the hopes of using their research to advocate for policy changes to modernize APRN practice authority regulations. Through historical perspectives from the pandemic, the visibility surrounding DEI issues, the available research, and the need for stronger collaboration, as well as a thorough understanding of new technologies entering our healthcare systems such as AI, humanitarianism will remain at the forefront of progress.

APP LEADERSHIP AND SUPPORT

There are various operational and progressive leadership models for healthcare-related professions. An APP leadership structure lends itself to both small and large institutions and can support diverse populations of APPs (Proulx, 2021). APP leadership can be quantified in a variety of ways, and organizations need to identify how APP leaders can best work within the organization's culture and leadership structure to make an impact, all while remaining vigilant to new innovations and visionary for the future. An important concept that should cross all leadership models in the future is ensuring a high-reliability organization to maintain high levels of safety. This takes leadership commitment to achieving zero patient harm, adopting a fully functional culture of safety throughout the organization, and the widespread deployment of effective process improvement tools (Chassin & Loeb, 2013).

Trying to capture what healthcare leadership structures will look like in the future, especially in the face of the multitude of issues facing the industry, should be viewed through a lens of openness and collaboration. Hierarchical environments have not served the healthcare industry well. Territorial issues over scope creep, and fear of stopping the line, potentially could in turn cause harm to the very people every healthcare profession has educated themselves to serve. Teams, working together, supporting and allowing all professions to practice to the top of license and education could improve our healthcare outcomes simply by eliminating power struggles and taking the focus off the hierarchy and onto what is right for the patients. Having an understanding and respect for all the disciplines and knowing what it takes to operationalize a highly successful and functional healthcare organization should be a future priority to ultimately deliver safe care to patients. Using resources within organizations; pulling in expertise; and educating about scope of practice, educational pathways, and partnerships all play into the future success of operationalizing highly functioning teams. This includes being seen as a unified front with legislation and practice barriers, payer barriers, and leadership issues. Problem-solving for a better healthcare future in the best interest of the patients can help guide solutions.

REGULATORY BARRIERS

APRNs with specialty board certification in adult gerontological primary and acute care certification are instrumental in the care of the geriatric population but face issues that limit the ability to serve and function in medical leadership roles. Nursing home care is one example where APRNs could impact quality outcomes and optimize practice through serving in director leadership roles and removing policy and regulatory barriers to practice (Bakerjian, 2022).

If universal full practice authority, full billing authority, or specialty APRN certification recognized by payers were a reality, APRNs could serve as medical directors and progress could be made in the nursing home, skilled nursing, and long-term care setting. There is ample evidence to demonstrate that policymakers must strengthen the APRN in these settings (Bakerjian, 2022).

FUTURE WORKFORCE

Universal access to high-quality healthcare in the United States goes beyond ensuring coverage, efficient delivery systems, and affordability (Butkus et al., 2020). There are many ways that APPs will impact healthcare over the next decade. Great opportunity exists to improve care by better utilizing APPs in underserved areas. Nearly 20% of US residents, an estimated 65 million people, live in small towns and sparsely populated areas designated as rural by the Census Bureau, where workforce shortages are a persistent challenge and rural residents do not have adequate access to healthcare and comparatively worse health status (Kozhimannil & Henning-Smith, 2021). Recruiting and retaining rural primary care providers will continue to be challenging in the future. Filling this gap requires strategy with the available workforce. There are pockets of patient populations where APPs are poised to meet the needs in providing access, leadership, and quality healthcare, and this will require a strategic, unified, persistent voice to hold legislators, payers, and all interested parties accountable.

Well-being, burnout, violence, and compassion fatigue are phenomena that impact every aspect of the workplace. Literature suggests that improving leadership and operations and promoting APP well-being can mitigate provider burnout (Klein et al., 2020). One study found that APPs are experiencing moderate levels of burnout linked to the

COVID-19 pandemic (Stallter & Gustin, 2021). The American Psychological Association (APA) released the results of their *2022 Work and Well-Being Survey*, which indicated 81% of survey respondents said that employers' support for mental health will be an important consideration when they look for work in the future, including 30% of workers who strongly agreed that employer support for mental health will factor into their future job decisions (APA, 2022). Organizations should develop a strategy and resources for provider well-being and ensure that APPs are included in the programming. This should be a common theme in the future to ensure APPs are included in all strategies that support well-being initiatives.

With low unemployment rates and continued shortages of certain healthcare workers, leadership in healthcare systems should continue to strategize how to combat turnover and ensure a stable and skilled workforce. The overall nursing and medical assistant shortages are also of concern for operations, as turnover and vacancy in these areas impact the care team and ultimately patient access. APRN and PA academic institutions are growing to meet the potential provider demand. Succession planning is a strategic effort to ensure future continuity when turnover, expected or unexpected, inevitably occurs (Pastores et al., 2019).

SUMMARY

The literature continues to evolve related to not only the future of APPs but also the future of our healthcare delivery systems. The more we can prepare APPs for what is expected from an operations perspective beyond their educational preparations, and assist all providers in best practices, the better for everyone. APPs are a growing workforce, and what was once about the scope creep and turf wars over patient population should now be about the APP role as a chosen profession, supporting colleagues, caring for vulnerable populations, optimizing the work APPs can do, and identifying ways to measure impact and patient outcomes.

REFERENCES

American Psychological Association. (2022, July). *Workers appreciate and seek mental health support in the workplace: APA's 2022 Work and Well-being Survey results.* https://www.apa.org/pubs/reports/work-well-being/2022-mental-health-support

Bakerjian, D. (2022). The advanced practice registered nurse leadership role in nursing homes: Leading efforts toward high quality and safe care. *Nursing Clinics of North America, 57*(2), 245–258. https://doi.org/10.1016/j.cnur.2022.02.011

Bourke, J., & Titus, A. (2019, March 29). Why inclusive leaders are good for organizations, and how to become one. *Harvard Business Review.* https://hbr.org/2019/03/why-inclusive-leaders-are-good-for-organizations-and-how-to-become-one

Butkus, R., Rapp, K., Cooney, T. G., Engel, L. S., & Health & Public Policy Committee of the American College of Physicians. (2020). Envisioning a better US health care system for all: Reducing barriers to care and addressing social determinants of health. *Annals of Internal Medicine, 172*(S2), S50–S59. https://doi.org/10.7326/M19-2410

Chassin, M. R., & Loeb, J. M. (2013). High-reliability health care: Getting there from here. *The Milbank Quarterly, 91*(3), 459–490. https://doi.org/10.1111/1468-0009.12023

Chen, Y., Moreira, P., Liu, W. W., Monachino, M., Nguyen, T. L. H., & Wang, A. (2022). Is there a gap between artificial intelligence applications and priorities in health care and nursing management? *Journal of Nursing Management, 30*(8), 3736–3742. https://doi.org/10.1111/jonm.13851

Corley, J. (2017, March 16). Advanced-practice providers are key to America's healthcare future [Editorial]. *Forbes.* https://www.forbes.com/sites/realspin/2017/03/16/advanced-practice-providers-are-key-to-americas-healthcare-future/?sh=491d14425998

Davenport, D., Alvarez, A., Natesan, S., Caldwell, M. T., Gallegos, M., Landry, A., Parsons, M., & Gottlieb, M. (2022). Faculty recruitment, retention, and representation in leadership: An evidence-based guide to best practices for diversity, equity, and inclusion from the Council of Residency Directors in Emergency Medicine. *Western Journal of Emergency Medicine, 23*(1), 62–71. https://doi.org/10.5811/westjem.2021.8.53754

Grunberg, N. E., McManigle, J. E., Schoomaker, E. B., & Barry, E. S. (2023). Leading change in health care. *Clinics in Sports Medicine, 42*(2), 249–260. https://doi.org/10.1016/j.csm.2022.11.007

Ingram J. (2023, January 10). *U.S. News* ranks the best jobs of 2023. *US News & World Report.* https://money.usnews.com/careers/articles/u-s-news-ranks-the-best-jobs

Klein, C. J., Dalstrom, M., Lizer, S., Cooling, M., Pierce, L., & Weinzimmer, L. G. (2020). Advanced practice provider perspectives on organizational strategies for work stress reduction. *Western Journal of Nursing Research, 42*(9), 708–717. https://doi.org/10.1177/0193945919896606

Kleinpell, R., Myers, C. R., Schorn, M. N., & Likes, W. (2021). Impact of COVID-19 pandemic on APRN practice: Results from a national survey. *Nursing Outlook, 69*(5), 783–792. https://doi.org/10.1016/j.outlook.2021.05.002

Kozhimannil, K. B., & Henning-Smith, C. (2021, March 16). Improving health among rural residents in the US [Editorial]. *JAMA: Journal of the American Medical Association, 325*(11), 1033–1034. https://doi.org/10.1001/jama.2020.26372

Marcelin, J. R., Siraj, D. S., Victor, R., Kotadia, S., & Maldonado, Y. (2019). The impact of unconscious bias in healthcare: How to recognize and mitigate it. *The Journal of Infectious Diseases, 220*(S2), S62–S73. https://doi.org/10.1093/infdis/jiz214

National Academies of Sciences, Engineering, & Medicine. (2021). *The future of nursing 2020-2030: Charting a path to achieve health equity.* National Academies Press. https://doi.org/10.17226/25982

Pastores, S. M., Kvetan, V., Coopersmith, C. M., Farmer, J. C., Sessler, C., Christman, J. W., D'Agostino, R., Diaz-Gomez, J., Gregg, S. R., Khan, R. A., Kapu, A. N., Masur, H., Mehta, G., Moore, J., Oropello, J. M., Price, K., & Academic Leaders in Critical Care Medicine Task Force of the Society of the Critical Care Medicine. (2019). Workforce, workload, and burnout among intensivists and advanced practice providers: A narrative review. *Critical Care Medicine, 47*(4), 550–557. https://journals.lww.com/ccmjournal/Fulltext/2019/04000/Workforce,_Workload,_and_Burnout_Among.8.aspx

Poon, Y. S. R., Lin, Y. P., Griffiths, P., Yong, K. K., Seah, B., & Liaw, S. Y. (2022). A global overview of healthcare workers' turnover intention amid COVID-19 pandemic: A systematic review with future directions. *Human Resources for Health, 20*(70). https://doi.org/10.1186/s12960-022-00764-7

Proulx, B. (2021). Advance practice provider transformational leadership structure: A model for change. *JONA: The Journal of Nursing Administration, 51*(6), 340–346. https://doi.org/10.1097/nna.0000000000001024

Rosenkranz, K. M., Arora, T. K., Termuhlen, P. M., Stain, S. C., Misra, S., Dent, D., & Nfonsam, V. (2021). Diversity, equity, and inclusion in medicine: Why it matters and how do we achieve it? *Journal of Surgical Education, 78*(4), 1058–1065. https://doi.org/10.1016/j.jsurg.2020.11.013

Stallter, C., & Gustin, T. S. (2021). Evaluating advanced practice nurses' burnout and potential helping modalities. *The Journal for Nurse Practitioners, 17*(10), 1297–1299. https://doi.org/10.1016/j.nurpra.2021.07.003

Stanford, F. C. (2020). The importance of diversity and inclusion in the healthcare workforce. *Journal of the National Medical Association, 112*(3), 247–249. https://doi.org/10.1016/j.jnma.2020.03.014

Young, S., & Guo, K. L. (2020). Cultural diversity training: The necessity of cultural competence for health care providers and in nursing practice. *The Health Care Manager, 39*(2), 100–108. https://doi.org/10.1097/hcm.0000000000000294

APPENDIX A

APP LICENSE AND BOARD CERTIFICATION REQUIREMENTS

PA (BOTH REQUIRED TO PRACTICE; MUST BE ACTIVE AT ALL TIMES)

1. PA License

2. PA Board Certification

   - National Commission on Certification of Physician Assistants (NCCPA)

APRN (ALL THREE REQUIRED TO PRACTICE; MUST BE ACTIVE AT ALL TIMES)

1. RN License

2. APRN License

3. Board Certification (based on patient population, renewal cycles vary, active certifying agencies listed below)

FNP (FAMILY NURSE PRACTITIONER)

- American Nurses Credentialing Center (ANCC)
- American Academy of Nurse Practitioners (AANP)

PNP (PEDIATRIC NURSE PRACTITIONER; ACUTE CARE OR PRIMARY CARE)

- Pediatric Nursing Certification Board (PNCB; acute or primary)

AGNP (ADULT/GERONTOLOGY NURSE PRACTITIONER; ACUTE CARE OR PRIMARY CARE)

- American Nurses Credentialing Center (ANCC; acute or primary)
- American Association of Critical-Care Nurses (AACN; acute)
- American Academy of Nurse Practitioners (AANP; primary)

PMHNP (PSYCH MENTAL HEALTH NURSE PRACTITIONER)

- American Nurses Credentialing Center (ANCC)

NNP (NEONATAL NURSE PRACTITIONER)

- National Certification Corporation (NCC)

WHNP (WOMEN'S HEALTH NURSE PRACTITIONER)

- National Certification Corporation (NCC)

CRNA (CERTIFIED REGISTERED NURSE ANESTHETIST)

- National Board of Certification and Recertification for Nurse Anesthetists (NBCRNA)

CNM (CERTIFIED NURSE MIDWIFE)

- American Midwifery Certification Board (AMCB)

CNS (CLINICAL NURSE SPECIALIST)

- American Nurses Credentialing Center (ANCC)
- American Association of Critical-Care Nurses (AACN)

APPENDIX B

PREPARING FOR YOUR NEW APP

The following guide has been developed to assist department leadership in preparing for onboarding advanced practice providers (APPs).

PREPARING FOR A NEW APP

This checklist suggests steps you may take before each new APP's first day. Review the list at least two weeks before new APP's start date to allow sufficient time to complete all the tasks.

- ❑ Confirm start date with HR and monitor status of credentialing and privileging
- ❑ Mail department welcome letter to new APP's home one to two weeks before start date
- ❑ Call new hire one week before start date:
    - ❑ Congratulate new APP and welcome to the team
    - ❑ Provide an overview of the first week (schedule, tasks, dress code, etc.)
    - ❑ Ensure new APP understands instructions for the first day (directions, parking, where to report, identification to bring, etc.)
    - ❑ Provide a contact for additional questions/issues that arise before start date
- ❑ Assign mentor/preceptor, schedule first and recurring meetings
- ❑ Prior to start date verify the following:
    - ❑ New hire ID/badge and schedule time for photo
    - ❑ Computer access
    - ❑ Email account
    - ❑ Voicemail account
    - ❑ Workspace/office assignment
    - ❑ Lab coat
- ❑ Add new APP to department organizational chart, telephone/email directory, find-a-provider
- ❑ Announce new APP's position and scheduled start date to department staff at staff meeting and via email

❑ Prepare new APP's workspace (ensure completion of all applicable tasks):

  ❑ Clean work area

  ❑ Order/install telephone and confirm phone is working and extension is correct

  ❑ Assign departmental mailbox

  ❑ Order supplies, business cards, and name plate

  ❑ Arrange for keys or passcode access

  ❑ Set up cellphone or pager account (if applicable)

❑ Arrange for department first day welcome gestures (welcome sign on new APP's workstation, snack/luncheon welcoming new APP to department, etc.)

APPENDIX C

INPATIENT SCHEDULING GUIDELINES

METRICS	APP SCHEDULING GUIDELINE	DATA SOURCE
Scheduling Guiding Principle	In a clinical environment, scheduling APPs to ensure adequate staffing for patient care demands is the priority. Shared responsibility and equitable scheduling among APPs are desired. When possible and the above criteria are met, consideration will be given for APPs' schedule preferences.	
Work Schedules	Work schedules will be established based on the needs of the clinical unit and with consideration for employees' preferences. Alternate work schedules may be established by mutual agreement.	
Hours per Week	APPs should be scheduled to work their full fte during the designated work week (40 hours/1.0 fte, pro-rated for part-time).	
Average Days per Week	Inpatient work weeks for 1.0 fte are typically five (5) days of eight-hour (8) shifts, four (4) days of ten-hour (10) shifts, or any other combination of shifts that equals forty (40) hours with at least two days off during the work week. Exceptions and alternate schedules may apply to meet patient care demands.	
Weekend/Holiday Scheduling Time-off Requests (vacation)	Departments/units shall establish holiday/weekend and vacation/ time off coverage protocols considering equitable and shared responsibility whenever possible. Patient care demands and coverage needs will take priority in scheduling.	Epic/Qgenda
Clinical Documentation	Departments/units shall establish documentation protocols and guidelines to ensure timely, accurate, and thorough documentation.	Epic

Scheduling: Establishing Guidelines

- Patient care needs are the top priority and consideration when creating a schedule.

- Consideration for shared responsibility for shift coverage among APP staff and equitable scheduling.

- When possible and the above criteria are met, consideration will be given for APPs' schedule preferences.

Time-off Requests

- Consider internal equity when approving days off for high-demand days/weeks. Examples include spring break week, holidays, Fridays, and weekends.

- Develop department or unit time-off request guidelines, including the time frame for requests and when requests are approved.

- Time-off requests submitted significantly in advance may be held (not yet approved) until the actual schedule is initiated so that all requests may be considered at the same time (example: future vacation requests, recurring days off).

Self-Scheduling

- Departments and units utilizing self-scheduling should establish guidelines to ensure adequate coverage.

- APPs who self-schedule should schedule their full fte each work week (pro-rated for part time).

- APPs scheduling > 8-hour shifts are encouraged not to schedule themselves more than four days in a row unless otherwise approved by APP lead or designee.

- All self-scheduling shifts must be approved in advance to ensure full clinical coverage is met.

- An APP lead or designee will adjust schedules according to the needs of unit if there are gaps in coverage prior to schedule finalization date.

- Generally, self-scheduling works well when team members work together cooperatively to ensure all shifts are covered and are respectful and considerate of others' schedule requests. In the event of ongoing scheduling challenges or conflicts among the team, a schedule template may be assigned.

Shift Changes/Trades/Unplanned Absences

- Shift trades must be requested in writing and require advance approval from lead APP or designee.

- Unit guidelines may suggest that APPs find their own coverage for unplanned absences. The APP lead may be contacted for additional assistance when clinical duties or other reasons hinder this process.

- Notification of unplanned absence should be communicated with the APP lead and other pertinent members of the healthcare team per unit guidelines.

Scheduling Practices:

- Nonpatient care (NPC) time (including time for projects) must be approved in advance and will be permitted only if all shifts are staffed, and patient census and acuity allows. NPC time may be canceled at any time if patient needs arise before or during a scheduled shift.

- Although employee preferences and requests will be considered, ultimately patient care needs will take priority in forming a schedule.

- Schedules require approval from the APP lead or designee before going live. Once the schedule is finalized and published, adjustments to the schedule need to be approved by the lead APP or designee.

- Schedule blocks should not be used as visual placeholders (comments on a template, also known as "soft blocks"). All block settings will release at a minimum of five days.

APPENDIX D

AMBULATORY SAMPLE
SCHEDULES

METRICS	APP BEST PRACTICE (BASED ON 1.0 FTE)	DATA SOURCE
# Sessions per Week	8–9 (four hour) sessions	Manually tracked through Epic or Qgenda
Average worked RVU per APP (wRVU)	At or above 65th Percentile MGMA Benchmark	Epic/Tableau
Average Patients per Session	8-10 Patients Per Session	Epic/Tableau
Slot Utilization Rate (Schedule Filled%)	Above 85% Filled	Epic/Tableau
Schedule Template Rate Unavailable/Private/Held %	< 10% of Template Schedule	Epic/Tableau
Facilitated Access Rate (% Patients Seen Within 10 Days, from defined group)	> 90%	Epic/Tableau
Care Provider Mean Score	At or above 96.00	Press Ganey Patient Satisfaction

SCHEDULING: BUILDING TEMPLATES

- Schedule templates will be built to be consistent with clinical FTE needs of the department and organization.

- Clinic session templates will be four hours in length.

- Provider schedules will be available to schedule into on a 13-month rolling calendar.

- Template slot lengths will be built to the lowest common denominator of the visit types for that area (e.g., new patient = 60 minutes, return = 20 min; slot lengths will be built in increments of 20 min).

- Breaks in the schedule will not be built to support "catch up" or documentation time.

MANAGING TEMPLATE BLOCKS

- Blocks are used to drive a particular visit type to a specified slot in the provider template. Templates should be restricted as infrequently as possible by blocks to promote patient choice in date/time of service.

- Blocks should be used when specific resources are needed for a visit and are only available at certain times of the day.

- All block settings will release at a minimum of five days.

- Blocks should not be used as visual placeholders (comments on a template, also known as "soft blocks").

HELD/UNAVAILABLE/PRIVATE TIME SLOTS

- Held Time – A tentative period of time when the provider may not be able to see patients in clinic. Should be used for a limited window of time, then released once availability is determined.

- Unavailable Time – A confirmed period of time when the provider cannot see patients in clinic, to be used for exceptions only.

- Private Slots – Time slots requiring elevated security for scheduling access; should be used as infrequently as possible as these limit patient and require escalation.

SCHEDULING PRACTICES:

- Provider schedules should be level-loaded across a typical work week and within a division/service to allow for efficient use of clinic resources and staffing.

- All providers will follow the Cancellation Policy.

- All appointments will be scheduled in negotiation (ear to ear, face to face or MyChart) with the patient and according to the patient's health needs and will be coordinated with other appointments when possible.

- A wait list will be used by all clinics to fill open slots and cancellations.

- All licensed practitioners providing care to patients in ambulatory clinics must have a rolling schedule session template open and available for scheduling 13 months in advance.

- A scheduled four-hour clinic session will not be canceled within eight weeks of the planned session due to a provider-driven absence.

SAMPLE SCHEDULE: 10-HOUR SHIFT
(EIGHT CLINICAL SESSIONS PER WEEK)
SAMPLE SCHEDULE (10.5-HOUR WORKDAY/FOUR PER WEEK; EIGHT CLINICAL SESSIONS)

	Schedule	Day 1	Day 2	Day 3	Day 4	Day 5	Weekly Total
Week 1	0700 - 0800	Documentation/Admin	Documentation/Admin	Off	Documentation/Admin	Documentation/Admin	
	0800 - 1200	Patient Care (4 hours)	Patient Care (4 hours)	(or rotate day off)	Patient Care (4 hours)	Patient Care (4 hours)	
	1200 - 1230	Break*	Break*		Break*	Break*	
	1230 - 1300	Documentation/Admin	Documentation/Admin		Documentation/Admin	Documentation/Admin	
	1300 - 1700	Patient Care (4 hours)	Patient Care (4 hours)		Patient Care (4 hours)	Patient Care (4 hours)	
	1700 - 1730	Documentation/Admin	Documentation/Admin		Documentation/Admin	Documentation/Admin	
	Total Worked Hours	10	10	0	10	10	40

	Schedule	Day 1	Day 2	Day 3	Day 4	Day 5	Weekly Total
Week 2	0700 - 0800	Documentation/Admin	Documentation/Admin	Off	Documentation/Admin	Documentation/Admin	
	0800 - 1200	Patient Care (4 hours)	Patient Care (4 hours)	(or rotate day off)	Patient Care (4 hours)	Patient Care (4 hours)	
	1200 - 1230	Break*	Break*		Break*	Break*	
	1230 - 1300	Documentation/Admin	Documentation/Admin		Documentation/Admin	Documentation/Admin	
	1300 - 1700	Patient Care (4 hours)	Patient Care (4 hours)		Patient Care (4 hours)	Patient Care (4 hours)	
	1700 - 1730	Documentation/Admin	Documentation/Admin		Documentation/Admin	Documentation/Admin	
	Total Worked Hours	10	10	0	10	10	40

	Schedule	Day 1	Day 2	Day 3	Day 4	Day 5	Weekly Total
Week 3	0700 - 0800	Documentation/Admin	Documentation/Admin	Off	Documentation/Admin	Documentation/Admin	
	0800 - 1200	Patient Care (4 hours)	Patient Care (4 hours)	(or rotate day off)	Patient Care (4 hours)	Patient Care (4 hours)	
	1200 - 1230	Break*	Break*		Break*	Break*	
	1230 - 1300	Documentation/Admin	Documentation/Admin		Documentation/Admin	Documentation/Admin	
	1300 - 1700	Patient Care (4 hours)	Patient Care (4 hours)		Patient Care (4 hours)	Patient Care (4 hours)	
	1700 - 1730	Documentation/Admin	Documentation/Admin		Documentation/Admin	Documentation/Admin	
	Total Worked Hours	10	10	0	10	10	40

	Schedule	Day 1	Day 2	Day 3	Day 4	Day 5	Weekly Total
Week 4	0700 - 0800	Documentation/Admin	Documentation/Admin	Off	Documentation/Admin	Documentation/Admin	
	0800 - 1200	Patient Care (4 hours)	Patient Care (4 hours)	(or rotate day off)	Patient Care (4 hours)	Patient Care (4 hours)	
	1200 - 1230	Break*	Break*		Break*	Break*	
	1230 - 1300	Documentation/Admin	Documentation/Admin		Documentation/Admin	Documentation/Admin	
	1300 - 1700	Patient Care (4 hours)	Patient Care (4 hours)		Patient Care (4 hours)	Patient Care (4 hours)	
	1700 - 1730	Documentation/Admin	Documentation/Admin		Documentation/Admin	Documentation/Admin	
	Total Worked Hours	10	10	0	10	10	40

Grand Total	160

SAMPLE SCHEDULE: 8 -HOUR SHIFTS
(EIGHT CLINICAL SESSIONS PER WEEK)
SAMPLE SCHEDULE (8.5-HOUR WORKDAY/FIVE PER WEEK; EIGHT CLINICAL SESSIONS)

Week 1

Schedule	Day 1	Day 2	Day 3	Day 4	Day 5	Weekly Total
0800 - 1200	Patient Care (4 hours)	Documentation/Admin	Patient Care (4 hours)	Patient Care (4 hours)	Patient Care (4 hours)	
1200 - 1230	Break	Break	Break	Break	Break	
1230 - 1630	Patient Care (4 hours)	Patient Care (4 hours)	Patient Care (4 hours)	Documentation/Admin	Patient Care (4 hours)	
Total Worked Hours	8	8	8	8	8	40

Week 2

Schedule	Day 1	Day 2	Day 3	Day 4	Day 5	Weekly Total
0800 - 1200	Patient Care (4 hours)	Patient Care (4 hours)	Patient Care (4 hours)	Documentation/Admin	Patient Care (4 hours)	
1200 - 1230	Break	Break	Break	Break	Break	
1230 - 1630	Patient Care (4 hours)	Documentation/Admin	Patient Care (4 hours)	Patient Care (4 hours)	Patient Care (4 hours)	
Total Worked Hours	8	8	8	8	8	40

Week 3

Schedule	Day 1	Day 2	Day 3	Day 4	Day 5	Weekly Total
0800 - 1200	Patient Care (4 hours)	Documentation/Admin	Patient Care (4 hours)	Patient Care (4 hours)	Patient Care (4 hours)	
1200 - 1230	Break	Break	Break	Break	Break	
1230 - 1630	Patient Care (4 hours)	Patient Care (4 hours)	Patient Care (4 hours)	Documentation/Admin	Patient Care (4 hours)	
Total Worked Hours	8	8	8	8	8	40

Week 4

Schedule	Day 1	Day 2	Day 3	Day 4	Day 5	Weekly Total
0800 - 1200	Patient Care (4 hours)	Patient Care (4 hours)	Patient Care (4 hours)	Documentation/Admin	Patient Care (4 hours)	
1200 - 1230	Break	Break	Break	Break	Break	
1230 - 1630	Patient Care (4 hours)	Documentation/Admin	Patient Care (4 hours)	Patient Care (4 hours)	Patient Care (4 hours)	
Total Worked Hours	8	8	8	8	8	40

Grand Total	160

SAMPLE SCHEDULE: 8-HOUR SHIFTS
(EIGHT CLINICAL SESSIONS PER WEEK; ONE ADMIN. DAY)
SAMPLE SCHEDULE (8.5-HOUR WORKDAY/FIVE PER WEEK; EIGHT CLINICAL SESSIONS, ROTATING ADMIN/DOCUMENTATION DAY)

Week 1

Schedule	Day 1	Day 2	Day 3	Day 4	Day 5	Weekly Total
0800 - 1200	Patient Care (4 hours)	Patient Care (4 hours)	Patient Care (4 hours)	Documentation/Admin	Patient Care (4 hours)	
1200 - 1230	Break	Break	Break	Break	Break	
1230 - 1630	Patient Care (4 hours)	Patient Care (4 hours)	Patient Care (4 hours)	Documentation/Admin	Patient Care (4 hours)	
Total Worked Hours	8	8	8	8	8	40

Week 2

Schedule	Day 1	Day 2	Day 3	Day 4	Day 5	Weekly Total
0800 - 1200	Patient Care (4 hours)	Documentation/Admin	Patient Care (4 hours)	Patient Care (4 hours)	Patient Care (4 hours)	
1200 - 1230	Break	Break	Break	Break	Break	
1230 - 1630	Patient Care (4 hours)	Documentation/Admin	Patient Care (4 hours)	Patient Care (4 hours)	Patient Care (4 hours)	
Total Worked Hours	8	8	8	8	8	40

Week 3

Schedule	Day 1	Day 2	Day 3	Day 4	Day 5	Weekly Total
0800 - 1200	Patient Care (4 hours)	Patient Care (4 hours)	Patient Care (4 hours)	Documentation/Admin	Patient Care (4 hours)	
1200 - 1230	Break	Break	Break	Break	Break	
1230 - 1630	Patient Care (4 hours)	Patient Care (4 hours)	Patient Care (4 hours)	Documentation/Admin	Patient Care (4 hours)	
Total Worked Hours	8	8	8	8	8	40

Week 4

Schedule	Day 1	Day 2	Day 3	Day 4	Day 5	Weekly Total
0800 - 1200	Patient Care (4 hours)	Documentation/Admin	Patient Care (4 hours)	Patient Care (4 hours)	Patient Care (4 hours)	
1200 - 1230	Break	Break	Break	Break	Break	
1230 - 1630	Patient Care (4 hours)	Documentation/Admin	Patient Care (4 hours)	Patient Care (4 hours)	Patient Care (4 hours)	
Total Worked Hours	8	8	8	8	8	40

Grand Total	160

SAMPLE SCHEDULE: 8-HOUR SHIFTS
(NINE CLINICAL SESSIONS PER WEEK)
SAMPLE SCHEDULE (8.5-HOUR WORKDAY/FIVE PER WEEK; NINE CLINICAL SESSIONS

	Schedule	Day 1	Day 2	Day 3	Day 4	Day 5	Weekly Total
Week 1	0800 - 1200	Patient Care (4 hours)	Patient Care (4 hours)	Patient Care (4 hours)	Patient Care (4 hours)	Patient Care (4 hours)	
	1200 - 1230	Break	Break	Break	Break	Break	
	1230 - 1630	Patient Care (4 hours)	Documentation/Admin	Patient Care (4 hours)	Patient Care (4 hours)	Patient Care (4 hours)	
	Total Worked Hours	8	8	8	8	8	40

	Schedule	Day 1	Day 2	Day 3	Day 4	Day 5	Weekly Total
Week 2	0800 - 1200	Patient Care (4 hours)	Patient Care (4 hours)	Patient Care (4 hours)	Patient Care (4 hours)	Patient Care (4 hours)	
	1200 - 1230	Break	Break	Break	Break	Break	
	1230 - 1630	Patient Care (4 hours)	Patient Care (4 hours)	Patient Care (4 hours)	Documentation/Admin	Patient Care (4 hours)	
	Total Worked Hours	8	8	8	8	8	40

	Schedule	Day 1	Day 2	Day 3	Day 4	Day 5	Weekly Total
Week 3	0800 - 1200	Patient Care (4 hours)	Patient Care (4 hours)	Patient Care (4 hours)	Patient Care (4 hours)	Patient Care (4 hours)	
	1200 - 1230	Break	Break	Break	Break	Break	
	1230 - 1630	Patient Care (4 hours)	Patient Care (4 hours)	Documentation/Admin	Patient Care (4 hours)	Patient Care (4 hours)	
	Total Worked Hours	8	8	8	8	8	40

	Schedule	Day 1	Day 2	Day 3	Day 4	Day 5	Weekly Total
Week 4	0800 - 1200	Patient Care (4 hours)	Patient Care (4 hours)	Patient Care (4 hours)	Patient Care (4 hours)	Patient Care (4 hours)	
	1200 - 1230	Break	Break	Break	Break	Break	
	1230 - 1630	Patient Care (4 hours)	Documentation/Admin	Patient Care (4 hours)	Patient Care (4 hours)	Patient Care (4 hours)	
	Total Worked Hours	8	8	8	8	8	40

Grand Total	160

SAMPLE SCHEDULE: 8-HOUR SHIFTS
(IP/OP SPLIT: SIX CLINICAL SESSIONS PER WEEK)
SAMPLE SCHEDULE (8.5-HOUR WORKDAY/FIVE PER WEEK; SIX CLINICAL SESSIONS, REMAINING INPATIENT)

Week 1

Schedule	Day 1	Day 2	Day 3	Day 4	Day 5	Weekly Total
0800 - 1200	Patient Care (4 hours)	Inpatient	Inpatient	Patient Care (4 hours)	Patient Care (4 hours)	
1200 - 1230	Break	Break	Break	Break	Break	
1230 - 1630	Patient Care (4 hours)	Documentation/Admin	Inpatient	Patient Care (4 hours)	Patient Care (4 hours)	
Total Worked Hours	8	8	8	8	8	40

Week 2

Schedule	Day 1	Day 2	Day 3	Day 4	Day 5	Weekly Total
0800 - 1200	Patient Care (4 hours)	Inpatient	Inpatient	Patient Care (4 hours)	Patient Care (4 hours)	
1200 - 1230	Break	Break	Break	Break	Break	
1230 - 1630	Patient Care (4 hours)	Documentation/Admin	Inpatient	Patient Care (4 hours)	Patient Care (4 hours)	
Total Worked Hours	8	8	8	8	8	40

Week 3

Schedule	Day 1	Day 2	Day 3	Day 4	Day 5	Weekly Total
0800 - 1200	Patient Care (4 hours)	Inpatient	Inpatient	Patient Care (4 hours)	Patient Care (4 hours)	
1200 - 1230	Break	Break	Break	Break	Break	
1230 - 1630	Patient Care (4 hours)	Documentation/Admin	Inpatient	Patient Care (4 hours)	Patient Care (4 hours)	
Total Worked Hours	8	8	8	8	8	40

Week 4

Schedule	Patient Care (4 hours)	Inpatient	Inpatient	Patient Care (4 hours)	Patient Care (4 hours)	Weekly Total
0800 - 1200	Break	Break	Break	Break	Break	
1200 - 1230	Patient Care (4 hours)	Documentation/Admin	Inpatient	Patient Care (4 hours)	Patient Care (4 hours)	
1230 - 1630	Patient Care (4 hours)	Documentation/Admin	Patient Care (4 hours)	Patient Care (4 hours)	Patient Care (4 hours)	
Total Worked Hours	8	8	8	8	8	40

Grand Total	160

SAMPLE SCHEDULE: 8-HOUR SHIFTS
(SPLIT: CLINIC A.M./IP P.M.)
SAMPLE SCHEDULE (8.5-HOUR WORKDAY/FIVE PER WEEK; A.M. CLINIC/P.M. INPATIENT)

Week 1

Schedule	Day 1	Day 2	Day 3	Day 4	Day 5	Weekly Total
0800 - 1200	Patient Care (4 hours)	Patient Care (4 hours)	Patient Care (4 hours)	Patient Care (4 hours)	Patient Care (4 hours)	
1200 - 1230	Break	Break	Break	Break	Break	
1230 - 1600	Inpatient	Inpatient	Inpatient	Inpatient	Inpatient	
1600 - 1630	Documentation/Admin	Documentation/Admin	Documentation/Admin	Documentation/Admin	Documentation/Admin	
Total Worked Hours	8	8	8	8	8	40

Week 2

Schedule	Day 1	Day 2	Day 3	Day 4	Day 5	Weekly Total
0800 - 1200	Patient Care (4 hours)	Patient Care (4 hours)	Patient Care (4 hours)	Patient Care (4 hours)	Patient Care (4 hours)	
1200 - 1230	Break	Break	Break	Break	Break	
1230 - 1600	Inpatient	Inpatient	Inpatient	Inpatient	Inpatient	
1600 - 1630	Documentation/Admin	Documentation/Admin	Documentation/Admin	Documentation/Admin	Documentation/Admin	
Total Worked Hours	8	8	8	8	8	40

	Grand Total	160

Week 3

Schedule	Day 1	Day 2	Day 3	Day 4	Day 5	Weekly Total
0800 - 1200	Patient Care (4 hours)	Patient Care (4 hours)	Patient Care (4 hours)	Patient Care (4 hours)	Patient Care (4 hours)	
1200 - 1230	Break	Break	Break	Break	Break	
1230 - 1600	Inpatient	Inpatient	Inpatient	Inpatient	Inpatient	
1600 - 1630	Documentation/Admin	Documentation/Admin	Documentation/Admin	Documentation/Admin	Documentation/Admin	
Total Worked Hours	8	8	8	8	8	40

Week 4

Schedule	Day 1	Day 2	Day 3	Day 4	Day 5	Weekly Total
0800 - 1200	Patient Care (4 hours)	Patient Care (4 hours)	Patient Care (4 hours)	Patient Care (4 hours)	Patient Care (4 hours)	
1200 - 1230	Break	Break	Break	Break	Break	
1230 - 1600	Inpatient	Inpatient	Inpatient	Inpatient	Inpatient	
1600 - 1630	Documentation/Admin	Documentation/Admin	Documentation/Admin	Documentation/Admin	Documentation/Admin	
Total Worked Hours	8	8	8	8	8	40

	Grand Total	160

APPENDIX E

GUIDE TO BEST PRACTICES FOR CLINICAL ONBOARDING

The following guide has been developed to assist department leadership in onboarding advanced practice providers (APPs).

DEVELOP A BUSINESS PLAN

HOW WILL THIS ROLE FUNCTION?

- Hours of work—consider resident schedule and other commitments (OR, off-site clinics)
- Weekend coverage, call, holiday coverage?
- Solely inpatient or mix of inpatient and outpatient?
- Working with other APPs or a new role in the department/division?

SCOPE OF NEW POSITION: PROVIDE TEMPLATE, FUNDING SOURCES

- Specific responsibilities (rounding, bed huddle, routine morning orders, cover calls from the floor, consults, documentation improvement goals)

DETAIL PRODUCTIVITY EXPECTATIONS AND TIMELINE

- Take into consideration the average census on the floor
- Acuity of patients
- Number and timing of admissions and discharges
- Number of providers

INCLUDE CASELOAD/SCHEDULE/OTHER METRICS

- Number of patients dependent on the acuity and patient turnover
- Consider the maximum number of patients/APP in ICU/non-ICU settings
- Customize productivity metrics based on the unique needs of the team

DEFINE WORK EFFORT TO SUPPORT TOP-OF-LICENSE PRACTICE

REVIEW OF SCHEDULING GUIDELINES/PATIENT PANEL TO OPTIMIZE PRODUCTIVITY

QUANTIFY HOW APP ROLE IS ESSENTIAL TO PATIENT ACCESS AND SCHEDULING GOALS

- Reduced length of stay
- Improved clinical documentation
- Increased patient satisfaction
- Increased nursing staff satisfaction
- Improved continuity of care
- Improved patient access

DISCUSS DURING INTERVIEW

- Credentialing and privileging process
- Productivity expectations
- General overview of onboarding/orientation timeline
- Expectations for full caseload (timing/metrics)
- Start date may be changed based on credentialing/privileging dates

SCHEDULE START DATE

- Review panel approval dates to anticipate date privileges granted
- Schedule start date/orientation around this date
- Adjust start date if needed to align with privileges/orientation schedule

PLAN/OUTLINE ORIENTATION/ONBOARDING

- Create a calendar/schedule and provide to new APP at hire (or before)
- Customize based on skills/experience of new hire
- Include shadows with other specialties the APP will work with on a regular basis (Radiology, Endocrine, ICU, Palliative, OR, etc.)
- Discuss IPPE/FPPE/OPPE process
- Identify go-to point of contact during orientation/onboarding and schedule meetings

SCHEDULE INITIAL TRAINING

- Epic
- New hire orientation/New provider orientation/APP seminar
- CQ
- Coding and billing
- Documentation

ONBOARDING APP TOWARD FULL CASELOAD

- Identify primary preceptor/mentor with support from everyone in the department getting APP to full caseload
- Schedule created based on sub-specialties
- PAC scheduling template clearly defines patient population
- Provide additional coding/billing/documentation review/resources after an APP is functional
- Open-door approach for troubleshooting coding/billing/documentation issues post onboarding
- APP participates in grand rounds (includes key updates on coding, etc.) and departmental educational meetings such as morbidity and mortality, resident education, divisional meetings

- Allow up to four to six months to be fully productive (dependent on APP skill level and patient population)

- Request core privileges first; as APP becomes competent in additional procedures, request to modify privileges

- Frequent check-in with preceptor/mentor to gauge progress; combination of structured and informal check-ins

- Identify those who will monitor progress of new APP to identify and address issues early and provide any further training

APPENDIX F

GLOSSARY

APP CLINICAL PRACTICE

ACGME: Accreditation Council for Graduate Medical Education

AMC: Academic Medical Center

CARTS: Clinical, Administrative, Research, Teaching, Strategic (time allocation for providers)

CDI: Clinical Documentation Improvement

CMI: Case Mix Index

DRG: Diagnosis-Related Grouper

ECMO: Extracorporeal Membrane Oxygenation

HCAHPS: Hospital Consumer Assessment of Healthcare Providers and Systems

ICON: Iowa Course Management System

LOS: Length of Stay

NEDOCS: National Emergency Department Overcrowding Scale

PHI: Protected Health Information

DEPARTMENTS

COM: College of Medicine

CON: College of Nursing

CSO: Clinical Staff Office

CVICU: Cardiovascular Intensive Care Unit

CWS: Children's and Women's Services

DEI: Diversity, Equity, and Inclusion

EHC: Employee Health Clinic

ELR: Employee and Labor Relations

MICU: Medical Intensive Care Unit

OAPP: Office of Advanced Practice Providers

PICU: Pediatric Intensive Care Unit

SNICU: Surgical/Neurological Intensive Care Unit

JOB TITLES

AGNP: Adult Gerontology Nurse Practitioner (primary or acute)

APP: Advanced Practice Provider (PA or APRN)

APRN: Advanced Practice Registered Nurse

ARNP: Advanced Registered Nurse Practitioner

CDA: Clinical Department Administrator

CNM: Certified Nurse Midwife

CNP: Certified Nurse Practitioner

CNS: Clinical Nurse Specialist

CRNA: Certified Registered Nurse Anesthetist

DEO: Departmental Executive Officer

FNP: Family Nurse Practitioner

NNP: Neonatal Nurse Practitioner

PA-C: Physician Assistant-Certified

PMHNP: Psych Mental Health Nurse Practitioner

PNP: Pediatric Nurse Practitioner (primary or acute)

WHNP: Women's Health Nurse Practitioner

EMPLOYMENT & OFFICE

ELR: Employee and Labor Relations

HRIS: Human Resources Information Systems (aka self-service)

LDAC: Long Distance Access Code

MFK: Master File Key (accounting)

P Card: Procurement Card (credit card used for department purchases)

APPENDIX G

ADVANCED PRACTICE
PROVIDER RESOURCES

ORGANIZATION INFORMATION

- Org chart
- Strategic plan
- Provider directory
- Employee newsletters
- Employee directory

EDUCATION AND PROFESSIONAL DEVELOPMENT

- Medical library
- New hire staff orientation
- Provider orientation
- LinkedIn Learning
- Leadership training
- Social media policy
- Revenue cycle training

NEW HIRE INFORMATION

- Parking
- Orientation
- Employee health clinic
- Employee intranet
- Payroll self-service
- Email web access

- Human resources
- Benefits
- Department directory

LICENSE & CERTIFICATION

- State licensing (PA & NP)
- Board certification links

YOUR APP PRACTICE

- APP website
- Professional portraits
- Update your provider profile
- Pager
- Medical library
- BLS/ACLS/PALS resources
- Scheduling
- EMR training
- DEA link
- CME/CE resources
- Skills lab
- Compliance helpline
- Safety resources
- Interpreter resources
- Conflict of interest

INTRANET

- APP intranet
- Remote access
- Incident reporting
- Sharps/needlestick protocol
- Recommended reading list

YOUR WELL-BEING

- Health coach
- Wellness site
- EAP program
- Mindfulness program resources
- Mental health hotline
- Child care resources

APPENDIX H

CASE STUDY: DEVELOPING
AN APP ONBOARDING
PROGRAM

UI Health Care initiated a project to examine the current state of APP onboarding, identify gaps, and design a more comprehensive process. APPs recently hired were asked to provide feedback on the time to complete onboarding, their understanding of the steps involved, and use of tools and resources available during the onboarding process. The data indicated that APPs were receiving an inconsistent onboarding experience in both time and content.

From the data it was determined that a key deliverable would be to develop and implement a new APP onboarding education session designed to be general enough to add value to any new APP, regardless of experience, specialty, and work site. Clear goals for the session were identified as:

1. Build a sense of community among APPs.

2. Discuss role transition.

3. Connect to valuable internal resources.

4. Network with other APPs to grow and strengthen connections.

5. Provide role clarity and productivity metrics.

Input from a cross-functional project team was critical in ensuring that the program met organizational expectations and needs. This group formed the agenda for the session based on an analysis in each of the five areas to identify the gap between current onboarding practices for APPs and the goals sought by the new APP onboarding session. A gap analysis is one of many tools available to healthcare leaders to assess an organization's readiness to change and identify priorities for improvement. The following table illustrates the gap analysis used in analyzing the need for a structured onboarding program.

GAP ANALYSIS FOR STRUCTURED ONBOARDING PROGRAM

PROJECT DELIVERA-BLES	GOALS: WHAT ARE WE FOCUSED ON?	DESIRED FUTURE STATE: WHERE DO WE WANT TO BE? (NEEDS)	CURRENT STATE: WHERE ARE WE NOW?	IDENTIFIED GAP: DIFFERENCE BETWEEN CURRENT STATE AND FUTURE STATE	POSSIBLE REMEDIES: WHAT ARE SOME IDEAS OF THINGS WE CAN DO?
Develop and implement a new APP Onboarding Education Session	Build a sense of community.	Need to do a better job bringing us together, allowing us to feel similar. Will build satisfaction.	APP Council not well attended, new hires not aware.	Lack of defined community that takes into consideration what's meaningful to the APPs, helping them identify as part of a group.	Welcome email/letter from OAPP upon hire or transfer to APP role.
			APPs not brought together formally as new employees.		Include APP Council (and other APP specific activities) as part of onboarding session education.
			APPs not defined as their own unique community.	New employees not made aware of or do not recall knowing about APP Council.	Create infographic/distribute infographic with UI APP stats (numbers, where working, fun facts).
			Lack of a sense of belonging and cohesiveness, which can impact job satisfaction.	New hires welcomed into their department/division. Not formally welcomed uniquely as APPs.	
	Network with other APPs to grow and strengthen connections.	Need to build relationships across the spectrum.	Limited opportunities to make contacts in outside areas.	No opportunities to network with APPs in other areas. Difficult to make connections. Some APPs do not know how to network, are not given the chance to practice networking, are unaware of the benefits, or find it uncomfortable.	Set aside time for structured networking during session.
		APPs need a sense of "I belong," need to meet others. Currently feel siloed.	Learning from other APPs occurs generally within their own work unit.		Provide networking guide and tips.
		APPs need to have contacts in outside areas, other areas.	No formal peer-to-peer support as new APP.		

PROJECT DELIVERABLES	GOALS: WHAT ARE WE FOCUSED ON?	DESIRED FUTURE STATE: WHERE DO WE WANT TO BE? (NEEDS)	CURRENT STATE: WHERE ARE WE NOW?	IDENTIFIED GAP: DIFFERENCE BETWEEN CURRENT STATE AND FUTURE STATE	POSSIBLE REMEDIES: WHAT ARE SOME IDEAS OF THINGS WE CAN DO?
	Connect to resources, know where to go for help.	Master list of resources would be helpful, where to connect with resources/questions, where to get more help (such as library, HR, etc.). Mentors are used within certain departments; do we need a mentorship program system-wide? Need to communicate that there are many ways/methods that an APP can meet with preceptor—in person, text, phone, etc.	Mentors are used within certain departments. Not every APP has a lead. Varying methods used within departments/divisions, due to differences in hiring volumes and resources.	APPs do not know who to contact if onboarding is not going well. No standardized resource list. No system-wide mentoring program. Some departments have formal preceptor education, and others do not. No standardized preceptor format.	Review APP intranet site. Develop list of APP resources. Develop onboarding roadmap so APP knows what to expect and who to contact.
	Role clarity, understand what is expected of me.	Leadership expectations for APPs include clear role expectations and tracks/metrics; number of clinic sessions, decreasing length of stay, patient satisfaction, etc. Need for good business plan prior to APP position being approved, with clearly defined expectations.	Role clarity can be an issue, with some APPs not clear on how they are to be utilized within a work group.	APPs need to have a clear understanding of their tasks, responsibilities, and what's expected of them. Clarity is an essential element of productivity and when lacking it can cause stress, confusion, and job dissatisfaction. Understanding expectations and setting goals are part of being successful.	Provide leadership expectations for APP including clear role expectations and tracks/metrics; number of clinic sessions, decreasing length of stay, patient satisfaction, etc. Q & A panel of experienced APPs. How do you do it? How are you so productive? How do you achieve results? Goal setting.

| Role transition and professional identity. | Need to address the typical evolution into role. Transition from novice to expert Setting into your role, realistic timelines. | APPs are high achievers, striving to do well and exceed expectations. May struggle with being a novice in a new role and unaware this is common. | Lack of awareness/discussion of the novice-to-expert continuum and common issues surrounding this transition. | Discuss and address this in Q & A panel. |

Solutions and remedies were brainstormed by the project team and documented, which led to the development and implementation of the program "APP Seminar: Introduction to Your Role." The program encourages round table discussions and reflection. Bringing APPs together as part of a professional community early in the role and offering professional development curriculum helps strengthen engagement and job satisfaction. Feedback from the session was favorable, with 86% of attendees giving the program the highest ranking of excellent, and 96% of attendees indicating the program was completely or mostly beneficial to them.

A sample agenda follows.

APP SEMINAR: INTRODUCTION TO YOUR ROLE

WELCOME TO YOUR APP PROFESSIONAL COMMUNITY

Welcome/Opening Remarks/Agenda/Introductions

- APP Professional Community
- Role Transition and Professional Identity
- Resources Available to APPs
- Professional Networking to Grow and Strengthen Connections

Break

- Office of Advanced Practice Providers Overview
- APP Role Expectations
- Efficient Practice Responsibilities

- How Experienced APPs Practice
- Round Table Discussion, Your Transition to Practice

- Course Evaluation
- Closing Remarks; Welcome to Your APP Professional Community!

APP SEMINAR FEEDBACK

- "I really appreciated the course and found it very valuable and meaningful to my growth in the APP role."

- "Highly recommend APP seminar before beginning practice."

- "Having a course like this earlier on just to meet other new APPs starting at the same time as me would have been beneficial."

- "Nice to meet other new APPs, and I appreciate getting more details on expectations. Role transition was helpful since I am new to the APP role. I love the resources provided. Always good to have a network of support."

- "Seminar gave resources on connecting with other APPs, with emphasis on practicing top of license. Good encouragement for continuing to set goals post-graduation. The internal website is a good resource. It's always good to have examples of others in a similar position be successful."

- "Very helpful session [which] makes the experience of being new to the organization seem relatable and less overwhelming. Would recommend for all APPs."

- "Role Expectations section was very helpful as my orientation is more general than specific. Gave me ideas to guide this."

- "It was very interesting to learn how many APPs currently employed. It's great to learn about all the helpful resources as I start as an APP new grad."

- "Helpful presentation. Brought lots of things to light and encouraged to start asking questions for myself and others."

- "Great seminar. Thanks for all you do and for advocating for APPs."

- "This class was exceptional! Truthfully, I did not expect to enjoy it as much as I did."

- "I felt that this was very valuable in getting me thinking about what questions I need to ask about my APP role and the need for advocacy for ourselves."

APPENDIX I

ACADEMIC CLINICAL PARTNERSHIP CASE STUDY

The UI Health Care APP central office partnered with multiple constituents in changing the process for priority and placement of APP students into practicum experiences. The proposed structure, which was supported by executive leadership, specified an exclusive partnership for clinical placement between the healthcare organization and their own affiliated PA/APRN educational programs.

Part of the new process was ensuring that employees who are enrolled in programs at outside schools who were close to graduating be able to finish their clinicals if placement could be accommodated. A list of these employees was compiled, and a cutoff date was established based on the majority of the employees' expected graduation dates. This ensured that students would have adequate notice for the change. This change was made knowing that some employees would choose to attend outside schools; however, aligning limited preceptor resources with preferred education programs ensured that students could be served for years to come.

The change was communicated internally and externally. All outside programs were notified of this change with solid rationale explaining the demand versus capacity was too taxing. It was clearly stated that the partnership with other schools was appreciated and respected, and the change was specifically limited to APRN and PA students and not RN, RN to BSN, or MSN students desiring clinicals in any other health-related profession.

HIGHLIGHTS FROM THE PROJECT

- Executive leadership from both UI Health Care and University of Iowa education programs supported this partnership

- Exclusive partnership with the affiliated APRN and PA education programs at the University of Iowa for clinical placements and projects

- UI Health Care no longer accepted any students (even their own employees) attending outside schools for APRN or PA clinical placements or projects after the cutoff date

- Exceptions were available for students enrolled in programs not offered by affiliated University of Iowa programs

- No other education preparation applied to the changes—i.e., RN, RN to BSN, or MSN students—and was strictly aligned with APRN and PA

- Ensured prospective students and schools were aware of the criteria
  - Letter sent to all non-exclusive schools informing them of priorities
  - Website updated with new process
  - Partner with department of nursing to ensure consistent messaging when students or schools inquire
  - Communicate priorities to nursing leadership and APP leads
  - Email sent to all APPs with scripting on how to respond if/when students contact them directly to request preceptorship
  - Timeline for application deadline, committee meeting, and placement schedule

APPENDIX J

APP CLINICAL OPERATING
GUIDE: BEST PRACTICE
TRACKS AND MEASURES

APP Clinical Operating Guide - Best Practice _Tracks and Measures_
CDA to work with Lead APP to estimate FTE % in each track

	Ambulatory	Hospitalist Non-ICU	Hospitalist ICU	Surgical/Procedural
Setting Definition	Outpatient clinic setting	Inpatient hospital or consult services, skilled or long-term care	NICU, PICU, CVICU, SNICU, MICU	OR, cath lab, infusion suites
Scope of Practice	Primary care or specialty certification/license		Acute care or specialty certification/license	
Patient Population Patient caseload expectations should be in alignment with patient population benchmarking. For the purposes of this document these are generalized per track.	An ambulatory service provides delivery of care in an outpatient setting. Based on best practices, the department will document and define which patients will be seen by APP independently) and which patients to be seen with APP/MD.	Hospitalist inpatient or step-down units provide delivery of comprehensive healthcare to hospitalized non-ICU patients with a range of complex and comorbid disease conditions and across a variety of specialties. Patient caseload ranges from one APP to 8-15 patients based on patient specific acuity and patient population. Caseload expectations often increase to one APP to 16-36 patients overnight or on off shifts.	ICUs provide care to patients with severe or life-threatening illnesses and injuries, which require constant care, close supervision from life support equipment, and medication to ensure normal bodily functions. Patient caseload ranges from one APP to 4-7 patients based on patient-specific acuity and patient population. Caseload expectations often increase to one APP to 10 patients overnight or on off shifts.	The surgical/procedural patient undergoes operative procedures or infusions. Patient caseload ranges based on the procedure protocols within the specialty.
Schedule	8-9 half day clinic sessions per 1.0 FTE	Patient caseload ranges from one APP to 8-15 patients based on patient-specific acuity and patient population. Caseload expectations often increase to one APP to 16-36 patients overnight or on off-shifts.	May require 24/7 coverage (defined by clinical service area).	
Productivity Tracks/Metrics **What will be measured?** (examples provided)	**Measure & Track:** * Split percentages (i.e., 50/50) used for internal APP productivity benchmarking and tracking purposes, not for compensation incentive and subject to change/adjustements as determined by executive leadership. APP and physician practice as a team (see patients together, i.e. half direct): Divide RVUs equally (*50/50 split) between APP and physician who see patients together to provide a benchmark for APP productivity for internal benchmarking. Combine RVU target goals when APPs and physicians practice as a team that increases physician productivity. APP practices independently (sees non-RVU visits): Calculate additional physician productivity when APP is seeing their non-RVU visits (i.e. pre- and post-op visits). APP practicing independently (sees RVU generating visits, billing indirect): Attribute all RVUs to APP. 8-9 clinic sessions per 1.0 FTE. Track patient satisfaction scores, measure improvement. Patient access: patients to be seen within 10 days of request, tracked and measured.	**Measure & Track:** Improved length of stay (LOS): Identify metric to measure length of time between admission and discharge to optimize CMS incentives and benchmarking data. Improved discharge time: Compare time discharge order placed to actual discharge time to quantify discrepancy with goals. Improved CC/MCC documentation (UHC CDI provides tracking and improvement measurement) Secondary diagnosis of Complicating Co-Morbidity (CC) and Major Complicating (MCC) will document the increased resources required to adequately care for the patient. As the patient's severity increases based on accurate documentation of CC/MCC, Case Mix Index (CMI) increases proportionately. Improve team communication surrounding plan of care. (Provider/RN/patient/team). Expectations set by department. Track patient satisfaction scores Measure improvement.	**Measure & Track:** Improved CC/MCC documentation (UHC CDI provides tracking and improvement measurement) Secondary diagnosis of Complicating Co-Morbidity (CC) and Major Complicating Co-Morbidity (MCC) will document the increased resources required to adequately care for the patient. As the patient's severity increases based on accurate documentation of CC/MCC, Case Mix Index (CMI) increases proportionately. Improve team communication surrounding plan of care. (Provider/RN/patient/team). Expectations set by department. Measure improvement. Track patient satisfaction scores Measure improvement. Department establishes admission stabilization length to adhere to golden hour methodology. Measure admissions stabilization length to adhere to golden hour methodology. Improve team communication surrounding plan of care. (Provider/RN/patient/team). Expectations set by department. Track patient satisfaction scores, measure improvement.	**Measure & Track:** Procedural time: Total scheduled FTE in procedures vs. non-procedure time. Procedural volume Number of procedures completed per scheduled procedure shift. Department metrics Specific to patient population Procedure completion time duration Measured and tracked for improvement

*APPs involved in research will have funding source adequately aligned with FTE.

APPENDIX K

BUSINESS PRO FORMA

APP Pro Forma Feeder Tab

		NOTES:
Total APP FTE projected:		
Projected cbFTE:		
Projected wRVUs for APP billing independently (at full capacity, adjusted for cbFTE):		
Projected wRVUs generated by the APP but billed by physician (at full capacity, adjusted for cbFTE):		*If RVUs cannot be projected, please submit info on fully onboarded APP poductivity metrics at full caseload.
MGMA APP specialty:		
MGMA APP %tile (standard APP is 50%/median):		
MGMA median RVUs for APP specialty (adjusted for projected cbFTE)		
Base salary:		
MGMA total compensation benchmark (- %tile):		
Division:		This drives the $/RVU in the pro forma.
Position type:		
University job code/job title:		
Fringe rate pool:		
MD FTE for specialty/subspecialty (immediate area):		
APP FTE for specialty/subspecialty (immediate area):		
Ratio MD FTE/APP FTE specialty/subspecialty (immediate area):		

Figure K.1   APP proforma, page 1

APP Workforce – Financial Pro Forma
Pro Forma Should Represent the Individual APP Position

	YEAR 1 80% wRVU Target	YEAR 2 100% wRVU Target	YEAR 3 100% wRVU Target	Notes:
DIRECT REVENUE				
Projected cbFTE	0%	0%	0%	
wRVU Target to (MGMA)				Rampups for NEW providers are 50/75/100. Replacement providers are 80/100/100.
Projected wRVUs for APP billing independently	-	-	-	
Proj. wRVUs generated by the APP, billed by physician	-	-	-	
Net Payment per wRVU for APP	$0.00	$0.00	$0.00	% of division $/RVU. Based on division actual NPR/wRVU.
Net Payment per wRVU for physician	$0.00	$0.00	$0.00	100% of division $/RVU. Based on division actual NPR/wRVU.
Net Patient Revenue	$0	$0	$0	
Extramural Grant Support	$0	$0	$0	
Other Revenue (describe below)	$0	$0	$0	
TOTAL NET REVENUE	$0	$0	$0	
EXPENSES				
APP Base Salary Expense	$0	$0	$0	Inflated by % each year.
APP Fringe Benefits	$0	$0	$0	
Professional Development Support	$0	$0	$0	
Malpractice	$0	$0	$0	
Relocation	$0			
Dept Incremental Staff Salary And Fringe (describe below)	$0	$0	$0	Inflated by % each year.
Start-Up Expenses: Computer, Office Revov., etc..	$0	$0	$0	
Other Expenses and/or Dept Overhead (describe below)	$0	$0	$0	
TOTAL EXPENSES (Before Group Practice Overheads)	$0	$0	$0	
DEPT INCREMENTAL NET INCOME BEFORE OVERHEADS	$0	$0	$0	
GROUP PRACTICE OVERHEADS				
University Overhead	$0	$0	$0	
Office Rent	$0	$0	$0	
Dean's Tax (% of Total Net Revenue)	$0	$0	$0	
UIP Overhead (% of Total Net Revenue)	$0	$0	$0	
Collection Service Overhead (% of NPR)	$0	$0	$0	
CID Overhead (% of NPR)	$0	$0	$0	
PAC Overhead (% of NPR)	$0	$0	$0	
Outreach Clinic Operations	$0	$0	$0	
Outreach Joint Office	$0	$0	$0	
TOTAL GROUP PRACTICE OVERHEADS	$0	$0	$0	
NET INCOME/(LOSS) TO DEPT PRIOR TO FUNDS FLOW	$0	$0	$0	
Funds Flow Support				
$ per wRVU	$0	$0	$0	This is the funds flow supplement to the collected $/RVU on row 16 above.
TOTAL FUNDS FLOW SUPPORT	$0	$0	$0	
NET INCOME/ (LOSS) AFTER FUNDS FLOW SUPPORT	$0	$0	$0	If a loss in any year, please describe below how the department will budget.

Other Revenue, Expenses, Profit/(Loss) description:

Pale gray cells – users type in data
Dark gray cells – re-populated but can override
White cells – totals

Figure K.2   APP proforma, page 2

APPENDIX L

COMPETENCY-BASED PROFESSIONAL PRACTICE EVALUATION

COMPETENCY-BASED PROFESSIONAL PRACTICE EVALUATION
Department of *(add your department here)*

Practitioner Name: _____
Department: _____
Division: _____
Date Privileges Granted: _____
Proctor/Preceptor: _____
Proctor/Preceptor: _____
Proctor/Preceptor: _____

NA = Not applicable	**CR** = Chart review
PE = Previous experience	**S** = Simulation
D = Discussed in orientation	**CA** = Competency achieved
E = Unit experience/clinical practice	

Core Areas of Competency	DATA SOURCE						

Patient Care
Provides care that is compassionate, appropriate, and effective for the promotion of health, prevention of illness, treatment of disease, and care at the end of life.

	NA	PE	D	E	CR	S	CA

Medical/Clinical Knowledge
Demonstrates knowledge of established and evolving biomedical, clinical, and social sciences, and applies this knowledge to patient care and education of others.

	NA	PE	D	E	CR	S	CA

Practice-Based Learning & Improvement
Uses scientific evidence and methods to investigate, evaluate, and improve patient care practices.

	NA	PE	D	E	CR	S	CA

Interpersonal & Communication Skills

Demonstrates interpersonal and communication skills that enable him/her to establish and maintain professional relationships with patients, families, and other members of healthcare teams.

	NA	PE	D	E	CR	S	CA

Professionalism

Demonstrates behaviors that reflect a commitment to continuous professional development, ethical practice, understanding and sensitivity to diversity, and a responsible attitude toward patients, their profession, and society.

	NA	PE	D	E	CR	S	CA

Systems-Based Practice

Understands the contexts and systems in which healthcare is provided, and applies this knowledge to improve and optimize healthcare.	NA	PE	D	E	CR	S	CA

Based upon my review and assessment of the results of the monitoring and evaluation activities, it is determined that:

☐ Initial Professional Practice Evaluation Plan (IPPE) has been satisfactorily completed (comments optional)

Comments: _____

☐ Initial Professional Practice Evaluation Plan (IPPE) has been **unsatisfactorily** completed (comments required)

Comments: _____

_____   _____
ORIENTEE   Date

_____
Print ORIENTEE'S Name

_____   _____
PROCTOR/PRECEPTOR   Date

_____
Print PROCTOR/PRECEPTOR'S Name

_____   _____
Medical Director Responsible   Date

_____
Print Medical Director's Name

APPENDIX M

ADVANCED PRACTICE PROVIDER PEER CHART REVIEW

Five charts must be reviewed for credit.

Therefore, this survey must be filled out five times—once per note being reviewed.

Advanced Practice Provider being reviewed:

***this is not the patient or your name**

Format – last name, first name

Medical Record Number being reviewed:

Date of encounter being reviewed:
(mm/dd/yyyy)

For the following questions, *Yes* **and** *n/a* **will score 1 and** *No* **will score 0.**

*If an inpatient progress note is being reviewed, several notes may need to be reviewed for accuracy.

*Answering ***n/a*** *is suitable when the question being asked truly is not applicable to the particular note being reviewed.*

1. Adequate history?

   o   1 – Yes
   o   0 – No
   o   1 – n/a

2. Does the exam relate to the history?

   o   1 – Yes
   o   0 – No
   o   1 – n/a

3. Are lab or other tests ordered, discontinued, or purposefully not ordered as appropriate for the history and exam?

- o   1 – Yes
- o   0 – No
- o   1 – n/a

4. Are pertinent problems listed on the patient's problem list?

- o   1 – Yes
- o   0 – No
- o   1 – n/a

5. Is the plan of care appropriate for diagnosis?

- o   1 – Yes
- o   0 – No
- o   1 – n/a

6. Is there appropriate follow-up noted in the plan of care?

- o   1 – Yes
- o   0 – No
- o   1 – n/a

From the six questions above, place the **Total** chart review score below, with 6 being the maximum score.

*Reminder that **n/a** also receives a score of 1.*

By typing my name below, I certify that I have read and reviewed the above information to the best of my ability.

Format – last name, first name

APPENDIX N

ADVANCED PRACTICE
PROVIDERS IOWA
STATEWIDE UNIVERSAL
PRACTITIONER
CREDENTIALING
APPLICATION (ISUPA) GUIDE

Advanced Practice Providers (APPs) ISUPA Guide

Note: If you have previously held privileges, this form may be pre-populated with your information.

Degree is not needed here (You'll enter it in section F).

Title (list one of the following):
PA-C
CNM/ARNP
CNP/ARNP
CNS/ARNP
CRNA/ARNP

Use your **full legal name**. Should match your name in all other areas of this form. Must match name on Social Security Card, Professional License, and NPI.

HR/Credentialing Contact will pre-populate both Position/Rank and Start Date.

Position/Rank should list both job classification and title. Example: *PVE2 PA/ARNP Hospitalist*.

Note: **Start date** may be adjusted based on status of Credentialing/Privileging.

Primary Practice: List your primary board certification (i.e. PA-C, FNP, PNP, etc.) (also mark "no" if board cert is pending (i.e. new grads)).

Secondary Practice: List any extra/additional board certifications you may have (i.e., FNP, PNP, etc.) (also mark "no" if board cert is pending (i.e. new grads)).

Skip this section. Your **HR/Credentialing Coordinator** pre-populates this section with their contact information.

IOWA STATEWIDE UNIVERSAL PRACTITIONER CREDENTIALING APPLICATION

NAME - Last: First: Middle: Title/Degree:

- Type or print responses in ink.
- Complete this form in its entirety and attach all requested documentation and explanations.
- A CV or "See CV" may not be used in lieu of completing any answers on this application.
- If a question does not apply to you, answer with "Non-Applicable" or "NA".
- If additional space is necessary to provide answers, attach additional sheet(s) of paper.
- All dates must be formatted as: Month/Date/Year (MM/DD/YEAR). Type/print "present" in Ending Date year for current status of activity, if applicable.

THIS APPLICATION MUST BE SIGNED AND DATED WHERE INDICATED

POSITION/RANK: ANTICIPATED START DATE:

PRIMARY PRACTICE SPECIALTY: BOARD CERTIFIED: ☐ YES ☐ NO

SECONDARY PRACTICE SPECIALTY(IES):
BOARD CERTIFIED: ☐ YES ☐ NO
BOARD CERTIFIED: ☐ YES ☐ NO
BOARD CERTIFIED: ☐ YES ☐ NO
BOARD CERTIFIED: ☐ YES ☐ NO

PERSON/ENTITY TO CONTACT REGARDING THIS APPLICATION:
NAME:
ENTITY/GROUP AFFILIATION:
ADDRESS:
CITY: STATE: ZIP:
PHONE NUMBER: FAX NUMBER:
E-MAIL:

Office of Advanced Practice Providers UI Health Care (2021)

Advanced Practice Providers (APPs) ISUPA Guide

Your full legal name and **Title** should match what was listed at the top of page 1.

If you will be **changing your name** in the near future with a known date (such as for an upcoming marriage), please indicate your current legal name at the time of the application is completed and enter your new married name and/or other maiden name(s) in the "Other Names" section along with the effective and end date for each name.

Thoroughly complete this section as applicable to you.

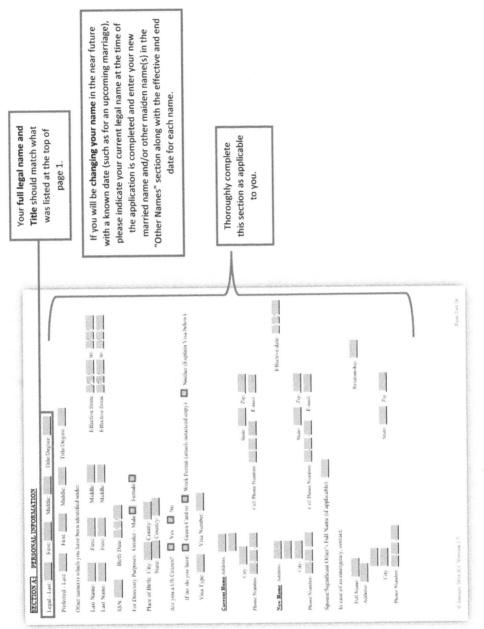

Office of Advanced Practice Providers UI Health Care (2021)

Advanced Practice Providers (APPs) ISUPA Guide

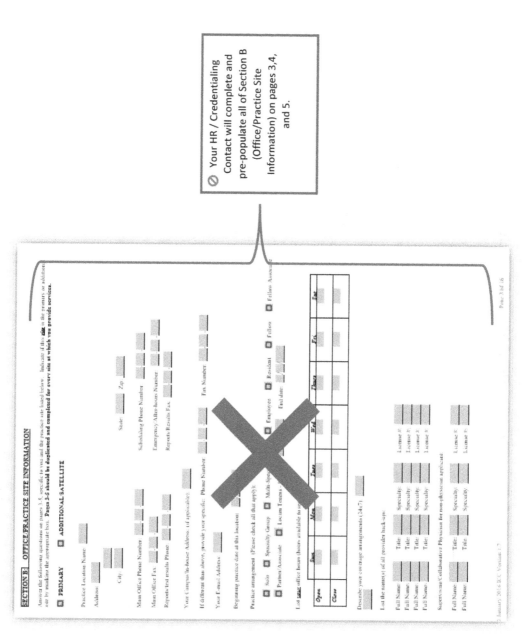

Advanced Practice Providers (APPs) ISUPA Guide

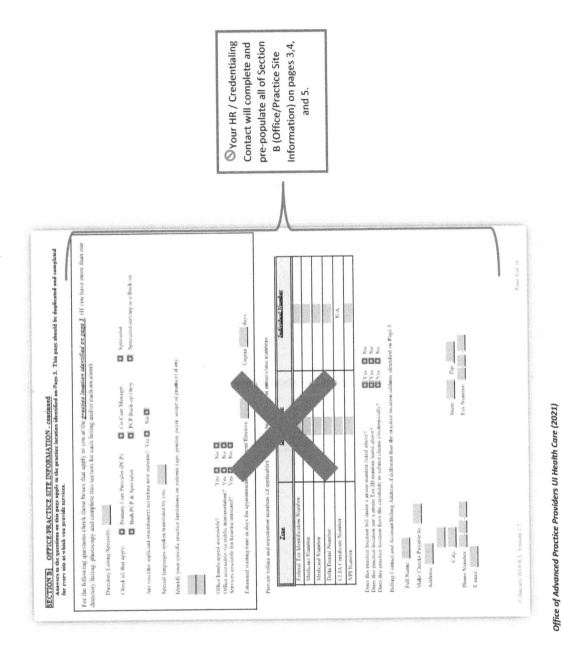

⊘ Your HR / Credentialing Contact will complete and pre-populate all of Section B (Office/Practice Site Information) on pages 3,4, and 5.

Office of Advanced Practice Providers UI Health Care (2021)

Advanced Practice Providers (APPs) ISUPA Guide

⊘ Your HR / Credentialing Contact will complete and pre-populate all of Section B (Office/Practice Site Information) on pages 3,4, and 5.

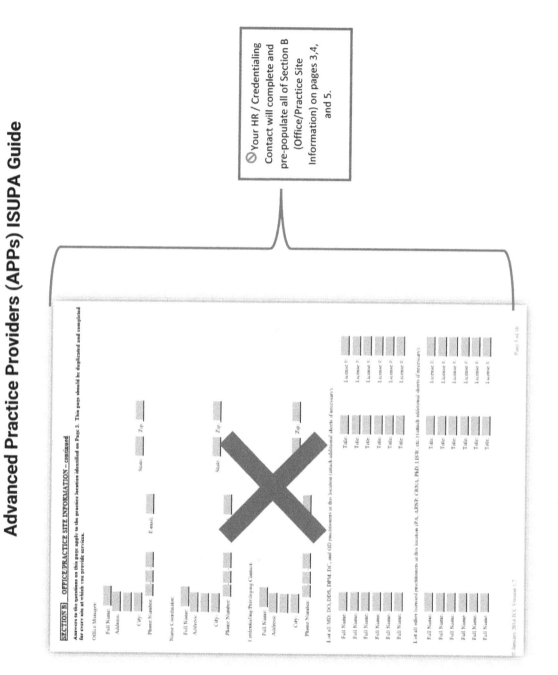

Advanced Practice Providers (APPs) ISUPA Guide

Check *"Reciprocity"* if you hold a Compact State License from a state other than Iowa.

ECFMG applies to Physicians only. APPs may disregard.

If you do not yet have your DEA or SCSC please mark "No" (such as for new APPs).

Explanations may include *"Application submitted on MM/DD/YY, pending approval"*, or, *"Have not applied"*.

Both DEA and SCSC are required for privileges to be granted. Applications should be submitted as soon as possible to avoid delays.

You will need to provide copies of your state issued license verification or print screens from their website verifications, and copies of your DEA and SCSC Certificates.

Links below:

- Link to IBON (for NP License)
- Link to IDPH (for PA License)
- Federal DEA
- Iowa Pharmacy Board (State Controlled Substance Certificate) SCSC or CDS

List **ALL your professional license information** (current and expired) in this section (example: Nursing licenses from IBON, PA License from DPH). Do NOT include your board certification.

Be sure to include all states you have been licensed and your RN license (if applicable).

SECTION C: LICENSURE INFORMATION

Professional License #	Degree	Name on License	State Issued	Country	Issue Date	Expiration Date

Certificate	State Issued	Certificate Number	Issue Date	Expiration Date
Federal DEA				
Federal DEA				
State CSC				
State CSC				

Advanced Practice Providers (APPs) ISUPA Guide

Complete Section D if you currently have non-UIHC provided **Professional Liability Coverage (malpractice)**. If you are currently employed and practicing as an APP, you will likely have this through your employment. You will need to provide a copy of this coverage certificate.

If you are employed by UIHC and covered by UI Malpractice you may leave this section blank, as we would already have this information.

Brand new APPs (new grads, or those not currently practicing as an APP) will likely not have coverage and thus will leave this section blank.

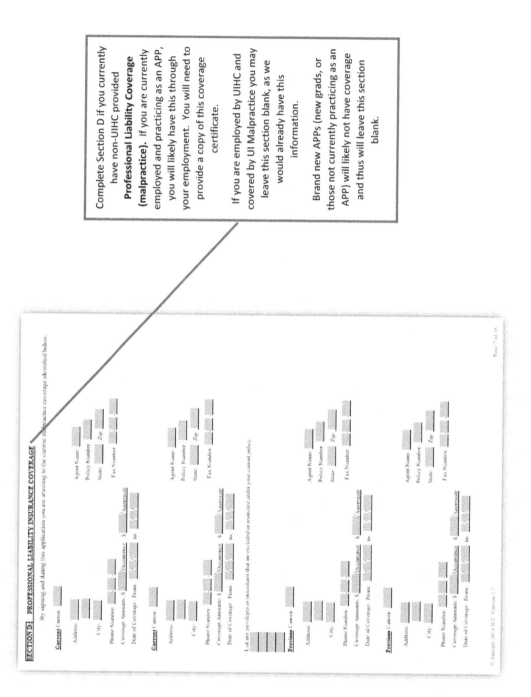

Advanced Practice Providers (APPs) ISUPA Guide

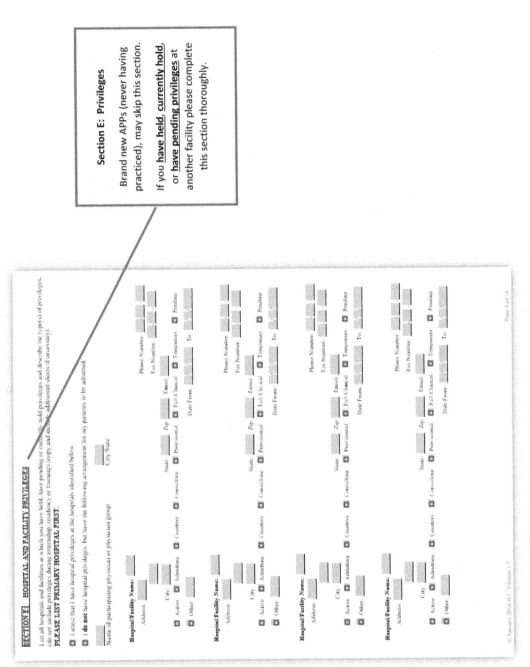

Advanced Practice Providers (APPs) ISUPA Guide

Tip: Have your educational transcripts handy when completing this section

Section F (Education) is required for all. Please carefully and specifically answer all questions.

Be very specific with the **ending date** (MM/DD/YYYY). You'll find this on your diploma or transcript.

The **phone/fax/email** of your school are optional, provided you have listed the Institutional name/address/city/state information accurately.

This is a critical section, and often overlooked. You **MUST list and explain** any gaps in your education continuous enrollment greater than 6 months in length (including month and year). (Tip: if you are unsure whether to list a gap, list it anyway. We'll disregard any gap that is not relevant)

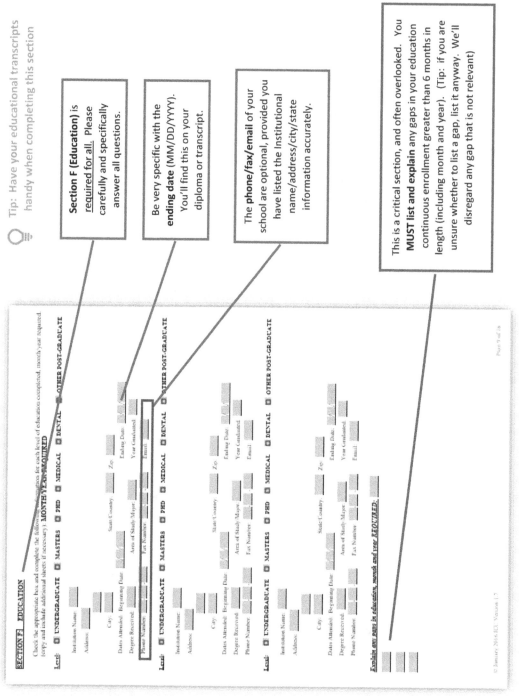

©The Iowa Credentialing Coalition. Reprinted with permission.

Office of Advanced Practice Providers UI Health Care (2021)

Advanced Practice Providers (APPs) ISUPA Guide

Section G: Training

APPs may skip this section.

©The Iowa Credentialing Coalition. Reprinted with permission.

Office of Advanced Practice Providers UI Health Care (2021)

Advanced Practice Providers (APPs) ISUPA Guide

Be very specific with the name of the agency issuing your board certification from the list below:

NCCPA: PA-C
AANP-CP: American Academy of Nurse Practitioners Certification Program
AACN: American Association of Critical Care Nurses
AMCB: American Midwifery Certification Board
NBCRNA: National Board of Certification & Recertification for Nurse Anesthetists
NCC: National Certification Corporation
PNCB: Pediatric Nursing Certification Board

Address, Phone and Fax number are not needed. Leave blank.

Do not list CPR certification here.

(but you will need to provide copies of your CPR ecards)

Complete this section if your board exams / certification is pending

You will need to provide copies of Board Certifications (can be print screens from their website verifications), and copies of your CPR Certifications (BLS, ACLS, PALS, NRP, etc.).

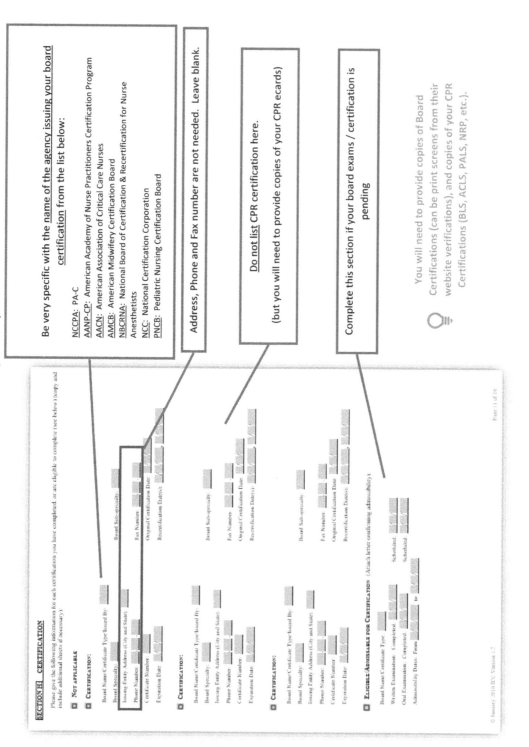

©The Iowa Credentialing Coalition. Reprinted with permission.

Advanced Practice Providers (APPs) ISUPA Guide

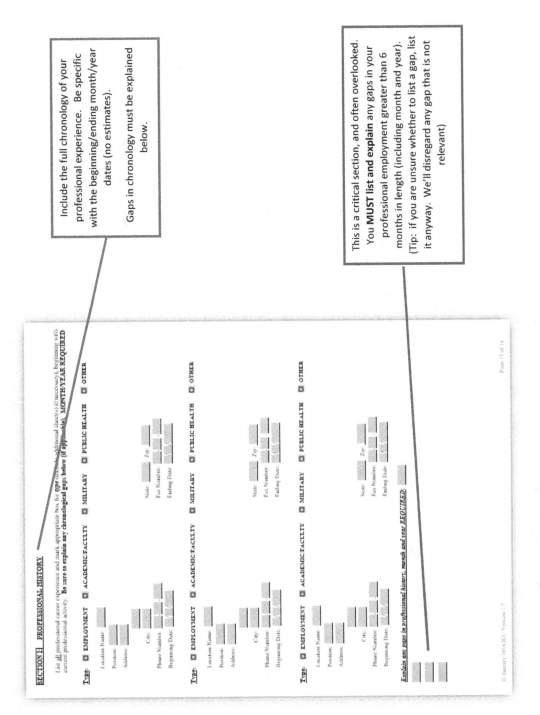

Include the full chronology of your professional experience. Be specific with the beginning/ending month/year dates (no estimates).

Gaps in chronology must be explained below.

This is a critical section, and often overlooked. You **MUST list and explain** any gaps in your professional employment greater than 6 months in length (including month and year). (Tip: if you are unsure whether to list a gap, list it anyway. We'll disregard any gap that is not relevant)

Office of Advanced Practice Providers UI Health Care (2021)

Advanced Practice Providers (APPs) ISUPA Guide

Section J: Professional References

This is the section that when missing/inaccurate info is provided *causes the most delays in issuing privileges.*

Below are some tips:

1. You **must list 4** professional peer references.

2. References must be at **your professional level or above** who are familiar with and can attest to your **clinical competency.** Do not list an RN as a reference, as they are not at your professional level or above.

3. References must have current knowledge of your clinical skills from **within the past 2 years.**

4. **Do not list family or fellow students.** Your best references are professors, practitioners in the same specialty, or department chairs.

5. **Valid email is an absolute requirement for all 4 references.** Also list phone and fax (if applicable), but email is the best and preferred method of contact.

6. **Contact your references in advance** and ask them or let them know you have already listed them as a reference and **validate their email.**

7. Also graciously request that your references **respond within 24 hours** of being contacted.

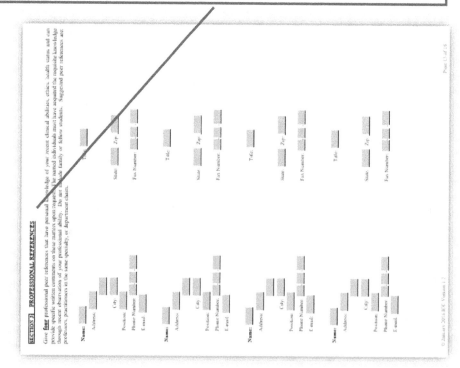

Office of Advanced Practice Providers UI Health Care (2021)

Advanced Practice Providers (APPs) ISUPA Guide

14

Section K: Quality Focused Questions

Must explain any "Yes" responses on page 15

Please be sure to carefully read and answer each question below, and explain any "yes" answers on page 15.
* Note - A special form is attached for Malpractice Claim History on Addendum C →

SECTION K   QUALITY FOCUSED QUESTIONS

1. Have you ever voluntarily or involuntarily surrendered or relinquished a state, district or federal professional license or registration (DEA or State Controlled Substance Certificate), board certification or any other certification? ☐YES ☐NO

2. Have you ever voluntarily or involuntarily had a state, district or federal professional license or registration (DEA or State Controlled Substance Certificate) board certification or any other certification revoked, suspended, limited, denied or refused by an Iowa licensing, state or federal drug administration, certifying board, or by such an entity in any other state(s)? ☐YES ☐NO

3. Have there been any previously successful or are there any currently pending challenges, complaints(s), sanction(s), disciplinary action(s), investigations or demials recommended or taken against your state, district or federal professional license(s), registrations (DEA or State Controlled Substance Certificate), board certification or any other certification(s)? ☐YES ☐NO

4. Have you ever voluntarily or involuntarily withdrawn from a clinical, medical, dental or professional staff? ☐YES ☐NO

5. Have you ever voluntarily or involuntarily withdrawn a request for an increase in privileges? ☐YES ☐NO

6. Have you ever been refused membership on a clinical, medical, dental or professional staff (either than for a general closure of that staff to providers of your specialty)? ☐YES ☐NO

7. Have you ever had a hospital, health care facility, or other health care organization invoke probation, issue a reprimand, impose proctoring (other than proctoring when privileges are initially granted), require a second opinion or initiate an investigation of your professional conduct or competency? ☐YES ☐NO

8. Are you currently performing or do you plan to perform any procedures for which you have ever been refused or lost privileges? ☐YES ☐NO

9. Have you ever been the subject of a formal or public citation or warning or ever had a sanction of any kind imposed by any health care institution, health care organization, licensing authority or other governmental entity, or voluntarily or involuntarily resigned under threat of the same? ☐YES ☐NO

10. Have your employment, medical staff appointment/membership, or clinical privileges ever been challenged or voluntarily or involuntarily suspended, reduced, revoked, refused, denied, relinquished/not terminated, limited or lost at any hospital, healthcare plan or other healthcare facility or organization? ☐YES ☐NO

11. Have you ever been convicted of any crime related to your clinical, medical, dental or professional practice? ☐YES ☐NO

12. Regarding Medicare, Medicaid, or any other governmental health-related program, have you ever been convicted of a crime or been subjected to civil penalties, disciplinary proceedings, investigations, denial of or suspension from participation, or had any type of sanction? ☐YES ☐NO

13. Do you have any felony, grand jury indictment, or other criminal charges pending? ☐YES ☐NO

14. Have you ever been convicted of, found guilty of or pled no contest to a felony, grand jury indictment or crime, other than a minor traffic violation? ☐YES ☐NO

15. Do you presently have a physical, mental or emotional condition (including alcohol or drug dependence), or do you presently engage in the use of illegal substances that affects or is reasonably likely to affect your ability to perform your professional duties appropriately or which could adversely affect the quality of care rendered by you to patients or jeopardize the safety of patients? ☐YES ☐NO

16. Has your malpractice insurance ever been denied, suspended, limited, not renewed or terminated by a carrier? ☐YES ☐NO

© January 2016 ICC Version 1/3   Page 14 of 16

Office of Advanced Practice Providers UI Health Care (2021)

Advanced Practice Providers (APPs) ISUPA Guide

15

SECTION K: QUALITY FOCUSED QUESTIONS...continued...

17. Have you ever had a malpractice case filed against you? (If yes, explain on Addendum C) ....   ☐ YES ☐ NO

18. Have you ever had a malpractice judgment entered against you? (If yes, explain on Addendum C) ....   ☐ YES ☐ NO

19. Have any malpractice settlements ever been made on your behalf? (If yes, explain on Addendum C) ....   ☐ YES ☐ NO

20. Are there any open claims or pending malpractice cases presently filed against you? (If yes, explain on Addendum C) ....   ☐ YES ☐ NO

21. Has/have any adverse action(s) or malpractice report(s) about you been made to the National Practitioner Data Bank, or any other database? ......   ☐ YES ☐ NO

22. Have you ever been denied membership in or voluntarily or involuntarily been terminated by any professional organization? ....   ☐ YES ☐ NO

23. Have you ever had any sanctions or disciplinary action executed against you by a Professional Standards Review Organization (PSRO), utilization or quality control Peer Review Organization (PRO), or any professional organization? ....   ☐ YES ☐ NO

24. Has your participation in a managed care plan or healthcare organization been limited, denied or terminated, or have you been sanctioned by such an organization? ....   ☐ YES ☐ NO

For any "YES" answers to the Quality Focused Questions above, please provide detailed explanation here, with the exception of any Malpractice Claim History (for Malpractice Claim History provide detailed information on Addendum C).

Question #	Detailed Explanation

If there is additional information about you or your practice that you feel will have a bearing on the consideration of this application, please provide details: (attach an additional page if needed):

"Yes" answers on questions 17-20 require more information on Addendum C instead of below.

Explain any "Yes" answer here (except for questions 17-20, which are to be explained on Addendum C).

Be very detailed. When in doubt, give more information than less.

© January 2016 ICC Version 1.0

Page 15 of 16

Office of Advanced Practice Providers UI Health Care (2021)

Advanced Practice Providers (APPs) ISUPA Guide

16

AUTHORIZATION TO RELEASE INFORMATION

Authorization: I understand and agree that I, as an applicant for privileges at the University of Iowa Hospitals and Clinics (UIHC), have the burden of producing adequate information for proper evaluation of and for resolving any doubts about my professional competence, character, ethics, credentials, and other qualifications. I hereby authorize the University of Iowa and its agents, staff and representatives to:

- collect and review all records and documents, including but not limited to medical records from past employers, malpractice carriers and other institutions with whom I have been associated that may be material to an evaluation of my professional qualifications and competences, as well as my ethical qualifications, to carry out the clinical privileges requested;
- consult with medical staff of other hospitals or institutions and malpractice carriers with whom I have been associated with respect to my professional competence, character and ethical qualifications, to carry out the clinical privileges requested; and
- collect, review and assess responses from the National Practitioner Data Bank (NPDB), criminal background check providers, verification of provision education, training, licensure, and board certification status.

Release: I release from liability the University of Iowa and its agents, representatives, and clinical staff for their acts performed in good faith in connection with evaluation of my application, credentials, and qualifications. I further release from liability any individuals or organizations who provide information pursuant to my application, when released in good faith, concerning my professional competence, character, ethics, credentials and other qualifications for clinical privileges, and I hereby consent to the release of all such information provided. This authorization also includes the release of liability of those entities, including but not limited to persons, who must receive such information pursuant to delegated credentialing agreements.

Governing Rules: In making any application for clinical privileges, I acknowledge that I have received and read the Bylaws, Rules and Regulations of the University of Iowa Hospitals and Clinics and its Clinical Staff. I agree to be bound by the policies, procedures, and directives of the University of Iowa including those of the Clinical Systems Committee (CSC) and the rules and regulations of each Clinical Department in which I may be granted clinical privileges. With respect to the matters for whom I will care assist the privileges granted pursuant to my application, I pledge to provide or arrange for their continuous care.

Communication with Applicant: I understand and agree that I have the burden to provide sufficient information for the purpose of reviewing my application for clinical privileges. In that regard, I will receive various communications with regard to information about my application through various means, including but not limited to telephone, mail, and/or e-mail over the internet. Further, certain fields of data on my application contain time-sensitive information and must be updated from time to time, as required by specific requirements and/or credentialing criteria. I agree to respond to requests for information in a timely way and authorize the CSO to collect from me and other sources this information on an as-needed basis. If I fail to provide for requested information, my application for privileges may not be approved.

Use of Information: The information requested is for the purpose of reviewing and evaluating my application are clinical privileges at UIHC. Information contained in my application may be used to 1) satisfy delegated credentialing agreements with payors for purposes of facilitating my participation and credentialing with respect to these payors; 2) fulfill information requests from and communicate with credentialing boards, certification boards, or preferred employers or healthcare entities for the specification of UIHC. The information I provide, immediately am submitted or necessary, or 3) any other purposes reasonably necessary for the operation of UIHC. The information disclosed to third parties as required for purposes collected attachment or disclosure shall be treated as confidential, with information disclosed to third parties as required for purposes authorized in any of the following ways: 1) as authorized by this Agreement; 2) by me; or 3) as authorized by applicable state or federal law.

Rights of Applicant: As an applicant for privileges: 1) I may request to review the information submitted in support of my application; 2) I may request corrections to information found in my credentialing file; 3) I will be notified if any information received during the credentialing process varies substantially from the information I submitted; and 4) I may request to be informed about the status of my credentialing application.

Certification of Information: All information submitted by me in this application, including the attached curriculum vitae, is true to the best of my knowledge and belief. I understand that any information entered on this application which subsequently is aware to be false could result in the denial of my privileges, revocation of some or all of my privileges at UIHC, termination of my membership in UI Physicians, removal as a provider eligible for reimbursement from a payor, and/or termination of my employment from the University of Iowa. Further, any significant misstatements or omissions from this application and/or attached documents, shall constitute cause or denial or termination of clinical privileges.

I hereby certify that the information contained in this credentialing application is accurate and complete.

Practitioner's signature _____

Applicant's printed name _____

Date (mm/dd/yyyy) _____

© January 2016 ICC Version 3.0

Signature _____

Printed name (initials) _____

Page 16 of 16

Read, sign, and date.

Office of Advanced Practice Providers UI Health Care (2021)

Advanced Practice Providers (APPs) ISUPA Guide

17

> Read, sign, and date.

PRACTITIONER ACKNOWLEDGEMENT STATEMENT

MEDICARE / MEDICAID / CHAMPUS (TRI-CARE)

Medicare Medicaid and Champus (Tri-Care) payment to hospitals is based in part on each patient's principal and secondary diagnoses and the major procedures performed on the patient, as attested by the patient's attending physician by virtue of his or her signature in the medical record. Anyone who misrepresents, falsifies, or conceals essential information required for payment of Federal funds may be subject to fine, imprisonment or civil penalty under applicable Federal laws.

_____
Name (Please Print)

_____
Practitioner's Legal Signature

_____
Practitioner's signature as written on medical records

_____
Practitioner's initials

_____
Date

This statement must be signed, dated and returned with your completed application.

Medicare Medicaid and Champus (Tri-Care) payment applies to all hospitals.

© January 2016 ICC Version 1.7

Addendum A

©The Iowa Credentialing Coalition. Reprinted with permission.

Office of Advanced Practice Providers UI Health Care (2021)

Advanced Practice Providers (APPs) ISUPA Guide

18

Addendum B: Alternate Coverage

APPs may skip this section.

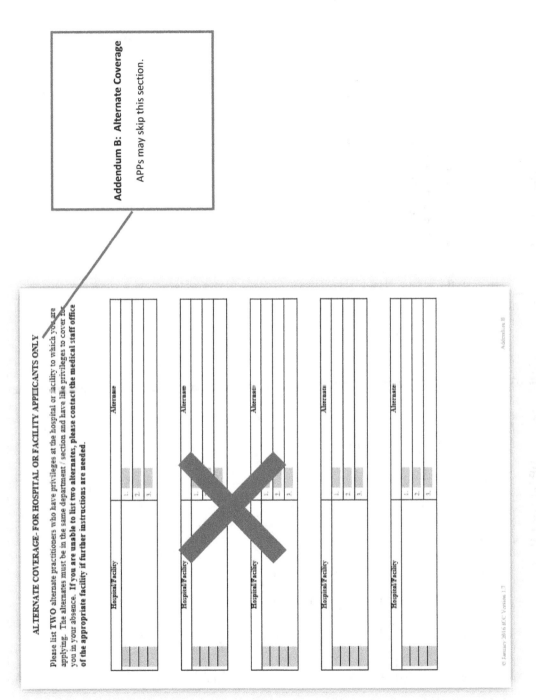

ALTERNATE COVERAGE - FOR HOSPITAL OR FACILITY APPLICANTS ONLY

Please list TWO alternate practitioners who have privileges at the hospital or facility to which you are applying. The alternates must be in the same department / section and have like privileges to cover for you in your absence. If you are unable to list two alternates, please contact the medical staff office of the appropriate facility if further instructions are needed.

Addendum B

© January 2016 ICC Version 1.7

Office of Advanced Practice Providers UI Health Care (2021)

Advanced Practice Providers (APPs) ISUPA Guide

Addendum C: Malpractice Claim History

Complete if you answered "Yes" to questions 17-20 on page 15.

If you have no malpractice activity to report, check the box at the top and sign below.

MALPRACTICE CLAIM HISTORY FORM

Practitioner Name:

☐ NO ACTIVITY TO REPORT (Proceed to Signature Line Below)

If you have any professional malpractice activity to report on this application, complete this page for each professional liability incident (copy and include additional sheets, if necessary).

Description of allegation or action taken:

Date of incident: Date of claim or suit filed:

Location of incident:

Insurance carrier name:

Insurance carrier address:

     City: State: Zip Code:

Phone Number: Fax Number:

Describe your involvement with the patient's care. Your narrative must include the following at a minimum.
1) Condition and diagnosis at time of incident
2) Dates and descriptions of treatment rendered
3) Condition of patient subsequent to treatment

Your Status: ☐ Primary Defendant   ☐ Co-Defendant   ☐ Other (specify):

Claim Status: ☐ Open   ☐ Pending   ☐ Closed

If closed, indicate the date closed and case outcome: Date Closed:

☐ Dismissed with Prejudice   ☐ Settled with Prejudice   ☐ Judgment for Defendant

☐ Dismissed without Prejudice   ☐ Settled without Prejudice   ☐ Judgment for Plaintiff

Amount of settlement or judgment paid on your behalf (if any): $ Date of payment:

I certify that the information in this document is correct and complete to the best of my knowledge.

Practitioner's Signature   Date

© January 2016 IUC Version 1.3   Addendum C

Advanced Practice Providers (APPs) ISUPA Guide

Iowa Statewide Universal Practitioner Application

Additional information here:

©The Iowa Credentialing Coalition. Reprinted with permission.

Advanced Practice Providers (APPs) ISUPA Guide

21

Answer Yes or No. Sign as noted here.

Answer Yes or No. Sign as noted here.

Ownership Disclosure

Do you or a family member own or have ownership in a healthcare facility or organization that provides health or medical services (lab, nursing home, pharmacy, radiology/imaging center, rehab, HMO, medical equipment supplier, etc.)? ☐ Yes ☐ No

If yes, complete information below:

Name of Facility/Entity:

Address: Street   City   **State**   **Zip Code**

Approximate percent of ownership: ☐ 1-5% ☐ 6-49% ☐ 50-100%

Is the entity or facility owned by: ☐ You as an individual ☐ Your family member
☐ Other organization with whom you are affiliated

Name of Organization:

Please document any current affiliations with other health care or health-related organizations (e.g. pharmaceutical companies, insurance carriers, nursing homes, etc.) If you receive regular compensation (e.g. salary board stipends, honorariums) from these organization, please indicate below (copy and include additional sheets if necessary).

Organization Name:

Address: Street   City   **State**   **Zip Code**

Starting Date: **Ending Date:**

Position Held:

Compensated: ☐ Yes ☐ No

Signature _____   Date _____

Printed Name _____

Misconduct

Have you ever been convicted of any crime involving sexual misconduct or do you have or have you had any licensure actions and/or sanctions brought against you involving sexual misconduct? ☐ Yes ☐ No

☐ Yes, please explain _____

Signature _____   Date _____

Printed Name _____

©The Iowa Credentialing Coalition. Reprinted with permission.

Advanced Practice Providers (APPs) ISUPA Guide

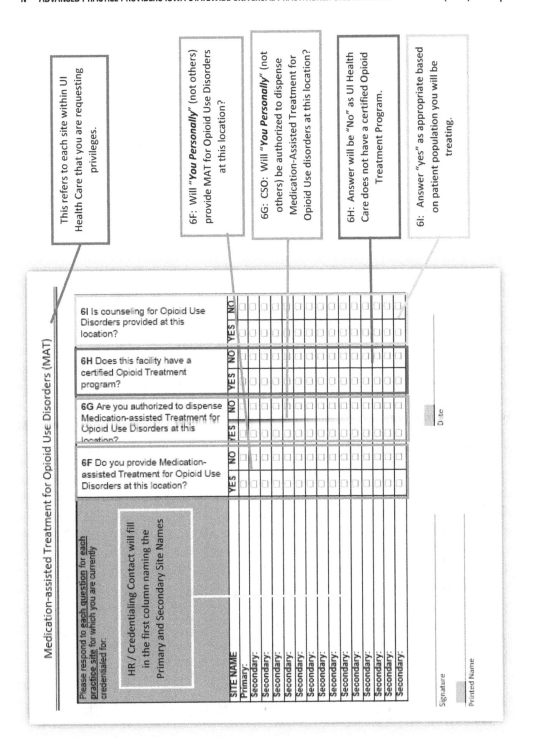

This refers to each site within UI Health Care that you are requesting privileges.

6F: Will **"You Personally"** (not others) provide MAT for Opioid Use Disorders at this location?

6G: CSO: Will **"You Personally"** (not others) be authorized to dispense Medication-Assisted Treatment for Opioid Use disorders at this location?

6H: Answer will be "No" as UI Health Care does not have a certified Opioid Treatment Program.

6I: Answer "yes" as appropriate based on patient population you will be treating.

Medication-assisted Treatment for Opioid Use Disorders (MAT)

Please respond to each question for each practice site for which you are currently credentialed for.

HR / Credentialing Contact will fill in the first column naming the Primary and Secondary Site Names

SITE NAME	6F Do you provide Medication-assisted Treatment for Opioid Use Disorders at this location?		6G Are you authorized to dispense Medication-assisted Treatment for Opioid Use Disorders at this location?		6H Does this facility have a certified Opioid Treatment program?		6I Is counseling for Opioid Use Disorders provided at this location?	
	YES	NO	YES	NO	YES	NO	YES	NO
Primary:								
Secondary:								
Secondary:								
Secondary:								
Secondary:								
Secondary:								
Secondary:								
Secondary:								
Secondary:								
Secondary:								
Secondary:								
Secondary:								
Secondary:								
Secondary:								

Signature _____   Date _____

Printed Name _____

Office of Advanced Practice Providers UI Health Care (2021)

22

Advanced Practice Providers (APPs) ISUPA Guide

Additional Documents Required

☐ Copy of Curriculum Vitae (CV)

☐ 2x3 Photo (headshot), jpeg format. Must be current photo. Please send via email.

☐ Documentation of your most recent TB Test and MMR Immunization records.

☐ Completed Collaborative Practice Agreement (NPs) or PA Addendum (PAs). You will receive this from your HR /Credentialing Contact, as this is a department specific form (also known as the Delineation of Privileges form).

☐ Copies of all State Issued Clinical Licenses (or printout from website). Examples: Nursing license (IBON) or PA License (IDPH).

☐ Copies of your board certification, which can be a printout from the board verification website.

☐ Copies of all current CPR certifications (ecard pdf format is acceptable). BLS, ACLS, PALS, NRP, etc.

☐ Copies of State Controlled Substance Certificate and current Federal DEA.

☐ If you have current malpractice insurance outside of UIHC (such as through another employer) as listed on page 7, Section D, please provide a copy. New APPs will likely not have this.

Note: Release of Information and Ownership Disclosure form are included in the ISUPA form on page 16 and Addendum D.

IOWA STATEWIDE
UNIVERSAL PRACTITIONER APPLICATION
ATTACHMENT CHECKLIST

☑ Privileges only, no billing

Applicant Name:
Applying to:
Department Division of:
Address:
City, State Zip:

Page 1 of this application indicates what the applicant is applying for.

The Credentialing Verification Organization processing this application for the above entity practitioner is as follows and should be continued for any questions regarding the application. The practitioner's original application will should be submitted to and will be maintained by the following office for future reference.

Documents required by UI Clinical Staff Office:	Enclosed	To Follow
Draft CCOM appointment and entry into UIHC HR Pre-Employment (UIHC only)		
Current photo, preferably 2 X 3 jpg file e-mailed to CSO (print ok if jpg is not available)		
Signed "Release of Information" and "Delineation of Privileges" forms		
Signed Ownership Disclosure form		
Copy of current professional state license(s)		
Health Service Provider Certificate (Psychologist only)		
Copy of current State Controlled Substance Certificate (if applicable)		
Copy of current Federal DEA (if applicable)		
Copy of ECFMG (if applicable)		
Copy of Medical/Dental Education Diploma		
Copy of current abbreviated Curriculum Vitae (CV) *		
Copy of board certificates or certification cards (including CPR or ACLS)		
Current certificate(s) for professional malpractice liability coverage (non-UIHC applicants only)		
Collaborative Practice Agreement or PA Addendum to ISUPA (UIHC ARNP PA's)		
Evidence of current TB /MMR		
DPC's for Psychiatry, Counseling & Health Promotion, Pediatric psychology & Center for Developmental Disabilities (Neuropsychologists and psychologists)		

Indicate if data on this file is/allowed to be sent to United Behavioral Health claims will be denied if the current indication is not made.

* A copy of your abbreviated CV is requested, however, it will NOT be accepted in lieu of completing any portion of this application. If it is current, it is used to support the necessary explanation of any gap history in education, training, or professional positions.

Advanced Practice Providers (APPs) ISUPA Guide

FAQ

How can a practitioner obtain a Federal DEA?

The DEA offers applications online. If the practitioner will only be practicing at a UI Hospitals & Clinics site, the fee should be exempt for this exemption. A department or division head may sign for this exemption.

Can a practitioner submit an ISUPA application before all the attachments are available?

Yes, after completing the entire Iowa Statewide Universal Practitioner (ISUPA) application, signing and dating, the application may be submitted along with a photo (2-inch x 3-inch .jpg) and the Cover-Checklist indicating which attachments will follow. For example, an Iowa License has not been issued yet. In the license section of the application, indicate this item is pending, on the Cover-Checklist indicate that the copy will follow, and send it as soon as it is received. By sending the application and photo before a license is issued, the CSO can begin processing to avoid delay. Please be sure to submit pending or missing required attachments as soon as possible to avoid continued delay application processing.

If a practitioner has moonlighted at a number of hospitals, should all hospitals be listed?

Yes, any and all hospital privileges should be listed on the application. The hospital privilege section of the application can be copied if additional space is needed or additional pages can be found on the application pages can be found on the application link on this website.

If the practitioner has already completed the application for another entity do they need to submit another one?

No. With the information in the database, the application can be preprinted and sent to the practitioner for renewal (review, updating, and signature).

If the practitioner will be getting married in the near future, which name is used?

Please indicate the current legal name at the time of the application completion and enter in the "Other Names" section the new married name and/or other maiden name(s) and the effective and end date for each name.

What is an NPI?

National Provider Identifier -the NPI is part of the Administrative Simplification Provisions of HIPAA 1996. This number should eventually replace other practitioner numbers such as the UPIN, Medicare/Medicaid, and payor specific numbers. You can search for NPI numbers online.

25

Advanced Practice Providers (APPs) ISUPA Guide

Related Links

Federal DEA

Iowa Pharmacy Board (State Controlled Substance Certificate) SCSC or CDS

Iowa Board of Nursing

Iowa Department of Public Health, Professional Licensure

NPI Registry

Office of Advanced Practice Providers UI Health Care (2021)

©The Iowa Credentialing Coalition. Reprinted with permission.

APPENDIX O

ADVANCED PRACTICE PROVIDERS BILLING PACKET GUIDE

Advanced Practice Providers (APPs) Billing Packet Guide

Use your **full legal name**. Should match your name on Social Security Card, Professional License, and NPI.

List any other names/alias you may have used and describe.

Example: maiden name or nickname (i.e. Jennifer/Jenny, Barbara/Barb, Michael/Mike)

List **your State of Iowa professional license information** (ARNP license from IBON, PA License from IDPH).

- Link to IBON (for NP License)
- Link to IDPH (for PA License)

Board Certification Certifying Entity will be one of the following:

NCCPA: PA-C
AANP-CP: American Academy of Nurse Practitioners Certification Program
AACN: American Association of Critical Care Nurses
AMCB: American Midwifery Certification Board
NBCRNA: National Board of Certification & Recertification for Nurse Anesthetists
NCC: National Certification Corporation
PNCB: Pediatric Nursing Certification Board

Contact your Credentialing Contact to obtain your University ID# or if assistance is needed applying for NPI

Practice information will be pre-populated. Please review this information and add any additional practice sites not listed.

Please add your practice phone/fax numbers, if known.

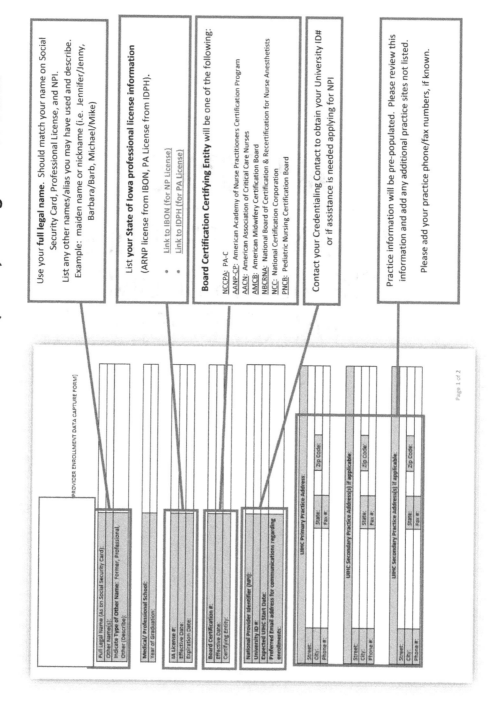

[PROVIDER ENROLLMENT DATA CAPTURE FORM]

Full Legal Name (As on Social Security Card):
Other Name(s):
Indicate Type of Other Name: Former, Professional, Other (Describe):

Medical/ Professional School:
Year of Graduation:

IA License #:
Effective Date:
Expiration Date:

Board Certification #:
Effective Date:
Certifying Entity:

National Provider Identifier (NPI):
University ID #:
Expected UIHC Start Date:
Preferred Email address for communications regarding enrollments:

UIHC Primary Practice Address:
Street:
City: | State: | Zip Code:
Phone #: | Fax #:

UIHC Secondary Practice Address(s) if applicable:
Street:
City: | State: | Zip Code:
Phone #: | Fax #:

UIHC Secondary Practice Address(s) if applicable:
Street:
City: | State: | Zip Code:
Phone #: | Fax #:

Advanced Practice Providers (APPs) Billing Packet Guide

Please carefully review this section, in particular if you have worked for another facility. For billing accuracy, your primary facility must be noted correctly.

APPs may skip residency questions

Will you maintain a practice with another facility?   Yes ☐   No ☐

If yes, please list the address of that practice:

Street: _____ State: _____ Zip Code: _____
City: _____

Will UHC become primary once you are approved for privileges here?   Yes ☐   No ☐

Are you currently in a residency program?   Yes ☐   No ☐

If YES, please list facility name and address where you are in residency:

Name of Facility: _____
Street: _____ State: _____ Zip Code: _____
City: _____

Current Home Address (Needed for Illinois Medicaid Enrollment)

Street: _____ State: _____ Zip Code: _____
City: _____

Has there ever been disciplinary action against your license by a licensing board in any state?

Yes ☐   No ☐   If YES, please attach an explanation

Have you ever been sanctioned by Medicare or any state health program?

Yes ☐   No ☐   If YES, please attach an explanation

Have you ever been convicted of any criminal offense?

Yes ☐   No ☐   If YES, please attach an explanation

Are you currently enrolled in another state's Medicaid/CHIP program?

Yes ☐   No ☐   If YES, please list the state and program you are enrolled in:

Signature: _____   Date: _____

Page 2 of 2

Advanced Practice Providers (APPs) Billing Packet Guide

Surrogate Approvals

Provider Name: _____

NPI: _____

The Center for Medicare & Medicaid Services (CMS) allows providers to elect a surrogate to update their online Medicare enrollment (PECOS), National Provider Identifier (NPI) and Electronic Health Record (EHR) Incentive registration and attestation.

UIHC Patient Financial Services (PFS) encourages all billing providers to approve surrogacy for provider enrollment specialists for quick and accurate enrolling/updating online. Please indicate (by signing below) if you approve PFS Provider Enrollment staff as your surrogate to complete these enrollments/updates on your behalf.

If you do not yet have an NPI, please indicate if you will be applying yourself or will approve PFS surrogate to apply on your behalf.

Please select an option:

I approve PFS Provider Enrollment staff to act as my surrogate to enroll and maintain my information online for:

- Medicare
- National Provider Identifier
- EHR Incentive Program

Signature: _____   **Date:** _____

You will be contacted via email when the online connection requests in the Identity and Access Management (I&A) system are ready for your approval.

Please indicate on the following page which Taxonomy Code(s) should be listed on your NPI.

If you elect to not approve surrogate for these tasks, you will be responsible for:

- Completing Medicare enrollment application via paper (will be sent to you to complete)
- Updating your NPI online
- UIHC will not be able to submit your meaningful use data to CMS

Surrogate Approval

Most UI Health Care Providers have signed this form to allow UI Patient Financial Services to enroll/update your CMS information

You are **strongly encouraged to sign and allow surrogacy on your behalf from our provider enrollment specialists**

Advanced Practice Providers (APPs) Billing Packet Guide

Carefully review this list and mark one code as primary (which is the closest match to your board specialty) and as many others as secondary as applicable

Taxonomy Codes

Taxonomy codes are CMS administrative **codes** set for identifying the **provider** type and area of specialization for health care providers

Each **taxonomy code** is a unique ten-character alphanumeric **code** that enables providers to identify their specialty at the claim level.

A **provider** can have more than one **taxonomy code**

To become a Medicare provider and file Medicare claims, you must Identify the taxonomy code that reflects your classification and specialization

You should identify the taxonomy code that most closely describes your provider type, classification, or specialization

You may select more than one code or code description, but you must indicate one of them as the primary code

Department	Code	P=Primary	S=Secondary
Nurse Practitioner	363L00000X		
Acute Care	363LA2100X		
Adult Health	363LA2200X		
Community Health	363LC1500X		
Critical Care Medicine	363LC0200X		
Family	363LF0000X		
Gerontology	363LG0600X		
Neonatal	363LN0000X		
Neonatal, Critical Care	363LN0005X		
Obstetrics & Gynecology	363LX0001X		
Occupational Health	363LX0106X		
Pediatrics	363LP0200X		
Pediatrics, Critical Care	363LP0222X		
Perinatal	363LP1700X		
Primary Care	363LP2300X		
Psychiatric/Mental Health	363LP0808X		
School	363LS0200X		
Women's Health	363LW0102X		

PA-Cs:

Department	Code	P=Primary	S=Secondary
Physician Assistant	363A00000X		
Medical	363AM0700X		
Surgical	363AS0400X		

Advanced Practice Providers (APPs) Billing Packet Guide

Read, answer Yes or No. If yes, provide additional information as requested

SECTION 3: FINAL ADVERSE LEGAL ACTIONS

This section captures information regarding final adverse legal actions, such as convictions, exclusions, license revocations and license suspensions. All applicable final adverse legal actions must be reported, regardless of whether any records were expunged or of any appeals are pending.

NOTE: To satisfy the reporting requirement, section 3 must be filled out in its entirety, and all applicable attachments must be included.

A. CONVICTIONS (AS DEFINED IN 42 C.F.R. SECTION 1001.2) WITHIN THE PRECEDING 10 YEARS

1. Any federal or state felony conviction(s).

2. Any misdemeanor conviction, under federal or state law, related to: (a) the delivery of an item or service under Medicare or a state health care program, or (b) the abuse or neglect of a patient in connection with the delivery of a health care item or service.

3. Any misdemeanor conviction, under federal or state law, related to the theft, fraud, embezzlement, breach of fiduciary duty, or other financial misconduct in connection with the delivery of a health care item or service.

4. Any misdemeanor conviction, under federal or state law, related to the interference with or obstruction of any investigation into any criminal offense described in 42 C.F.R. section 1001.101 or 1001.201.

5. Any misdemeanor conviction, under federal or state law, related to the unlawful manufacture, distribution, prescription, or dispensing of a controlled substance.

B. EXCLUSIONS, REVOCATIONS OR SUSPENSIONS

1. Any current or past revocation or suspension of medical license.

2. Any current or past revocation or suspension of accreditation.

3. Any current or past suspension or exclusion imposed by the U.S. Department of Health and Human Service's Office of Inspector General (OIG).

4. Any current or past debarment from participation in any Federal Executive Branch procurement or non-procurement program.

5. Any other current or past Federal Sanctions.

6. Any Medicaid exclusion, revocation, or termination of any billing number.

C. FINAL ADVERSE LEGAL ACTION HISTORY

1. Have you, under any current or former name, ever had a final adverse legal action listed above imposed against you?

☐ YES - continue below

☐ NO - skip to section 4

2. If yes, report each final adverse legal action, when it occurred, and the federal or state agency or the court/administrative body that imposed the action.

FINAL ADVERSE LEGAL ACTION	DATE	ACTION TAKEN BY

CMS-855A (12/18)

11

Advanced Practice Providers (APPs) Billing Packet Guide

Read, sign and date

Remember to contact Patient Financial Services if payment for services are ever inadvertently sent to you directly

UNIVERSITY of IOWA
HEALTH CARE

Patient Financial Services

Memorandum

To: Clinical Staff Providers
From: Director, Patient Financial Services

When statements and bills for professional services to private patients are mailed from the Medical Services section of Patient Financial Services, we ask that the check be made payable to Medical Services. In spite of this request, a good number of checks are still received made payable to the provider, which in turn requires that we route the check to that provider for endorsement.

This delay and inconvenience can be avoided if you will sign the form below which authorizes our office to sign your name, with a restricted endorsement, to those checks from patients, insurance companies, and other agencies which only are in payment of fees for professional services.

The Compensation Committee has reviewed and approved this procedure. If you have any questions, please let me know. Please return the signed form to this office. Thank you for your assistance.

I hereby authorize the office of Medical Services to endorse my name on checks, money orders, and bank drafts that are payable to my order and which payments I am required to deposit in the Iowa Medical Service Plan through the Treasurer of the State University of Iowa.

_____
Date

_____
Name (Signature)

_____
Name (Typed or Printed)

_____
Department

Advanced Practice Providers (APPs) Billing Packet Guide

Read/Initial

Additional Enrollment Documents/Actions

Out of state (OOS) Medicaid payers may require additional information as each state has its own process.

If you provide care (billing, ordering, referring and/or prescribing provider) for an OOS Medicaid patient the following MAY be required:

- Copy of SSN Card
- Copy of current driver's license
- Electronic signature completion
- Creation of online login IDs, Passwords and/or Business Profiles
- Assistance with adding/updating provider data in CAQH Credentialing System
- Assistance with contacting the payer via phone when information will only be released to the provider

You will be contacted if this information or any other unique items are required for enrollment. Some of the OOS payers have tight deadlines for timely enrollment/claims filing so your quick response is appreciated.

Please note that Illinois Medicaid requires your home address and that information is requested within the billing packet.

_____ Please initial here to verify you have read and understand these requirements.

_____
Printed Name

Advanced Practice Providers (APPs) Billing Packet Guide

All providers who bill will be sent the 20 page "Physicians Teaching Physician Billing Policy" to review. You'll need to acknowledge you've read this on the Attestation Form

Read/Sign/Date

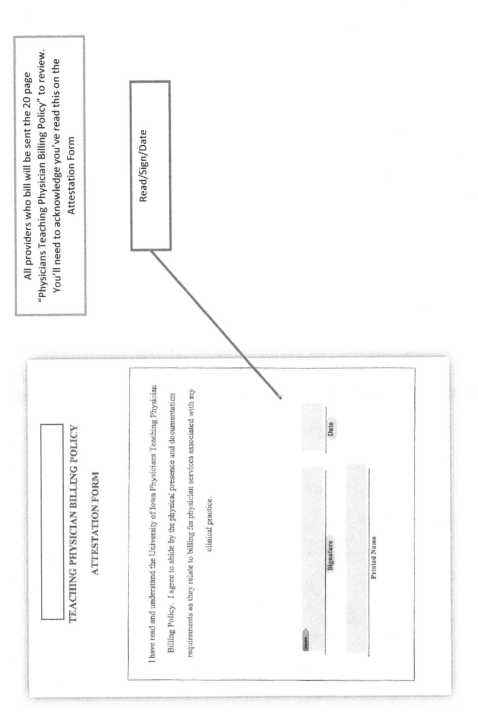

TEACHING PHYSICIAN BILLING POLICY

ATTESTATION FORM

I have read and understand the University of Iowa Physicians Teaching Physician Billing Policy. I agree to abide by the physical presence and documentation requirements as they relate to billing for physician services associated with my clinical practice.

Signature

Printed Name

Date

APPENDIX P

PEER EVALUATION
QUESTIONNAIRE

Peer Evaluation Questionnaire

Staff Name: _____ Department: _____

Are you aware of any health impairments that would affect this individual's ability to perform professional duties? Yes ☐ No ☐

Explain _____

Rate this individual's demonstrated performance compared with that reasonably expected of another practitioner having the same level of training, experience, and background:

Characteristics	Meets expectations	Does not meet expectations	Don't know
PATIENT CARE: Makes informed decisions about diagnostic and therapeutic interventions based on patient information and patient preferences, up-to-date scientific evidence, and clinical judgment. Communicates effectively with patients about the plan of care. Maintains clinical competency in the area for which re-privileging is sought.			
MEDICAL KNOWLEDGE: Demonstrates sound application of medical knowledge and an investigatory and analytic thinking approach to clinical situations.			
PRACTICE-BASED LEARNING AND IMPROVEMENT: Critically appraises clinical studies and literature on diagnostic and therapeutic effectiveness. Uses information technology to manage information and access online medical information. Facilitates the learning of students and other healthcare professionals.			
INTERPERSONAL AND COMMUNICATION SKILLS: Works effectively with others as a member or leader of a healthcare team or other professional group.			
PROFESSIONALISM: Demonstrates respect, compassion, and integrity. Demonstrates a commitment to ethical principles pertaining to provision or withholding of clinical care, confidentiality of patient information, informed consent, and business practices.			
SYSTEMS-BASED PRACTICE: Practices cost-effective healthcare and resource allocation that does not compromise quality of care. Partners with healthcare managers and healthcare providers to assess, coordinate, and improve healthcare and knows how these activities can affect system performance.			

Do you have any reservations about recommending this individual to be re-privileged? ☐ Yes   ☐ No

Peer Signature _____ Title _____ Date _____

Printed or Typed Peer Name _____

APPENDIX Q

REQUEST FOR MODIFICATION OF PRIVILEGES

Request for Modification of Additional Privileges for
Advanced Practice Providers (APP)

Name of APP: _____

Department: _____

Division: _____

Name of procedure/skill: _____

Name of credentialing contact: _____

Date form submitted: _____
Date form received: _____

Provide the following documentation to the Clinical Staff Office (CSO) with this request to add additional privileges:

☐ Definitional statement and delineation of privilege form
☐ Documentation of competency with APP signature, proctor signatures, and Department Head signature
☐ Authorization to release form
☐ Current Curriculum Vitae (CV)

**Procedure/Skill Competency Documentation and IPPE
Advanced Practice Provider (APP)**

Name of APP obtaining privilege: _____

Name of procedure/skill: _____

A)   Documentation that the APP assisted/observed an expert performing procedure/skill

Date of assisting or observation	NAME OF EXPERT WHOM APP ASSISTED/OBSERVED
1)	
2)	
3)	

B)   Documentation that the APP performed the procedure/skill proctored by an expert

SIX CORE COMPETENCIES	PATIENT CARE: Based intervention on patient information and patient preferences, up-to-date scientific evidence, and clinical judgment, and communicates effectively with patients about the plan of care. MEDICAL KNOWLEDGE: Demonstrates sound application of medical knowledge and applies appropriately to the clinical situations. PRACTICE-BASED LEARNING AND IMPROVEMENT: Understands clinical studies and literature on diagnostic and therapeutic effectiveness. INTERPERSONAL AND COMMUNICATION SKILLS: Works effectively with others as a member of the healthcare team. PROFESSIONALISM: Demonstrates respect, compassion, and integrity. SYSTEMS-BASED PRACTICE: Practices cost-effective healthcare and resource allocation that does not compromise quality of care. OBSERVER: I attest that the applicant has performed the procedure/skill successfully based on the six core competencies for clinical practice. (Print name in left column and signature in right column—if observation requirements exceed three performances, please use the Procedure Skill Competency Form—Additional Signatures.)	
Date of performance	**NAME OF EXPERT WHO ASSISTED AND OBSERVED APP**	
1)		
2)		
3)		

I attest that I understand the risks and benefits associated with the procedure/skill and have successfully been educated based on the six core competencies for clinical practice.

Signature/Date of APP: _____   _____
                       (signature)   (date)

Signature of Department Head: _____   _____
                              (signature)   (date)

APPENDIX R

SAMPLE EMAILS FOR PEER MENTORING PROGRAM

Dear APP:

We are excited to support APPs new to the institution through an APP peer mentoring program. This program pairs new and experienced APPs and provides a structured year-long mentoring curriculum. Through this mentoring relationship the experienced APP will provide information, advice, support, and encouragement to guide the new APP by serving as a trusted advisor. Mentees have significantly benefited from this type of relationship and resources. Program materials are provided.

Working as an APP mentor or mentee will enhance your professional network and grow your leadership, coaching, and feedback skills. Please review the program highlights below and consider whether you would like to apply to participate in this program. If you are interested, please discuss this with your direct supervisor and secure their support for your participation in the program.

The year-long program requires at least eight mentoring sessions within a 12-month period.

A mentoring guide and curriculum have been developed with suggested topics and discussions for your meetings.

The program coordinators are assigned to oversee the program and offer support and guidance through any issues that may arise.

Mentors and mentees may be matched from different departments, and ARNP/PAs may be matched together in the program.

Sample Email Notifying Peer Mentoring Program Participants

Dear APP:

Congratulations! On behalf of the mentoring committee, we would like to confirm your acceptance into the APP mentoring program.

This program pairs new to the organization and experienced APPs and provides a structured year-long mentoring curriculum. Through this mentoring relationship the experienced APP will provide information, advice, support, and encouragement; guide the new APP by example through their expertise or success; and serve as a trusted advisor. Mentees benefit from this relationship and resources. Program materials, training, and curriculum are provided. The mentoring pairs (mentee and mentor) are listed below.

Program Details:

The year-long program requires at least eight mentoring sessions within a 12-month period.

A mentoring guide and curriculum have been developed so that each month has a structured topic and discussion questions.

The APP mentoring committee oversees the program and offers support and guidance through any issues that may arise.

Your supervisor and department leadership must approve of your participation in the program.

Next Steps:

A member of the mentoring program committee will schedule a brief orientation/overview to the program.

We encourage you both to seek out and introduce yourselves prior to your first meeting.

A mentorship agreement form is required to be completed to participate in the program and will be provided to you at your first meeting.

The mentoring committee is here to support you and to help you succeed. Thank you so much for partnering with us in this exciting endeavor.

APPENDIX S

MENTORING PROGRAM GUIDE

APP Mentoring Program Guide

This guide will provide a structured approach to facilitate discussion and dialogue for a mutually beneficial mentoring relationship. Suggested meeting frequency is monthly, with the sessions completed within 12 months of starting the program.

Session 1: Getting to Know Each Other

☐ **Discussion Topics**

What made you decide to become an APP? Share your career story. How did you get to where you are?

☐ **Mentor/Mentee Relationship Expectations**

What do you want to accomplish? What would a successful mentoring relationship look like?

☐ **Confidentiality**

Discuss expectations and guidelines for confidential discussions.

☐ **Mentoring Agreement Form**

Review and complete the Mentoring Agreement Form together.

☐ **Required Homework**

Submit signed agreement form.

☐ **Set up next meeting**

Determine how/when you will meet (in-person, phone, Zoom). Who will schedule this meeting?

Session 2: Goal Setting

☐ **Discussion Topics**

What goal have you reached that you are most proud of? What were some of the obstacles you overcame to reach that goal?

☐ **Goal Setting**

Discuss why goal setting is important. How do you remain accountable when committing to goals?

☐ **SMART Goal Worksheet (handout)**

Review and discuss the SMART Goal worksheet.

☐ **SMART Goal Setting Example**

Build confidence in giving presentations by volunteering to give two presentations to my area within the next six months.

☐ **Required Homework**

Mentee completes the SMART Goal worksheet.

☐ **Set up next meeting**

Determine how/when you will meet (in-person, phone, Zoom). Who will schedule this meeting?

APP Mentoring Program Guide (page 2)

Session 3: Involvement in Your Department/Unit

☐ Discussion Topics

Do you feel part of a community within your department/unit? How have you felt welcomed? What obstacles have there been to getting involved?

☐ Required Homework

Identify one way in which you can become more involved in your unit/department.

☐ Your Personal Brand

How would you describe your personal brand? What image do you want to project? How would that serve you? What interpersonal skills have been the most important in your profession?

☐ Set up next meeting

Determine how/when you will meet (in-person, phone, Zoom). Who will schedule this meeting?

Session 4: Involvement in Professional Organizations & Networking

☐ Discussion Topics

Are you currently involved in any professional organizations? What organizations would help support your practice? What can you gain from being involved in your professional organization?

☐ Required Homework

Develop an action item related to your professional organization or networking.

☐ Networking

Why is networking important? What is your comfort level with professional networking? How have you grown your professional network? What types of people would you like to add?

☐ Set up next meeting

Determine how/when you will meet (in-person, phone, Zoom). Who will schedule this meeting?

APP Mentoring Program Guide (page 3)

Session 5: Work/Life Balance

☐ **Discussion Topics**

What does work/life balance mean to you? What self-care habits do you currently use? What would you like to add?

☐ **Required Homework**

Identify two or three actions that you could take right now that would positively impact your well-being.

☐ **Self-Care Resources**

Discuss strategies for coping with transitions. How have you bounced back from a setback? What department organizational resources are available? (Examples: EAP, Wellness, etc.)

☐ **Set up next meeting**

Determine how/when you will meet (in-person, phone, Zoom). Who will schedule this meeting?

Session 6: Goal Check-In

☐ **Discussion Topics**

How are you feeling about your professional growth and development? What lessons have you learned from your success and setbacks?

☐ **Required Homework**

Develop an action item related to your SMART goal.

☐ **Revisit SMART Goal**

Identify progress toward the SMART goal and determine if goal should be adjusted or if a new goal needs to be set.

☐ **Set up next meeting**

Determine how/when you will meet (in-person, phone, Zoom). Who will schedule this meeting?

APP Mentoring Program Guide (page 4)

Session 7: Scholarship and Skills Growth

☐ **Discussion Topics**

What scholarship activities are you involved with (writing, journal clubs)? How do you stay up to date on relevant practice changes? What have you done to stay competitive in your organization? What do you see as a trend over the next five years that you think you should pay attention to?

☐ **Required Homework**

Identify resources for expanding your scholarship or skills, such as presenting at a conference, training/teaching, or writing professionally.

☐ **Skills Inventory**

What new skills would you suggest for an APP? What skills do you want to acquire? What experiences do you want to have? What is an untapped strength of yours that you'd like to see the organization take greater advantage of? Discuss resources that support these skills.

☐ **Set up next meeting**

Determine how/when you will meet (in-person, phone, Zoom). Who will schedule this meeting?

Session 8: Wrap-Up and Review Accomplishments

☐ **Discussion Topics**

What career paths interest you? What changes will you have to make to pursue your interests? How do you see yourself growing in your profession?

☐ **Reflection**

How did you benefit from participation in the mentoring program? What did you find most valuable about the mentoring experience?

☐ **Revisit SMART Goal**

Identify progress toward the SMART goal. Recognize and celebrate the achievement of goals.

☐ **Required Homework**

Complete program completion survey/evaluation.

APPENDIX T

JOB AND FAMILY CAREER LADDER

Health Care (PV) Job Function Purpose	Contribute to providing and supporting health care services through leadership, management, clinical/technical specialty services, revenue cycle, support services, clinical education, and research programs.						
Patient Services (PVL) Job Family Purpose	Provide services related to access, scheduling, wayfinding and support to assure effective and efficient delivery of health care services striving toward an excellent patient experience. Positions in this job family are engaged in one or more activities related to scheduling patient appointments, serving as a patient advocate, handling patient access requests, handling service recovery incidents, ensuring appointments are scheduled appropriately, and using independent judgement to best ensure the patient has an excellent experience. Key areas of responsibility include providing patient access services, communicate/collaborate with internal and external constituents, operations and performance standards, human resource management, and financial management. This job family was last reviewed on 5/1/2018.						
	PVL1	PVL2	PVL3	PVL4	PVL5	PVL6	PVL7
Job Codes	3A	3A	4A	4A	5A	5A	6A
Pay Levels							
Key Areas of Responsibility	Patient Access Specialist	Clinic Services Specialist	Patient Access Coordinator	Clinic Services Coordinator	Patient Access Manager	Clinic Services Manager	Patient Access Director
Provide Patient Access Services to Clinical and Non-Clinical Departments	Provide centralized services to patients such as scheduling patient appointments for multiple clinics, support in obtaining care, navigating the health care systems, addressing care/service issues, ensuring the prerequisites to schedule are completed, and ensuring the patient is financially secured. Perform tasks to meet patient access, scheduling, and patient satisfaction goals. Follow and apply policies and procedures to meet patient scheduling and access requirements. Report variances and work to address them. Recommend policies and/or enhancements to new and improved processes	Provide frontline clinic operation support, such as the coordination of patient appointment scheduling, the preparation of pre-registration paperwork for patient visits, obtaining and verifying pre-authorizations, and the education of patients regarding billing process and additional financial responsibilities. Review patient charges to ensure accuracy and answer questions concerning billing procedures and charges.	Coordinate and provide centralized services for patient access, scheduling services, and support. Ensure compliance of tasks, compliance goals, and customer satisfaction expectations. Supervise the delivery of patient scheduling and access for multiple assigned areas of focus. May provide functional and/or administrative supervision of staff.	Coordinate and facilitate the flow of patient access activities of a department and/or clinic. Collaborate with clinic faculty and management regarding proposed scheduling guideline changes. Develop, analyze and maintain standards of excellence for patient registration, scheduling and check-in/check-out process within the department.	Supervise the work of staff. Analyze data and information to improve centralized patient access and scheduling services. Develop plans to meet compliance goals, patient/customer satisfaction expectations and quality of services provided	Supervise and coordinate activities of a clinic/department to include establishing and maintaining systems for patient flow through the clinic/department and the utilization of clinic resources. Direct and coordinate all scheduling, check-in, check-out, and financial services activities within the clinic/department. Enforces regulatory and compliance requirements and accountable for understanding, enforcing and following all internal controls. Positions at this level would typically be located in moderate to large scale clinics overseeing more than one patient support unit or function.	Direct department operations by providing resources and services to meet the needs of the department and hospital departments. Plan, organize, direct, control and evaluate administrative functions. Responsible for strategic planning, vision, and growth of the department.
Patient Satisfaction/ Service Excellence	Collaborate with peers and co-workers to enhance the delivery of health care. Assist with resolving issues from staff and customers.	Provide high level customer service with internal and external customers, including patients, visitors, physicians and other clinical staff. Ensure patient satisfaction and safety by ensuring calls and inquiries are documented and triaged appropriately. Address concerns of patients, provide service recovery, and escalate issues as needed.	Collaborate with peers, co-workers, customers, hospital departments, and external agencies to enhance the delivery of patient scheduling and access services. Implement strategies to resolve scheduling issues. Review, respond, and resolve requests and issues from staff and customers.	Practice and promote positive peer and patient relations. Manage and coordinate service recovery initiatives for patients. Initiate and implement processes to enhance patient and customer satisfaction. May develop scripting and provide coaching to staff members regarding service excellence behaviors. Work with departmental administrator, nurse manager, physicians or others in the clinic to enhance patient experience. Collaborate with the Office of Patient Experience regarding patient satisfaction results and recommend action as needed.	Collaborate with customers, external agencies, and hospital departments to enhance the delivery of patient access and scheduling services. Develop improved and new strategies to resolve issues.	Maintain interface with physicians, patients and administrative staff to provide information and to resolve problems relating to clinic services. Communicate with other units on a regular basis to promote effective and efficient operations within the clinic. Analyze patient satisfaction data and report results to management and report and staff	Serve as a liaison between staff, departments served, external agencies and healthcare leadership. Facilitate and maintain collaborative relationships between all internal and external stakeholders. Develop and implement strategies to resolve issues.

Category							
Operations and Quality Standards/ Improvement	Meets targets set by supervisor regarding assigned areas of patient access. Meets targets set by supervisor regarding volume and accuracy. Work in cooperation with medical staff on accurate scheduling. Work with clinic, department administration, and others regarding appropriate patient scheduling and access.	Recommend processes to enhance patient and customer satisfaction. Review scheduling templates and make recommendations for improvement opportunities related to patient access and clinical operations.	Perform quality assurance checks and productivity audits. Implement new processes and targets. Responsible for operational effectiveness of applicable scheduling processes. May make recommendations based on analysis of data.	Analyze scheduling and phone management data and recommend opportunities for improvement. Provide recommendations to department leadership on policies and procedures to improve patient care and utilization of clinic resources.	Develop goals for quality improvements and monitor key metrics. Use data to recommend and implement operational improvements. Analyze new scheduling protocols and develop processes to address changes. Assess and assist in planning technology to support operational needs and efficiency. Develop and/or implement programs, policies, and practices for department.	Develop goals for quality improvements and monitor key metrics. Coordinate activities of the clinic/department with services of other departments to ensure effective patient care and efficient service. Generate, analyze and/or interpret reports relating to clinic performance, staff performance, and financial performance. Execute appropriate action plans based on findings.	Develop goals for quality improvements and monitor key metrics. Use data to recommend and implement operational improvements. Analyze new scheduling protocols and implement changes. Implement technology to support operational needs and efficiency. Ensure that goals and objectives are met within the established time frames and hospital requirements, conduct and facilitate meetings, address any constraints and resolve problems.
Human Resources Management	May provide training or other aspects of the onboarding process for staff.	May provide training or other aspects of the onboarding process for students and other staff.	May hire, develop and manage the performance of Patient Access Specialists. Provide direction, assignments, feedback, coaching and counseling to assure outcomes are achieved. Develop new and current staff through training to improve patient scheduling and access.	May hire, develop and manage the performance of other administrative clinic personnel. Provide direction, assignments, feedback, coaching and counseling to assure outcomes are achieved. Develop new and current staff through training to improve frontline operations	Hire, develop and manage the performance of staff; assure staff are compliant with l policies and procedures. Provide direction, assignments, feedback, coaching and counseling to assure outcomes are achieved. Develop new and current staff through training to improve patient scheduling and access.	Hire, develop and manage the performance of staff; assure staff are compliant with policies and procedures. Provide direction, assignments, feedback, coaching and counseling to assure outcomes are achieved. Develop new and current staff through training to improve frontline operations. Ensure adequate staffing levels.	Provide operational leadership and oversight over department. Provide direct supervision of management level staff. Mentor, lead, and work to develop staff and the services they provide.
Financial Management	Follows the appropriate workflows to confirm the patient is financially secured for their visit.	Collaborate with others regarding the management of Pre-Access and Financial Counseling.	May make budget recommendations and manage expenses.	May make budget recommendations and manage expenses. Works with Patient Financial Services regarding the management of Pre-Access, Financial Counseling, or billing related activities.	May make budget recommendations and manage expenses. Play significant role in making recommendation and managing the personnel budget of the unit.	May make budget recommendations and manage expenses. Play significant role in making recommendation and managing the personnel budget of the clinic.	Assist with unit budget development. Recommend staffing levels. Analyze, monitor, and report financial data. Address budget discrepancies.

APPENDIX U

PAC LEAD/COORDINATOR COMPARISON

PAC Lead/Coordinator Comparison

P = "Primary" person responsible for the task
S = "Secondary" person responsible for the task
X = NA
Yes/No = Required Skill/Task

	Lead	Coordinator	Manager
Communication			
Communication of policy/procedure changes	Yes	Yes	Yes
Clinical Relationships - liaison/collaborate with all depts.	Yes	Yes	Yes
Host clinic meetings - work sessions, Data Packets, ad hoc meetings	X	S	P
Core Metrics			
Monitor Finesse and workdrivers on an ongoing basis; reassign staff as needed	P	P	P
Implement strategies to resolve service issues (SSAAP)	S	P	P
ELMS/Timekeeping			
Calendaring - Maintain division OOO calendar	X	P	S
ELMS - approve leave requests and OT	X	P	S
ELMS - final sign-off at pay period close	X	P	S
EPIC/Scheduling			
Respond to Scheduling Variances, Perform Variance Audits, Troubleshoot Errors	X	P	S
Templates - identify problems; look for efficiencies, subject matter expert	P	P	S
Work with clinic on access issues, workflow efficiencies	X	S	P
HR			
Participate on interview committees and assist with strengthening team dynamics	X	S	P
Assist with orientation of new staff	P	P	S
Administrative Supervisor – Primary/Lead supervisor with authority to hire, evaluate, discipline, and terminate. Full ePersonnel access (performance descriptor, appointment history, compensation history, etc.) completes performance appraisals, etc.	X		P
Functional Supervisor – Typically limited to the assignment/oversight of work and scheduling. HRIS view limited to education, training, and compliance.	X	X	P
Point of contact for manager absences (Staffing, etc)	X	P	Utilize a mngr. designate / X
Ensure compliance expectations are met in appropriate timeframe	X	P	P

PAC Lead/Coordinator Comparison

	Lead	Coordinator	Manager
Projects			
Special project work as assigned (dependent on scope and involvement)	Yes	Yes	Yes
Implement pilots, new projects, upgrades	S	P	P
Provide input and suggestions to improve services	P	P	P
Documentation Tracking for manager	X	P	S
Reports/Call Stats			
QA - Review calls sent by QA, add to staff monthly 1:1 stats	X	S	P
Scheduling Accuracy - Review calls sent by QA, add to staff monthly 1:1 stats; provide re-education as needed	X	S	P
Scheduling			
Schedule pt. appts- % Expectation of Clinic or PAC Departmental Productivity Benchmark	90% (Clinic)	50% (UI PAC)	S
Overbook appointments	P	S	S
Scheduling Questions - the clinic scheduling "expert"	P	S	S
Complaints - Address patient/department complaints	S	P	P
Resources - create and maintain division OneNote documents	P	P	S
Phone Coverage, Daily Work Assignments, Etc			
Orientation of new staff	P	P	S
Staff absences- Provide phone coverage	P	P	S
Assign and oversee daily work of staff, utilization and cross-training	S	P	P
Technology/Reporting			
Microsoft Suite (Excel, PowerPoint, Outlook, Word, OneNote)	Yes	Yes	Yes
Tableau - use for special projects, Data packets, etc.	X	Yes	Yes
Visio	X	Yes	Yes
CISCO - Pull reports from CUIC	X	Yes	Yes
Monthly Data Packets - pull data to create monthly presentations	X	P	S
Monthly Data Packets - present PPT to clinic	X	S	P

APPENDIX V

SAMPLE QUALITY SCORING MATRIX

Incoming/Outgoing Schedule

Scheduling Accuracy		Call Direction	Patient	Patient Rep	External Referring Provider	Internal Clinic/Nurse/Provider	Other	Point Value
Call Introduction								
Greeting: ex. Good Morning/Good Afternoon/Hello		I/O	x	x	x	x	x	5
Clinic Identification: ex. Dermatology scheduling		I/O	x	x	x	x	x	5
Self Identification: ex. My name is Kelly		I	x	x	x	x	x	5
Offer Assistance: How may I help you?		I	x	x	x	x	x	5
Reason for Outbound Call		O	x	x	x	x	x	5
Clinic Callback Number on Outbound voicemail		O	x	x	x	x	x	5
Patient Verification								
Patient Lookup (two patient identifiers: Name, DOB, and/or MRN)		I/O	x	x	x	x	x	10
Verify Patient Contacts (calls for minors, if caller is patient rep)		I/O	x	x			x	5
Verify Insurance		I/O	x	x			x	5
If Registration needed (new MRN, change in insurance, Self Pay) was reg completed before sched?		I/O						5
Scheduling								
Offer Appointment Notification (verify phone, text, email when appropriate)	VS	I/O	x	x	x	x	x	5
Was Appointment Notification entered into encounter field?		I/O	x	x	x	x	x	5
Verify If Accident Related (when scheduling appt only, not resched)		I/O	x	x	x	x	x	5
Was Accident Related entered into encounter field?	VS	I/O	x	x	x	x	x	5
Verify Referring Provider	VS	I/O	x	x	x	x	x	5
Was Referring Provider entered correctly into provider field?	VS	I/O	x	x	x	x	x	5
Verify Patient Care Team		I/O	x	x	x	x	x	5
Was Care Team entered correctly into provider field?	VS	I/O	x	x	x	x	x	5
Did scheduler use correct department to schedule appointment?	VS	I/O	x	x	x	x	x	5
Did scheduler use correct visit-type to schedule appointment?	VS	I/O	x	x	x	x	x	5
Did scheduler use correct provider to schedule appointment?	VS	I/O	x	x	x	x	x	10
Did scheduler use correct bill area to schedule appointment?	VS	I/O	x	x	x	x	x	5
Did scheduler complete attending field area correctly?	VS	I/O	x	x	x	x	x	5
Did scheduler clean up other worker drivers? (recalls, linked orders, assign referrals, etc)	VS	I/O	x	x	x	x	x	5
Did scheduler complete standard appointment note information?	VS	I/O	x	x	x	x	x	5
Did scheduler complete necessary follow through procedures? (ex. Add pt to waitlist, sent note to nurse, etc)	VS	I/O	x	x	x	x	x	5
Infection Screening	VS	I/O					x	5
PCP Screening	VS	I/O					x	5
Patient Verification Screening	VS	I/O					x	5
When Transferring calls (if no transfers, then answer N/A)								
Explained reason for hold		I/O					x	5
Explanation for transfer:		I/O					x	5
Provide caller with name/number of person being transferred to/instructions for VM:		I/O					x	5
Closing the Call (N/A only if caller disconnects before closing):								
Confirmation of appointment information/location/time		I/O	x	x	x	x	x	5
Asked Is There Anything Else I Can Do For You?/Do you have any questions?		I/O	x	x	x	x	x	5
Thanked the caller		I/O	x	x	x	x	x	5
Policy/Overall Performance								
Verified identity/authority of caller/Was PHI protected?		I/O	x	x	x	x	x	10
Did the call meet the minimum standards for Customer Service		I/O	x	x	x	x	x	10
Did they present themselves in a Professional manner		I/O	x	x	x	x	x	10
Total Call Score								215

APPENDIX W

ACCEPTABLE PHRASES

Acceptable Phrases

Accident Related *(If they get upset at this question, you may respond by saying, "I understand, we just need to ask because we want to make sure everything gets billed correctly"; if they say "yes," look for a claim)*

1. Will a workers' compensation or third-party payer insurance be covering the expenses for the visit we are scheduling today?
2. Is this the result of an accident or injury?
3. For billing purposes, is this accident or injury related?
4. This is not due to an accident or injury, correct?
5. For insurance purposes, is this related to an accident or injury?
6. We're not seeing you for anything accident related, is that correct?
7. Will anything related to an accident or injury be discussed at this appointment?
8. Is this appointment due to an accident or injury where we'd need to bill someone other than your insurance?
9. Will someone other than _ (name their insurance) be billed for this appointment?

Patient Care Team *(If someone asks what this is, you can tell them that this allows them access to see follow-up notes from their appointments)*

1. Is there anyone that you would like to receive notes for your visits?
2. Is there anyone you would like to add to your patient care team to receive notes for your visits?
3. Is there anyone else you would like to add to your patient care team?
4. I have _ (address), _ (address), _ (address) listed on your patient care team. Would you like to add anyone else?
5. For your continued care, we routinely share information with your healthcare team. Is this OK? Is there anyone else you would like to have added to receive notes from your visits?
6. Are the following providers (names & addresses) involved in your care? Is there anyone else you would like to add to your patient care team?
7. Are there any other providers you would like to know about your care here?
8. I am reviewing your patient care team. Is there anyone you would like to add?
9. Is there anyone else besides _ (doctor) and _ (doctor) that you would want us to share clinical notes with?

Patient Lookup

1. May I get your name and date of birth?
   If you get an internal call and are given an MRN, make sure to confirm first & last name.
   You may ask for their middle name or initial, but let them provide it to you.
   You still must get two identifiers, even if you find them by their phone number. Every call, every time!

Primary Care Provider (PCP)

1. Do you have a Primary Care Provider?
2. Is Dr. _ your Primary Care Provider?
3. I see Dr. _ at (address) listed as your Primary Care Provider. Is that correct?
4. Who would you like us to list as your Primary Care Provider?
5. I see we don't have a Primary Care Provider listed. Do you have someone you would like to list?
6. Unfortunately, I cannot list a facility, who do you usually see there?

Referring Provider

1. Has anyone referred you for this visit?
2. Did your Primary Care Provider refer you for the visit we are scheduling?
3. Is there anyone referring you/or the patient for this appointment?
4. We have Dr. _ as the person who referred you, is that correct?
5. I am reviewing your patient care team and see that Dr. _ is your Primary Care Provider, is that who referred you for this visit?
6. Is there a provider who referred you for this visit?
7. Would you like to add the referring provider to the patient care team to continue to receive notes on your care?

Combined Option

1. I'm reviewing your patient care team. It looks like Dr. _ is your Primary Care Provider and Dr. _ referred you here, is that correct? Are there any other providers who you would like to receive notes about your appointment?

***All phrasing must be presented as a question and receive a response for credit.
(i.e.: "I assume this was not an accident" would not be a question.)

APPENDIX X

DIFFICULT CALLERS &
DE-ESCALATION PROCESS

Difficult Callers & De-escalation Process

Objective:
To provide preliminary scripting statements intended to assist in de-escalating less offensive calls, with the final scripting in red intended for more highly offensive callers. As with all callers, the use of professional judgment and courtesy needs to be exercised by staff when determining the best course of action.

Suggestions for processing the information from caller:
1. **Make notes** – Listen to the caller very carefully and patiently. Make note of every detail, as you can make the caller increasingly irate if you make them repeat information.
2. **Don't interrupt** – Never interrupt the caller while they are explaining the issue. Let them pour out their aggression and get them ready to listen and understand what you are saying. Pause before you start.
3. **Watch your tone** – Be polite. What you say is important; however, how you say it is even more important.
4. **Smile** – It helps you not lose your patience and keep calm and will aid you in resolving issues more effectively.

Caller Types:
Vulgar, Threatening or Intimidating Caller: May use profanity (swearing directly at you), but also may use emotional or physical intimidation, may be a threat to themselves or others (if you or the institution are threatened in any way, report it to your manager immediately)
1. I do understand the inconvenience you have faced...
2. Let me see how I can help to fix this.
3. I am more than happy to help you (name)...
4. For the quickest resolution, I would request you to...
5. I am sorry you are so upset.
Escalated Response: "This is unacceptable behavior. This call is now finished."

Grievance Caller: We made a mistake. We have failed our customer. May need to send to our supervisor.
1. Thank you so much for letting us know about this...
2. I'm so sorry to hear about this...
3. I understand how you must feel...
4. I will take action on this right away...
5. Thank you so much for your patience while we can find a way to work through this.
Escalated Response: "I can refer you to the Office of Patient Experience."
Escalated Response: "Repeatedly calling back does not create other ways for us to help you."
Escalated Response: "Repeated callbacks slow down our ability to help your need."
Escalated Response: "I understand you're frustrated, but we are at a stalemate. I suggest we try again in a few minutes. Sometimes a break makes things clearer. I'll call you back in approximately (#) minutes."

Talkative Caller: Changes from one topic to another. Difficult to get a word or question into the conversation. Can be very specific and detailed.
1. Thanks for sharing. With that going on, how about we set up your appointment on...
2. (Name) I am glad to hear that you _ (or I'm sorry to hear that _). I know that you called for a reason, so let me see if I can help you set up that appointment.
Escalated Response: "It is apparent this conversation is going nowhere. I now need to end this call." **(This is for excessive call duration or no satisfactory resolution. If follow-up is needed, plan a call-back time.)**
Escalated Response: "I need to interrupt as you are telling me more than I need to know at this time. Your provider will want to hear all about your history during your visit."
Escalated Response: "I understand these details are important; however, I must ask about _ in order to get you appropriately scheduled."
Escalated Response: "These are issues that need to be discussed in person, not over the phone. I am limited on what information I am able to provide. Please discuss this during your appointment

APPENDIX Y
ADDITIONAL CALL SCRIPTS

International or ELL Caller: Apply the principles of good customer service. Speak slower, not louder. Ask them to repeat or slow down. Confirm understanding. Request interpreting services if needed.

1. I am not sure I know how to help. Do you want to see a doctor?
2. I am sorry. I am having trouble understanding. Would you mind helping me spell your last name?
3. I apologize, I'd like to try to help you. Do you have someone there I could speak to?

Escalated Response: "I would like to help you. Can I connect you with someone in our interpreting services?"

Frantic Caller: May not be listening due to their emergent request for access; however, there is a need to collect required information to process their call.

1. (If applicable) We have a triage process. To proceed, there is necessary information that we will need to collect from you.
2. Thank you for the details. I will need to collect some required information to proceed with your request.

Escalated Response: "I would like to help. Would there be a better time for us to have a conversation?"

Disappointed Caller:

Frustration displayed about not being able to obtain the desired appointment. *(Also see department's process for Access Facilitation).*

1. We can schedule this appointment and then add you to the waitlist if you would like.
2. Our medical staff triages each case according to urgent and emergent need. Would you like me to see if there is anything else we can provide? *(Use dept process to have patient remain on hold or provide a callback.)*
3. If this is something your referring provider feels is urgent, they can get in contact with us to discuss it.

Escalated Response: "We can appreciate your concern. We will contact you when our situation changes."

Escalated Response: "I understand you're frustrated, but we are at a stalemate. I suggest we try again in a few minutes. Sometimes a break makes things clearer. I'll call you back in approximately (#) minutes."

Escalated Response: "Repeated callbacks slow down our ability to help your need."

Escalated Response: "Repeatedly calling back does not create other ways for us to help you."

Escalated Response: "I understand you are concerned about obtaining an appointment; however, if you do not stop (name the behavior) I will hang up."

APPENDIX Z

BEST PRACTICES OUTBOUND CALL MANAGEMENT

Best Practices-Outbound Call Management

General Description

The following document describes manual outbound patient contact best practice and management for scheduling appointments, reminders, rescheduled appointments, and recalls. The scope of the document differentiates between types of contacts. Each may be handled slightly differently. <u>We must always identify who we are speaking with or whose device we are leaving a message on and plan our scripting accordingly.</u> Below are examples to help guide practice. Examples can be heard by clicking the .

Outbound calls

1. <u>Patient is positively identified.</u>
   - After collecting two patient identifiers, continue with normal (incoming) scheduling workflow, including insurance and demographic updates, if required. The following option may be used for phone verification: **"Is this the best number to reach you at?"**
   - Example scripting:
     - "Hello is (patient's name) available?" (**Once the patient identifies**) "This is (scheduler) from the (dept) Scheduling. To protect your privacy, may I get your full name and date of birth please?"

2. <u>Voice mailbox belongs to the patient you are calling.</u>
   "This is_____calling from Department of_____."*
   - "Please call us back at your earliest convenience at (telephone number)."
   - "Please call us at (telephone number) to schedule/reschedule your appointment. Thank you."
   - Calling to remind (patient name) you have a visit on (date) in the (clinic name) at (elevator/floor/location). Please arrive at (time) for your appointment at (time).

3. <u>Undetermined voice mailbox ownership or contact with someone other than the patient.</u>
   "This is_____calling from Department of_____."*
   - "Please have (patient name) call us at (telephone number) to schedule/reschedule your appointment. Thank you."
   - "We wanted to remind (patient name) of an upcoming appointment on (date). If you are unable to keep this appointment or have any other questions, please call us back at (telephone number)."
     (If you are in a sensitive clinic, look to your clinic guidelines for best practices.)

4. <u>Contacting patient regarding change due to a Bump List (all voicemail).</u>
   "This is_____from Healthcare Department of_____. (Name) has an appointment at (time & date) and we need to cancel. Please call us at (telephone number) and push the option for scheduling. If I am with a patient, any of our schedulers would be happy to assist you. Thank you."*

Additional Considerations:

* Some areas may not identify their department or services to protect patient confidentiality as it relates to sensitivity of condition or situation. Examples may include:
   - Clinical Cancer Center
   - Adult & Child Psychiatry
   - Others as identified (refer to your clinic guidelines)

INDEX

S

U

V

W